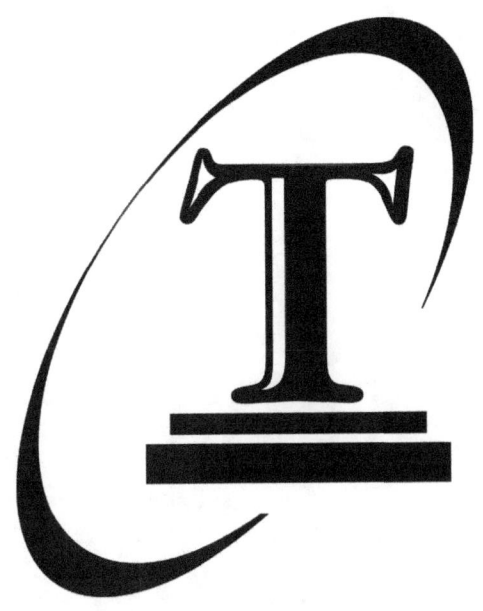

www.tennantinstitute.com

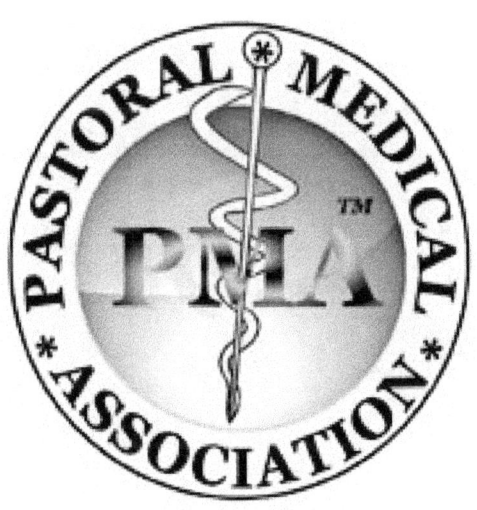

www.pmai.us

Table of Contents

LEGAL NOTICE:

The information provided in this book is intended to educate the reader about certain medical conditions and certain possible solutions. It is not a substitute for examination, diagnosis, and medical care provided by a licensed and qualified health professional. If you believe you or your child or someone you know suffer from the conditions described herein, please see your health care provider. Do not attempt to treat yourself, your child, or anyone else without proper medical supervision.

DISCLAIMER OF LIABILITY:

FOREWORD

My introduction to the concept of electromagnetic measurements in biological systems came while I was studying for my M.D. at Yale University School of Medicine. To graduate from this particular medical school, one must write a thesis. I chose, in 1959, Dr. Harold Saxton Burr, Professor of Neuro-anatomy, as my advisor for my thesis project. Dr. Burr, at that time, was acknowledged as a lead investigator and proponent of The Electromagnetic Field

Theory in Biology. During my studies with Dr. Burr, I was exposed to the concept of taking electronic measurements with a direct current potentiometer on various living organisms, including humans, to measure electrical changes that accompanied changes in those biological systems.

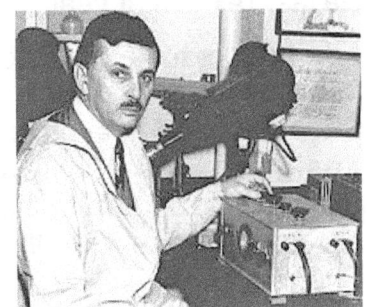

Subsequently, I became familiar with the knowledge that creating an electrical field, such as that reported by Dr. Robert O. Becker and Dr. Andrew Bassett, an orthopedic surgeon at Columbia University School of Medicine, could be of assistance for healing processes in the clinical condition of nonunion of orthopedic fractures. Therefore, I understood that electronics in living systems could not only be measured but, indeed, these systems could be modified by an electrical field.

With the information provided above as a background, I was, perhaps, more receptive than most physicians would be to accept the idea that electronic stimulation could be of benefit in certain clinical conditions. My first hand exposure to the benefit of electronic stimulus as therapy was a very rapid recovery from a previous knee injury after being treated with a Russian electronic device, called a SCENAR, utilized by Dr. Jerald Tennant, in January 2003.

I had met Dr. Tennant in the late 1970s and arranged, with assistance of Dr. John Corboy, for him to present the first intraocular lens course with hands on guidance ever taught in Honolulu, Hawaii. Our friendship had been established then and, therefore, I was interested in the Energetic Medicine workshop he was presenting at the Hawaii Meeting on Maui in 2003. My inquiry about the course at the Faculty dinner led to his treating me for the injury which I had acquired while indulging in my favorite sport of surfing. The dramatic improvement in my knee function led me to buy the Russian device and take Dr. Tennant's course taught in Dallas, Texas that year.

I do not presume to understand or profess all the concepts that are presented in this book authored by Dr. Tennant. The SCENAR, and the other electronic devices, subsequently designed by Dr. Tennant, such as the Tennant BioModulator®, are classified by the FDA as class 2 accepted devices for the relief of pain and inflammation. Over the past eight years, I have, in my ophthalmic practice personally treated with these devices over 275 patients who had painful ocular syndromes with approximately 85% success. The syndromes have included pain after corneal injury, iritis, migraine, and postoperative discomfort after strabismus and cataract surgery. The pain syndrome, known as post-herpetic neuralgia (pain after shingles), has been especially responsive. In some patients, the pain in the skin had plagued the patient for over 10 years. You can imagine the gratitude of these patients when there is a complete relief, after treatment by an electronic device, for a condition that has not responded to drugs and other modalities of treatment. I thank Dr. Tennant for introducing me to this new paradigm of medical treatment. We may not understand the mechanisms of healing at this point, but, ultimately, **results trump theory in any case**.

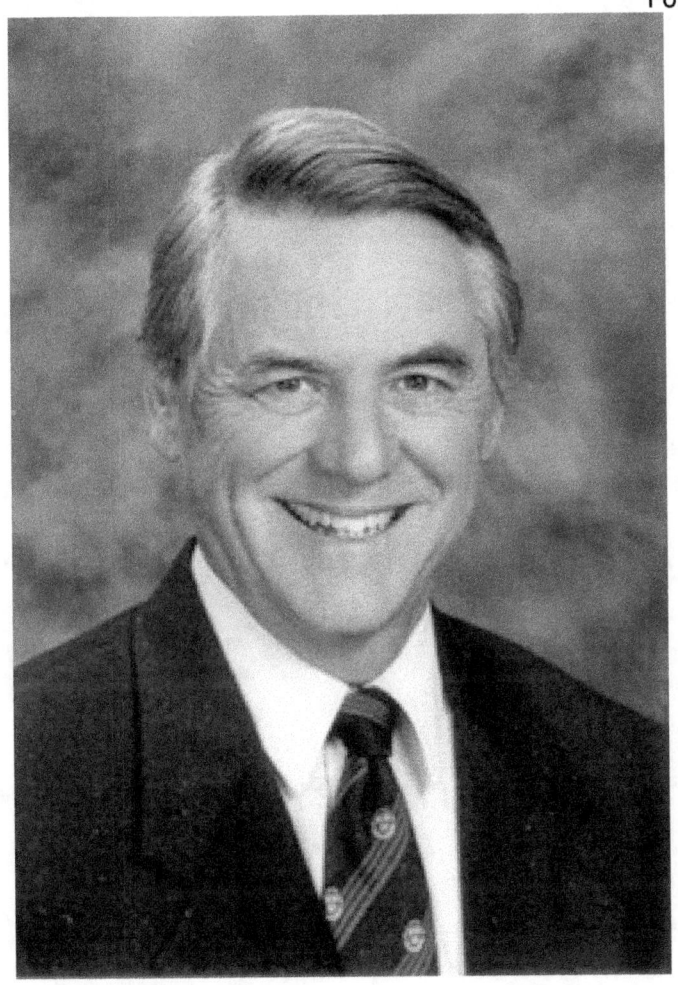

Malcolm R. Ing, MD

Clinical Professor of Surgery

Division of Ophthalmology, Department of Surgery

John A. Burns School of Medicine, University of Hawaii

While conventional medicine is a blessing beyond compare for many reasons, it is frankly undeniable that in the scientific quest to understand and control life, conventional ideas and drugs actually pose one of the leading threats to life. One needs only to review statistics to see that the entire world is facing a health care crisis never before known, and it should be obvious that if we continue on the same "scientific" path to resolve our health woes we will continue to get the same results. If the answer is not to continue the path that is clearly not working, perhaps it is to look back instead, to restore to health care the almighty's messages for health, to restore common sense and to focus on effective and safer solutions.

It will undoubtedly be difficult to change the medical paradigm but with organizations like the Pastoral Medical Association, along with caring and dedicated medical professionals like Dr. Jerry Tennant that are willing to "step outside" that paradigm and research effective and safer options, we will certainly give hope and perhaps life to some of the millions of suffering individuals. In his remarkable book – Healing is Voltage, Dr. Tennant shares a wealth of medical knowledge and it is a "must read" for health care professionals and laypersons alike. Thank you Dr. Tennant for bringing this invaluable resource to us....

Eric Carter, President
Pastoral Medical Association
http://www.pmai.us
866-206-8469

A note from the author:

First let me express my gratitude to the thousands that have bought my book and recommended it to others. I am grateful that I may be making a difference in how chronic disease is treated here and abroad.

I wanted to make a comment about grammar and formatting. When I wrote edition one, I started in Microsoft Word. Soon it was moving my images to different pages even though I told it to lock them in place with the text. Sometimes I would find the image 10-20 pages from where I left it. When I called Microsoft for help, the agent simply told me that hers wasn't doing that so it was my fault.

I then wrote the first edition in Mac Pages. At that time, Pages had a spell checker but not a grammar checker. I exported it from Pages to Word so I could use Word's grammar checker. Unfortunately it moved the graphics again. After correcting grammar and punctuation, I ported it back to Pages, repositioned the images and exported it to PDF, the format demanded by Amazon's printer. What I didn't realize was that porting it back and forth changed the spelling and punctuation. I also didn't realize that an image that looked great in color in Adobe PDF may be unreadable when printed in black and white.

I found that most authors of books and newspapers use Adobe InDesign for writing. I bought it and spent the time learning its quirks. I wrote the second edition in InDesign. I used its spell checker and grammar checker and used Adobe Photoshop to turn the color images into black and white. I exported it to Adobe PDF and it was printed by Amazon's printer.

I still got criticism for the formatting and grammar. I then had Amazon's printer staff edit it. Unfortunately and surprisingly, they don't work with Adobe InDesign but insisted on having it in---you guessed it---Microsoft Word for editing. Of course Adobe InDesign doesn't export into Microsoft Word but only Adobe Acrobat. I therefore had to export it to PDF and then use Adobe Acrobat to export it to Word. Amazon's editors edited it but removed all the graphics in the process--- uugggh! Now I had the text edited but Word keeps moving the graphics around and Microsoft doesn't know why.

Eventually I ported it back into Pages, put the graphics where they belong and had another editor review it. You guessed it---they changed some of the editing that Amazon's editors had made.

I taught English in the 1950s so I know the rules of punctuation that we used then. Back then, it was correct to say, "1950's" not "1950s". It was also correct to use a comma before the "and" when you say, "A, B, C, and D". Now we are supposed to omit the comma before the "and". Who had the authority to say that the way we used commas for the years before was incorrect? Why?

According to Wikipedia, Publishers' style guides establish house rules for language use, such as spelling, italics and punctuation; their major purpose is consistency. There are rulebooks for writers, ensuring consistent language. Authors are asked or required to use a style guide in preparing their work for publication; copy editors are charged with enforcing the publishing house's style.

I have discovered that there is no consistency in these rules from one editor to another.

I find all of this confusing and annoying. I am simply trying to communicate information to my audience but the message is being drowned out by those more interested in whether I followed their rulebook or someone else's.

I have spent a lot of time and resources dealing with editors, formatting and computer software deficiencies instead of science. Three editors have reviewed it. I have done the best I can do in trying to communicate my concepts to you. I hope you will try to understand the message and not worry too much about whether my comma is in the right or wrong place according to whatever rule book you follow.

Be Well!

Jerry Tennant, MD, MD(H), PSc.D

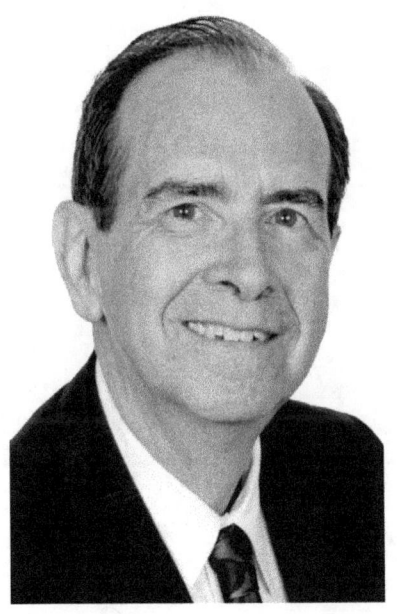

Prologue

NOTICE:

Tennant Institute for Pastoral Medicine is an Ecclesiastical Private Expressive Association, as defined by law, and is under the direction of Jerry Tennant, MD(P), a Pastoral Health Practitioner and Counsellor. Under this appointment, Dr. Tennant is ordained a minister and chaplain to minister to the sick and suffering under International Law and under Texas statue Sec. 503.054 (b)

Reading this book implies that the participant has given an acknowledgement of rights noted above and others recognized by law, and asserts First and Ninth Amendment rights. Participation means, "I voluntarily license Jerry Tennant, MD(P) to counsel me in his role as a Pastoral Health Practitioner and Counsellor."

Tennant Institute is a Private Expressive Association registered with the IRS and fulfills all the legal requirements of a Private Expressive Association.

COMMENTS by the author:

In the US, there is a separation of church and state. For example, when you apply for and sign your name to a driver's license, you are giving the state permission to control your operation of a vehicle. However, police officers have no authority in a church, registered as a Private Expressive Association, unless they are invited in by those ordained by the church. A Private Expressive Association is exempt from secular laws because secular laws apply to the public and members of the Association are private. The Supreme Court makes it clear that private members of a Private Expressive Association may do whatever they wish as long as what they do does not create a clear and present danger that rises to the level of a substantive evil. For example, you could create a boxing club. Boxing creates a clear and present danger but does not rise to the level of a substantive evil and thus the police or other governmental agencies cannot prevent the members from boxing.

Most churches operate under the rules governing Private Expressive Associations. Because of these laws, public agencies like the police cannot dictate to church members how they conduct themselves within the confines of the church property unless what they are doing is a clear and present danger that rises to the level of a substantive evil. Thus the police could enter a church if a judge feels that children are being sexually abused since this is a substantive evil.

Most attorneys are not familiar with the laws regarding Private Expressive Associations. Neither are regulatory officials of cities, states or the federal government. They should become familiar since if they violate these rights, they are personally liable for their actions and their governmental immunity does not apply.

There is a separate set of case law regarding the separation of church and state. These laws often overlap the rights given to Private Expressive Associations.

"In the United States, the term is an offshoot of the phrase, "wall of separation between church and state", as written in Thomas Jefferson's letter to the Danbury Baptist Association in 1802. The original text reads: "Believing with you that religion is a matter which lies solely between Man & his God, that he owes account to none other for his faith or his worship, that the legitimate powers of government reach actions only, & not opinions, I contemplate with sovereign reverence that act of the whole American people which declared that their legislature should 'make no law respecting an establishment of religion, or prohibiting the free exercise thereof,' thus building a wall of separation between Church and State." Jefferson reflected his frequent speaking theme that the government is not to interfere with religion. The phrase was quoted by the United States Supreme Court first in 1878, and then in a series of cases starting in 1947. The phrase "separation of church and state" itself does not appear in the United States Constitution.The First Amendment states that "Congress shall make no law respecting an establishment of religion, or prohibiting the free exercise thereof." The Supreme Court did not consider the question of how this applied to the states until 1947; when they did, in <u>Everson v. Board of Education</u>, the court determined that the first amendment applied to the states and that a law enabling reimbursement for busing to all schools (including parochial schools) was constitutional." wikipedia

Article 18 of the Universal Declaration of Human Rights states, "Everyone has the right to freedom of thought, conscience and religion; this right includes freedom to change his religion or belief, and freedom, either alone or in community with others and in public or private, to manifest his religion or belief in teaching, practice, worship and observance."

The First Amendment of the US Constitution is concerned with three areas of Freedom necessary for Religion. The Supreme Court links these all together as "expressive association..."

First, it guarantees the Freedoms of Association and Assembly, rights which are essential for the creation and continuance of religious bodies. Second, it forbids the "establishment" of any Church as the official government religion. Third, it forbids any "abridgment" of Religious Liberty -- of the right to believe as you will.

"...neither this court nor any branch of this government will consider the merits or fallacies of a religion. Nor will the court compare the beliefs, dogmas, and practices of a newly organized religion with those of an older, more established religion. Nor will the court praise or condemn a religion, however excellent or fanatical or preposterous it may seem. Were the court to do so, it would impinge upon the guarantee of the First Amendment." Judge Brattin, Eastern District of California, in Universal Life Church, Inc. vs. United States, 372 F. Supp. 770, 776 (E.D. Cal 1974)

In addition to such landmark cases as <u>Boy Scouts of America et al. v. Dale, 530 US 640 (2000)</u> which made it clear that Expressive Association activities are protected under First Amendment Private Association rights, other governmental actions have strengthened religious association rights.

Chief Justice William Rehnquist wrote the majority opinion. It relied heavily upon an earlier case, <u>Roberts v United States Jayceees, 468 U.S. 609, 622 (1984)</u>. In that decision the Supreme Court said: "Consequently, we have long understood as implicit in the right to engage in activities protected by the First Amendment a corresponding right to associate with others in pursuit of a wide variety of political, social, economic, educational, religious, and cultural ends." This right, the Roberts decision continues, is crucial in preventing the majority from imposing its views on groups that would rather express other, perhaps unpopular, ideas. "We are not, as we must not be, guided by our views of whether the Boy Scouts' teachings with respect to homosexual conduct are right or wrong; public or judicial disapproval of a tenet of an organization's expression does not justify the State's effort to compel the organization to accept members where such acceptance would derogate from the organization's expressive message. While the law is free to promote all sorts of conduct in place of harmful behavior, it is not free to interfere with speech for no better reason than promoting an approved message or discouraging a disfavored one, however enlightened either purpose may strike the government."

The Congress of the United States adopted the RFRA, the Religious Freedom Restoration Act of 1993 (P.L. 103-141). In this enactment Congress determined that "governments should not substantially burden religious exercise without compelling justification..." and that "laws 'neutral' toward religion may burden religious exercise..." Therefore Congress determined to protect the free exercise of religion as follows:

"Sect. 3. Free Exercise of Religion Protected. (a) In General. -- Government shall not substantially burden a person's exercise of religion, even if the burden results from a rule of general applicability, except as provided in subsection (b). (b) Exception. -- Government may substantially burden a person's exercise of religion only if it demonstrates that application of the burden to the person -- (1) is in the furtherance of a compelling governmental interest; and (2) is the least restrictive means of furthering that compelling governmental interest. (c) Judicial Relief. -- A person whose religious exercise has been burdened in violation of this section may assert that violation as a claim or defense in a judicial proceeding and obtain appropriate relief against a government..."

The Supreme Court has both limited this law (doesn't apply to the States) and reaffirmed it: "Restoration Act of 1993 (RFRA), 107 Stat. 1488, as amended, 42 U. S. C. §2000bb et seq., ... adopts a statutory rule .... Under RFRA, the Federal Government may not, as a statutory matter, substantially burden a person's exercise of religion..." Gonzales v O Centro, No. 04–1084 - February 21, 2006.

In the case of State v Biggs (46 SE Reporter 401, 1903) the North Carolina Supreme Court dealt with a person who was advising people as to diet, and administering massage, baths and physical culture. That Court held that there could be no "state system of healing" p.402 and while "Those who wish to be treated by practitioners of medicine and surgery had the guaranty that such practitioners had been duly examined...those who had faith in treatment by methods not included in the 'practice of medicine and surgery' as usually understood, had reserved to them the right to practice their faith and be treated, if they chose, by those who openly and avowedly did not use either surgery or drugs in the treatment of diseases..." (p.402). "Medicine is an experimental, not an exact science. All the law can do is to regulate and safeguard the use of powerful and dangerous remedies, like the knife and drugs, but it cannot forbid dispensing with them. When the Master, who was himself called the Good Physician, was told that other than his followers were casting out devils and curing diseases, he said, 'Forbid them not.'" (p.405).

In the Texas Supreme Court case: WESTBROOK JR v. PENLEY; C.L. WESTBROOK, JR., Petitioner, v. Peggy Lee PENLEY, Respondent.; No. 04-0838. Argued Sept. 26, 2006. -- June 29, 2007. They concluded: "The religion clauses are designed to "prevent, as far as possible, the intrusion of either [religion or government] into the precincts of the other," Lemon v. Kurtzman, 403 U.S. 602, 614, 91 S.Ct. 2105, 29 L.Ed.2d 745 (1971), and are premised on the notion that " 'both religion and government can best work to achieve their lofty aims if each is left free from the other within its respective sphere.' " Aguilar v. Felton, 473 U.S. 402, 410, 105 S.Ct. 3232, 87 L.Ed.2d 290 (1985) (quoting McCollum v. Bd. of Ed., 333 U.S. 203, 212, 68 S.Ct. 461, 92 L.Ed. 649 (1948)). The First Amendment's limitations on government extend to its judicial as well as its legislative branch. See Kreshik v. Saint Nicholas Cathedral, 363 U.S. 190, 191, 80 S.Ct. 1037, 4 L.Ed.2d 1140 (1960).

Government action may burden the free exercise of religion in two quite different ways: by interfering with an individual's observance or practice of a particular faith, see, e.g., Church of the Lukumi Babalu Aye, Inc. v. City of Hialeah, 508 U.S. 520, 532, 113 S.Ct. 2217, 124 L.Ed.2d 472 (1993), and by encroaching on the church's ability to manage its internal affairs, see, e.g., Kedroff v. St. Nicholas Cathedral, 344 U.S. 94, 116, 73 S.Ct. 143, 97 L.Ed. 120 (1952). See EEOC v. Catholic Univ. of Am., 83 F.3d 455, 460 (D.C.Cir.1996)."

"The right to organize voluntary religious associations to assist in the expression and dissemination of any religious doctrine and to create tribunals for the decision of controverted questions of faith within the association, and for the ecclesiastical government of all the individual members, congregations, and officers within the general association, is unquestioned. All who unite themselves to such a body do so with an implied consent to this government, and are bound to submit to it. But it would be a vain consent and would lead to the total subversion of such religious bodies, if any one aggrieved by one of their decisions could appeal to the secular courts and have them reversed. It is of the essence of these religious unions, and of their right to establish tribunals for the decision of questions arising among themselves, that those decisions should be binding in all cases of ecclesiastical cognizance, subject only to such appeals as the organism itself provides for.

Watson v. Jones, 80 U.S. (13 Wall.) 679, 728-29, 20 L.Ed. 666 (1872).5 Accordingly, the autonomy of a church in managing its affairs and deciding matters of "church discipline or the conformity of the members of the church to the standard of morals required of them" has long been afforded broad constitutional protection. Id. at 733.6 This Court, too, has long recognized a structural restraint on the constitutional power of civil courts to regulate matters of religion in general, Brown v. Clark, 102 Tex. 323, 116 S.W. 360, 363 (Tex.1909), and of church discipline in particular, Minton v. Leavell, 297 S.W. 615, 621-22 (Tex.Civ.App.-Galveston 1927, writ ref'd). The Minton court cogently explained why courts must decline jurisdiction over disputes concerning church membership."

"It seems to be settled law in this land of religious liberty that the civil courts have no power or jurisdiction to determine the regularity or validity of the judgment of a church tribunal expelling a member from further communion and fellowship in the church. Membership in a church creates a different relationship from that which exists in other voluntary societies formed for business, social, literary, or charitable purposes."

I am licensed as an M.D. in the state of Texas. Holding this license brings me privileges, responsibilities, and limitations placed upon me when I applied for a medical license and signed that I accepted that license. My activity as an MD may be controlled by state and federal laws. However, when I function as a Pastoral Health Practitioner and Counsellor, state law has no jurisdiction over me but instead I am responsible to the ecclesiastical organization that ordained me and by God. In the Private Expressive Association, Tennant Institute, I have been selected by its members to provide medical advice and therapies to our members free from comment or supervision by organizations created by state legislators and/or federal regulations as long as our members do not create a clear and present danger that rises to the level of a substantive evil.

MDs are no longer able to treat patients according to scientific literature, the experiences of the physician, or the desires of the patient. MD's are required to treat patients according to what are called "standards of care". These guidelines are not really guidelines at all, but are considered mandatory edicts by medical boards.

One of my patients was hospitalized. He developed constipation and requested that he be given vitamin C to solve the problem. He was told that the hospital could not give him vitamin C as it was not considered standard of care for constipation. He refused the pharmaceutical treatment for constipation, had his wife bring some vitamin C from home, and the problem was solved.

Another of my patients was hospitalized with a heart attack. The nurse brought him medication. He asked what one of the pills was. He was told it was to lower his blood pressure. He told the nurse that his blood pressure was 90/60 and that if they lowered it anymore he would pass out. She said, "it doesn't matter. All patients who enter the hospital with a heart attack must take blood pressure medicine." He asked about the second pill. She told him it was to lower his cholesterol. He asked what his cholesterol level was. She said, "I don't know, we haven't tested it." He asked why he must take a pill to lower it. The nurse said, "it doesn't matter. All patients who enter the hospital with a heart attack must take medication to lower their cholesterol. It's the standard of practice."

Most people have heard of Andrew Weil, MD, the

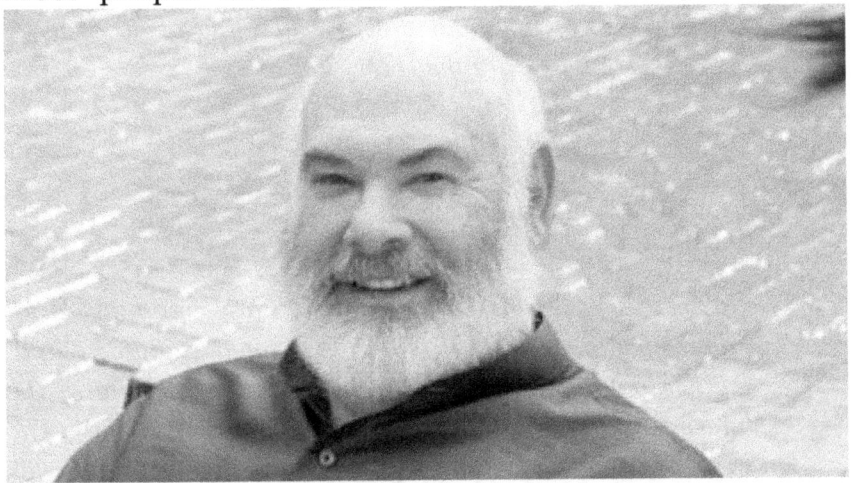

famous professor at the medical school in Tucson AZ. His teachings about the use of nutrition to support health is widely known, respected, and practiced. In spite of that, the FDA and the FTC told him that if he didn't stop suggesting that improving your immune system would help prevent you from getting the flu, he would be put in jail and fined!

UNITED STATES OF AMERICA
FEDERAL TRADE COMMISSION
BUREAU OF CONSUMER PROTECTION
WASHINGTON, D.C. 20580
DEPARTMENT OF HEALTH
AND HUMAN SERVICES
FOOD AND DRUG ADMINISTRATION

WASHINGTON, D.C. 20740

TO: ebenjamin@drweil.com
   www.drweil.com
FROM: The Food and Drug Administration and the Federal Trade Commission

RE: Unapproved/Uncleared/Unauthorized Products Related to the H1N1 Flu Virus; and
   Notice of Potential Illegal Marketing of Products to Prevent, Treat or Cure the H1N1 Virus

DATE: October 15, 2009

WARNING LETTER

This is to advise you that the United States Food and Drug Administration ("FDA") and the United States Federal Trade Commission ("FTC") reviewed your website at the Internet address www.drweil.com on October 13, 2009. The FDA has determined that your website offers a product for sale that is intended to diagnose, mitigate, prevent, treat or cure the H1N1 Flu Virus in people. This product has not been approved, cleared, or otherwise authorized by FDA for use in the diagnosis, mitigation, prevention, treatment, or cure of the H1N1 Flu Virus.

This product is your Immune Support Formula. The marketing of this product violates the Federal Food, Drug, and Cosmetic Act (FFDC Act). 21 U.S.C. §§ 331, 351, 352. We request that you immediately cease marketing unapproved, uncleared, or unauthorized products for the diagnosis, mitigation, prevention, treatment, or cure of the H1N1 Flu Virus.

10

In addition, FTC staff reminds you that the FTC Act, 15 U.S.C. § 41 et seq., requires that claims that a dietary supplement can prevent, treat, or cure human infection with the H1N1 virus, must be supported by well-controlled human clinical studies at the time the claims are made. More generally, it is against the law to make or exaggerate health claims, whether directly or indirectly, through the use of a product name, website name, metatags, or other means, without rigorous scientific evidence sufficient to substantiate the claims. Violations of the FTC Act may result in legal action in the form of a Federal District Court injunction or Administrative Order. An order also may require that you pay back money to consumers.

Some examples of the claims on your website include:

On a webpage entitled, "The Swine Flu - H1N1 ," with the subtitle "Swine Flu and You":

"[D]uring the flu season, I suggest taking a daily antioxidant, multivitamin-mineral supplement, as well as astragalus, a well-known immune-boosting herb that can help ward off colds and flu. You might also consider. .. the Weil Immune Support Formula[,] which contains both astragalus and immune-supportive polypore mushrooms ...."

On a product webpage describing the Immune Support Formula:

"The Immune Support Formula contains astragalus. . . . . Astragalus ... is used traditionally to ward off colds and flu and has been well studied for its antiviral and immunity-enhancing properties."

"Th[e] synergistic combination of immune modulators [found in the Immune Support Formula] is especially useful for those who tend to get every bug that goes around during the winter."

On the same webpage, under "Supplement Facts," describing the Astragalus supplement (which is one element of the Immune Support Formula):

"Astragalus ... is ... used traditionally to ward off colds and flu, and has demonstrated both antiviral and immune-boosting effects in scientific investigation."

On the website's home page, DrWeil.com:

"Worried About Flu? Dr. Weil's Immune Support Formula can help maintain a strong defense against the flu. It contains astragalus, a traditional herb that boosts immunity. Buy it now in one click, and start protecting your immune system against flu this season."

On the Dr. Weil Vitamins - Daily Vitamin Packs webpage:

"[L]earn more about Dr. Weil's Immune Support Formula, which contains astragalus - an herb Dr. Weil recommends to help ward off colds and flu."

The Secretary of Health and Human Services, under section 319 of the Public Health Service Act, 42 U.S.C. § 247d, has determined that a public health emergency exists nationwide involving the H1N1 Flu Virus that affects or has the significant potential to affect national security. Following this determination and in response to requests from the U.S. Centers for Disease Control and Prevention, FDA issued letters authorizing the emergency use of certain unapproved and uncleared products or unapproved or uncleared uses of approved or cleared products, provided certain criteria are met, under 21 U.S.C. § 360bbb-3. The marketing and sale of unapproved or uncleared H1N1 Flu Virus-related products that are not authorized by and used in accordance with the conditions of an Emergency Use Authorization, is a potentially significant threat to the public health. Therefore, FDA is taking urgent measures to protect consumers from products that, without approval or authorization by FDA, claim to diagnose, mitigate, prevent, treat or cure H1N1 Flu Virus in people.

You should take immediate action to ensure that your firm is not marketing, and does not market in the future, products intended to diagnose, mitigate, prevent, treat or cure the H1N1 Flu Virus that have not been approved, cleared, or authorized by the FDA. The above is not meant to be an all-inclusive list of violations. It is your responsibility to ensure that the products you market are in compliance with the FFDC Act and FDA's implementing regulations. We advise you to review your websites, product labels, and other labeling and promotional materials to ensure that the claims you make for your products do not adulterate or misbrand the products in violation of the FFDC Act. 21 U.S.C. §§ 331, 351, 352. Within 48 hours, please send an email to FDAFLUTASKFORCECFSAN@fda.hhs.gov., describing the actions that you have taken or plan to take to address your firm's violations. If your firm fails to take corrective action immediately, FDA may take enforcement action, such as seizure or injunction for violations of the FFDC Act without further notice. Firms that fail to take corrective action may also be referred to FDA's Office of Criminal Investigations for possible criminal prosecution for violations of the FFDC Act and other federal laws.

FDA is advising consumers not to purchase or use H1N1 Flu Virus-related products offered for sale that have not been approved, cleared, or authorized by FDA. Your firm will be added to a published list on FDA's website of firms and websites that have received warning letters from FDA concerning marketing unapproved, uncleared and unauthorized H1N1 Flu Virus-related products in violation of the FFDC Act. This list can be found at www.accessdata.fda.gov/scripts/h1n1flu. Once the violative claims and/or products have been removed from your website, and these corrective actions have been confirmed by the FDA, the published list will be' updated to indicate that your firm has taken appropriate corrective action.

If you are not located in the United States, please note that unapproved, uncleared, or unauthorized products intended to diagnose, mitigate, prevent, treat, or cure the H1N1 Flu Virus offered for importation into the United States are subject to detention and refusal of admission. We will advise the appropriate regulatory or law enforcement officials in the country from which you operate that FDA considers your product listed above to be an unapproved, uncleared, or unauthorized product that cannot be legally sold to consumers in the United States.

Please direct any inquiries to FDA at FDAFLUTASKFORCECFSAN@fda.hhs.gov or by contacting Kathleen Lewis at 301-436-2148.

It is also your responsibility to ensure that the products you market are in compliance with the FTC Act. FTC staff strongly urge you to review all claims for your products and ensure that those claims are supported by competent and reliable scientific evidence. The FTC also asks that you notify it via electronic mail at flu@ftc.gov within 48 hours of the specific actions you have taken to address the agency's concerns. If you have any questions regarding compliance with the FTC Act, please contact Karen Jagielski at 202-326-2509.

Very truly yours,
/S/
Mary K. Engle
Associate Director
Division of Advertising Practices
Federal Trade Commission

/S/
Roberta F. Wagner
Director
Office of Compliance
Center for Food Safety and Applied Nutrition
Food and Drug Administration

Thus we see that even in a medical school professor backed by reams of scientific literature proving the efficacy of herbs in improving immune function can be threatened with fines and imprisonment by our government.

Michael F. Holick, MD, PhD, a professor at Boston University, was asked to resign in from BU's Department of Dermatology because of a book he wrote in which he describes the importance of

> Thus we see that even in a medical school professor backed by reams of scientific literature proving the efficacy of herbs in improving immune function can be threatened with fines and imprisonment by our government.

sunlight in boosting vitamin D levels.   Holick is a talented, experienced and highly respected researcher. He is a professor of medicine and physiology, and formerly of dermatology, at Boston University School of Medicine, and (until 2000) chief of endocrinology, metabolism and nutrition. Since 1987 he has also been the program director of the University's General Clinical Research Center. Department chair Barbara Gilchrest, MD, told the Boston Globe that the book "is an embarrassment for this institution and an embarrassment for him."

In writing this book, I am not writing as an M.D. I am writing as a Licensed Pastoral Health Practitioner And Counselor under the Texas Occupational Code Section 503.054 and under rights guaranteed by the First and Ninth Amendments of the United States Constitution. This allows me to discuss medical concepts that my MD license prevents me from discussing.

Introduction

Although modern medicine provides ever-increasing efficiency in emergency medicine (once you get out of the waiting room and actually get care), the results of care for chronic disease in the US is on par with third world countries according to the World Health Organization.

This book suggests a different paradigm for the care of chronic disease based on the recognition that we must constantly make new cells to replace those that are worn out or damaged. Chronic disease occurs when we lose the ability to make new cells that work.

To reverse chronic disease we must look for the reasons that we have lost the ability to make new cells that work. Making new cells requires -50 millivolts of energy, amino acids to make the inside of cells, fats to make the outside of cells, vitamins and minerals to make the metabolic processes work, oxygen, a fuel system (fats and glucose), a sewage system to get rid of waste proteins (lymphatic system), a system to protect us from infections, and a way to get rid of toxic substances.

Almost all chronic diseases are characterized by low voltage. Just as a new Mercedes without a battery isn't going anywhere, a body without a functional electrical system doesn't work either. Therefore, the title of this book is Healing is Voltage.

The main things that control voltage are thyroid hormone, fulvic acid, dental infections, scars and exercise.

The body's primary source of amino acids is stomach acid breaking proteins into amino acids. You cannot be well without stomach acid.

The body's source of fats is bile from the liver/gall bladder system allowing fat to be absorbed. Surprisingly, production of bile is based on stomach acid.

Humic and fulvic acid are in control of vitamins and minerals as well as being a source of amino acids. Because of our farming practices there is little humic and fulvic left in our food supply.

Oxygen is dependent upon iron in hemoglobin to carry it to the cells. Again humic/fulvic are in control of minerals including iron. Vitamin C is also necessary to absorb iron. Circulation is also necessary for the blood to carry oxygen. Much of the circulation is controlled by nitric oxide.

Much of the digestive process that provides fats and glucose is controlled by stomach acid since it is stomach acid that tells the pancreas to make the enzymes necessary to digest our food.

Since we are a portable system we must have a battery system that provides voltage as we move about. Our muscles are voltage generators as well as rechargeable batteries. However this system only works when we are moving/exercising. Without exercise, our battery system goes dead. In addition, it is exercise that activates our lymphatic system to remove waste proteins from dead cells from our body. Without exercise, our sewage backs up.

This book begins the process of your understanding what things you must do to make new cells. Making new cells that work is the key to curing all chronic disease. You must stop thinking about having heart disease, indigestion, headaches, a gall bladder problem etc. and trying to find a solution for that particular disease/symptom. You must ask the question, "Why can't I make new cells that work?" When you find the answer, you know what to do to get well. It all starts when you start thinking like an electrician instead of a physician. Check the voltages in the wiring system of the body (the acupuncture system) and you will be on your way to finding the problem and its solution.

1 Who is Jerry Tennant?

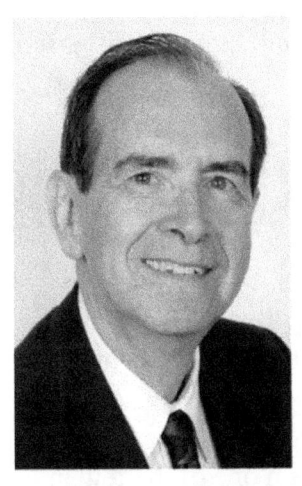

I graduated as valedictorian of high school at age sixteen. I completed my junior and senior years simultaneously by taking home study courses. I completed college except for three hours in two and a half years at Texas Tech University. I received the Phi Kappa Phi Award and the premed of the year award.

I attended the University of Houston School of Optometry before medical school. I was accepted into Southwestern Medical School at age nineteen. I graduated in the top ten at age twenty-three.

I completed a residency in ophthalmology at Harvard Medical School/Massachusetts Eye and Ear Infirmary and the Southwestern Medical School/Parkland Hospital system between 1965 and 1968.

I am board certified in ophthalmology and ophthalmic plastic surgery.

I was the director of the ophthalmic plastic surgery clinic at Parkland Hospital.

I was the founder/director of Dallas Eye

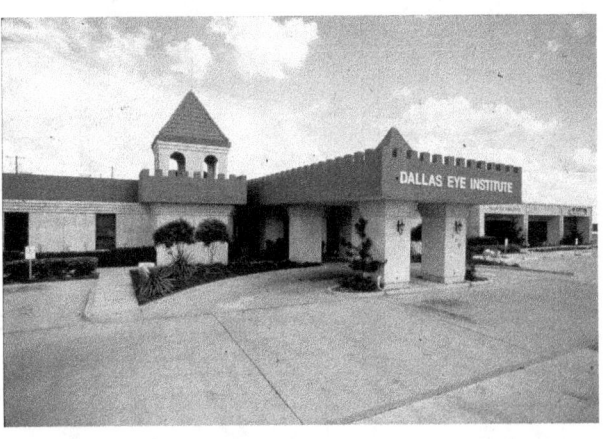

Institute. I have a doctorate of natural medicine license from the Pastoral Medical Association. I am licensed in Arizona by the Board of Homeopathic and Alternative Medicine.

I hold patents for medical devices including intraocular lenses, surgical instruments, etc.

I was co-founder of the Outpatient Ophthalmic Surgical Society, and I taught most of the ophthalmologists how to do outpatient eye surgery in the 1980s.

I was one of the first surgeons in the United States to place intraocular lenses in eyes after cataract surgery. I taught those techniques around the world.

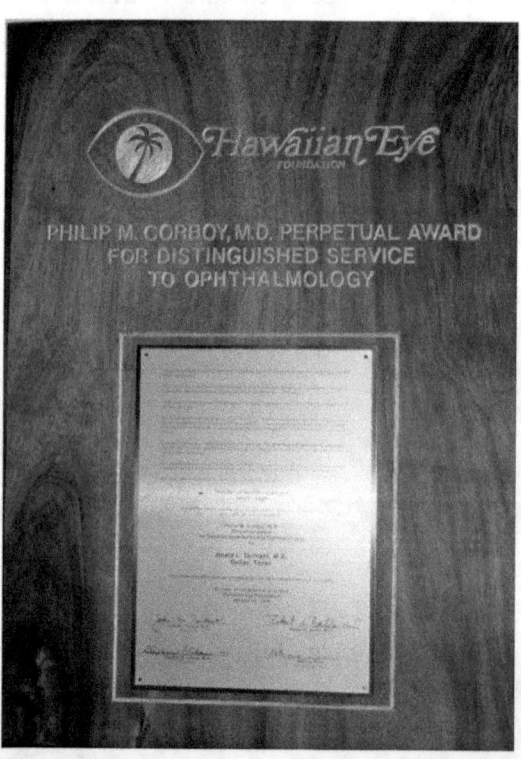

I am one of the few in the world to receive the Corboy Award for Advancements in Ophthalmology.

I received the American Academy of Ophthalmology Award for my contributions to ophthalmology.

I've written several books about cataract surgery and lifestyle management.

The Order of Saint Sylvester is intended to award Roman Catholic laymen who are actively involved in the life of the church, particularly as it is exemplified in the exercise of their professional duties and mastership of the different arts. It is also conferred on non-Catholics, but more rarely than the Order of Saint Gregory.

I am not Catholic. However, I was awarded the Order of Saint Sylvester by Pope Benedict XVI in July 2008 for my contributions to medicine.

I received a PhD (hon.) in anthropology and education from the ORDEN DE SANTIAGO APÓSTOL, an ancient religious order of Spain, under the priory of Monseñor Basilius Adao Pereira, Priorato Real de los Caballeros de Jerusalem, Pontífice Instituto de Estudios de la Religión under the Order of Santiago, more properly the Military Order of Saint James of the Sword.

I currently work at the Tennant Institute for Pastoral Medicine, an Ecclesiastical Private Expressive Association, as defined by law, and provide service as a pastoral health practitioner and counselor.

See www.tennantinstitute.com.

I practiced ophthalmology from 1964 to 1995. I did much of the FDA study for the VISX excimer laser. I performed about one thousand cases in the United States and about two thousand cases abroad from 1991 to 1995.

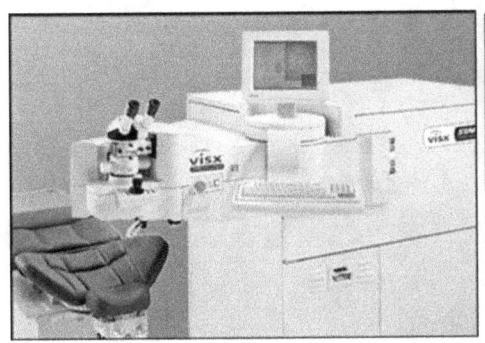
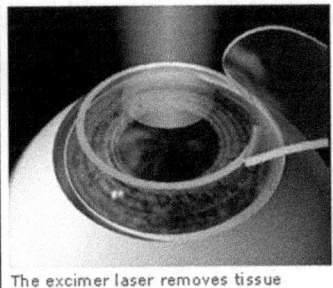

The excimer laser removes tissue from the cornea's internal layers.

http://www.ohsuhealth.com/cei/images/lasik_laser.jpg

23

What we didn't know at the time was that the laser did not kill viruses. The laser would strike the cornea, release viruses, and they would float upward through my mask into my nose and into my

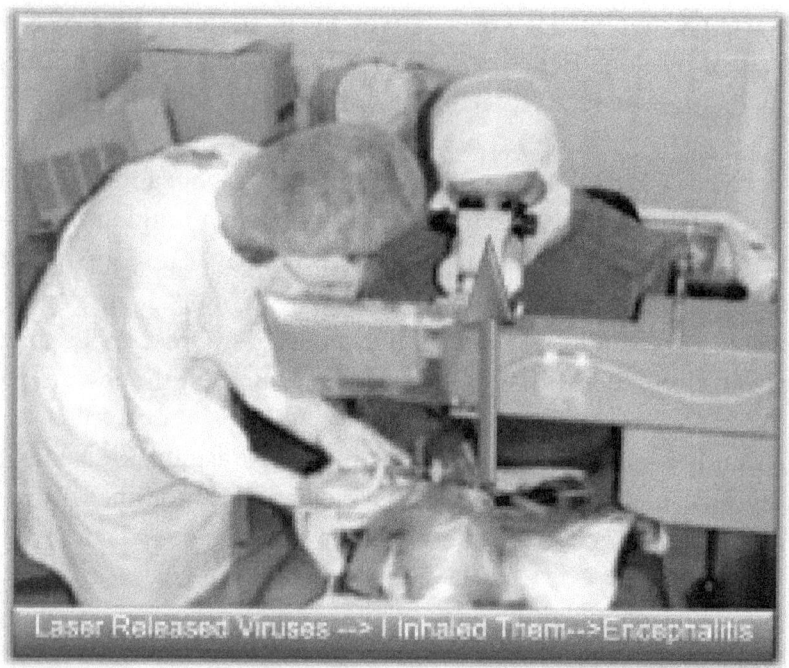

Laser Released Viruses --> I Inhaled Them-->Encephalitis

brain. I developed encephalitis, neuropathies, a low platelet count, and other nervous system defects in 1994. I could see a patient to diagnose what was wrong with them, but I couldn't remember how to write a prescription. I also developed spastic movements that prevented me from safely performing eye surgery. I had to quit

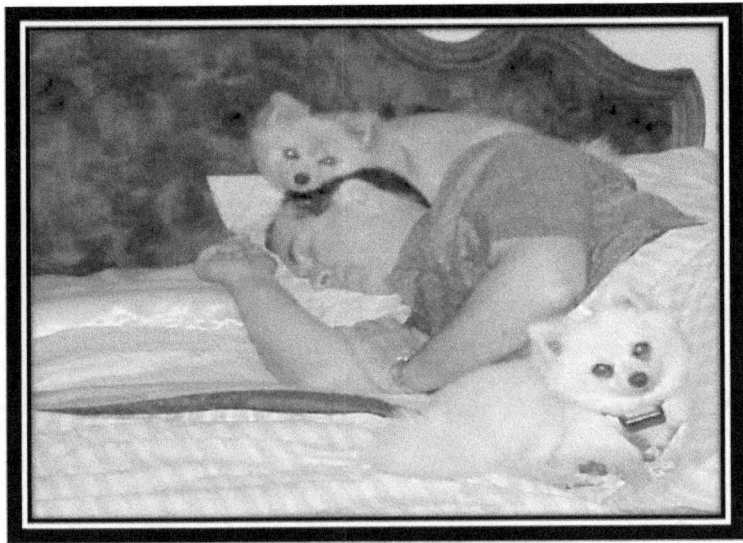

work on November 30, 1995.

For almost seven years, I slept about sixteen hours per day. Remember that I had viruses in my brain and viruses in my spleen. Note in the picture that my dog Tigger would sleep on my head, and my dog Pooh would curl up next to my spleen. They seemed to know where my voltage was low, and they were my constant "electron donors"!

2 We Need a New Medical Paradigm

The purpose of this book is to suggest a new paradigm for western medicine. Many think that the paradigm we have is the best in the world. That simply isn't true. Our health care system is a disaster, both in outcomes and affordability.

It is true that we have some amazing techniques to help people, such as trauma surgery, cataract surgery, imaging techniques, etc. But our results in chronic disease and cancer are a dismal failure at best.

par·a·digm (pār'ə-dīm', -dǐm') n.

1. One that serves as a pattern or model.
2. A set of assumptions, concepts, values, and practices that constitutes a way of viewing reality for the community that shares them, especially in an intellectual discipline.

Despite the popular myth that the United States has the best medical care in the world, the opposite is true. We are ranked thirty-seventh in the world by the World Health Organization! The World Health Organization's ranking of the world's health systems was last produced in 2000, and the WHO no longer produces such a ranking table, because of the complexity of the task.

The World Health Organization has carried out the first ever analysis of the world's health systems. Using five performance indicators to measure health systems in 191 member states, it found that France provides the best overall health care followed among major countries by Italy, Spain, Oman, Austria, and Japan.

The findings were published June 21, 2000, in "The World Health Report 2000 – Health Systems: Improving Performance."

The U. S. health system spends a higher portion of its gross domestic product than any other country but ranks 37 out of 191

1 France	2 Italy	3 San Marino	4 Andorra
5 Malta	6 Singapore	7 Spain	8 Oman
9 Austria	10 Japan	11 Norway	12 Portugal
13 Monaco	14 Greece	15 Iceland	16 Luxembourg
17 Netherlands	18 United Kingdom	19 Ireland	20 Switzerland
21 Belgium	22 Colombia	23 Sweden	24 Cyprus
25 Germany	26 Saudi Arabia	27 United Arab Emirates	28 Israel
29 Morocco	30 Canada	31 Finland	32 Australia
33 Chile	34 Denmark	35 Dominica	36 Costa Rica
37 USA	38 Slovenia	39 Cuba	40 Brunei
41 New Zealand	42 Bahrain	43 Croatia	44 Qatar
45 Kuwait	46 Barbados	47 Thailand	48 Czech Republic
49 Malaysia	50 Poland	51 Dominican Republic	52 Tunisia
53 Jamaica	54 Venezuela	55 Albania	56 Seychelles
57 Paraguay	58 South Korea	59 Senegal	60 Philippines
61 Mexico	62 Slovakia	63 Egypt	64 Kazakhstan
65 Uruguay	66 Hungary	67 Trinidad and Tobago	68 Saint Lucia
69 Belize	70 Turkey	71 Nicaragua	72 Belarus
73 Lithuania	74 Saint Vincent and the Grenadines	75 Argentina	76 Sri Lanka
77 Estonia	78 Guatemala	79 Ukraine	80 Solomon Islands
81 Algeria	82 Palau	83 Jordan	84 Mauritius
85 Grenada	86 Antigua & Barbuda	87 Libya	88 Bangladesh
89 Macedonia	90 Bosnia-Herzegovina	91 Lebanon	92 Indonesia
93 Iran	94 Bahamas	95 Panama	96 Fiji
97 Benin	98 Nauru	99 Romania	100 Saint Kitts and Nevis
101 Moldova	102 Bulgaria	103 Iraq	104 Armenia
105 Latvia	106 Yugoslavia	107 Cook Islands	108 Syria
109 Azerbaijan	110 Suriname	111 Ecuador	112 India
113 Cape Verde	114 Georgia	115 El Salvador	116 Tonga
117 Uzbekistan	118 Comoros	119 Samoa	120 Yemen
121 Niue	122 Pakistan	123 Micronesia	124 Bhutan
125 Brazil	126 Bolivia	127 Vanuatu	128 Guyana
129 Peru	130 Russia	131 Honduras	132 Burkina Faso
133 Sao Tome and Principe	134 Sudan	135 Ghana	136 Tuvalu
137 Ivory Coast	138 Haiti	139 Gabon	140 Kenya
141 Marshall Islands	142 Kiribati	143 Burundi	144 China
145 Mongolia	146 Gambia	147 Maldives	148 Papua New Guinea
149 Uganda	150 Nepal	151 Kyrgyzstan	152 Togo
153 Turkmenistan	154 Tajikistan	155 Zimbabwe	156 Tanzania
157 Djibouti	158 Eritrea	159 Madagascar	160 Vietnam
161 Guinea	162 Mauritania	163 Mali	164 Cameroon
165 Laos	166 Congo	167 North Korea	168 Namibia
169 Botswana	170 Niger	171 Equatorial Guinea	172 Rwanda
173 Afghanistan	174 Cambodia	175 South Africa	176 Guinea-Bissau
177 Swaziland	178 Chad	179 Somalia	180 Ethiopia
181 Angola	182 Zambia	183 Lesotho	184 Mozambique
185 Malawi	186 Liberia	187 Nigeria	188 Democratic Republic of the Congo
189 Central African Republic	190 Myanmar		

countries according to its performance, the report finds. The United Kingdom, which spends just six percent of gross domestic product (GDP) on health services, ranks eighteenth. Several small

28

countries—San Marino, Andorra, Malta, and Singapore—are rated close behind second-placed Italy.

WHO Director-General Dr. Gro Harlem Brundtland says: "The main message from this report is that the health and well-being of people around the world depend critically on the performance of the health systems that serve them. Yet there is wide variation in performance, even among countries with similar levels of income and health expenditure. It is essential for decision-makers to understand the underlying reasons so that system performance, and hence the health of populations, can be improved." See www.who.int.

Our western medical paradigm assumes that when an organ fails to perform adequately, it can only be corrected by finding a chemical (drug) to make it work or to remove it surgically. As we will discuss, the western medical paradigm is based in chemistry and on Newtonian concepts.

An often overlooked truth is that we tend to get well by making new cells, not by correcting those that are malfunctioning. We replace the rods and cones in our retina every forty-eight hours. The lining of our intestines is replaced every three days. We replace our skin every six weeks, our liver every eight weeks, our nervous system every eight months, and our bones every year. This brings nutrition into a clearer focus. If we are going to make good cells, we must have good raw materials to make them. In addition, we must not be missing necessary components.

If we build a new house from material taken from a house that was torn down because of termite damage, the new house will not be a very good one. If we build new cells from recycled materials, the new cells may not be any better than the ones that were worn out.

If we build a house but we don't have any shingles, the house won't be a good house. If we build a cell that is missing a critical component like vitamin C, it may not work correctly. To be healthy, we must eat quality food that is not filled with preservatives and toxins. When was the last time that your doctor told you about the dangers of trans fats, synthetic sweeteners, fluoride, etc.?

Many doctors are required to see fifty to sixty patients a day to have enough income to keep their offices open and pay the corporations that hire them. It is impossible to do much more than write a prescription and move on to the next patient.

When you go to a doctor he/she will likely order a complete blood count, a urinalysis, a comprehensive medical profile (tests for liver and kidney function, glucose, minerals, etc.), and a blood fat analysis. If these tests come back normal, the doctor will tell you that you are fine and that your complaints are all in your head. If you persist in complaining about your health, you will likely be sent to a psychiatrist!

Economics vs. Science

A major part of our medical dilemma in the United States is the goal of our medical system. It is a matter of making money vs. making people well. These are often conflicting goals. Let's look at an example:

> "Is Screening For Breast Cancer With Mammography Justifiable?" Gotzsche, P.C., and Olsen, O., *Lancet,* (2000 Jan 8), 355(9198): 129–34

> Abstract:
> BACKGROUND: A 1999 study found no decrease in breast cancer mortality in Sweden, where screening has been recommended since 1985. We therefore reviewed the methodological quality of the mammography trials and an influential Swedish meta-analysis, and did a meta-analysis

ourselves.

METHODS: We searched the Cochrane Library for trials and asked the investigators for further details. Meta-analyses were done with Review Manager (version 4.0).

FINDINGS: Baseline imbalances were shown for six of the eight identified trials, and inconsistencies in the number of women randomized were found in four. The two adequately randomized trials found no effect of screening on breast cancer mortality (pooled relative risk 1.04 [95% CI 0.84–1.27]) or on total mortality (0.99 [0.94–1.05]). The pooled relative risk for breast cancer mortality for the other trials was 0.75 (0.67– 0.83), which was significantly different (p=0.005) from that for the unbiased trials. The Swedish meta-analysis showed a decrease in breast cancer mortality but also an increase in total mortality (1.06 [1.04–1.08]); this increase disappeared after adjustment for an imbalance in age.

INTERPRETATION: Screening for breast cancer with mammography is unjustified. If the Swedish trials are judged to be unbiased, the data show that for every 1,000 women screened biennially throughout 12 years, one breast cancer death is avoided whereas the total number of deaths is increased by six. If the Swedish trials (apart from the Malmo trial) are judged to be biased, there is no reliable evidence that screening decreases breast cancer mortality.

So if mammography for breast cancer is unjustified and actually increases deaths from breast cancer, why are we still doing them? Why are our medical societies and governmental agencies insisting that American women get mammography? One can only conclude that it is because doctors and the corporations that hire them make so much money doing mammography.

Another example is the use of the hepatitis B vaccine for newborns. Infection with hepatitis B virus usually occurs in those using IV street drugs like heroin or with multiple sexual partners. It can also be a problem with blood transfusions. A mother with the disease can pass it to her unborn child and thus one must consider the health of that fetus.

However, most children born in the United States are not at risk for hepatitis B. It would be easy to identify those at risk by simply testing pregnant women for the virus. Instead, U.S. health policy requires that every newborn baby be given the vaccine for hepatitis B!

"The Vaccine Adverse Event Reporting System is a United States program for vaccine safety, co-sponsored by the Centers for Disease Control and Prevention (CDC) and the Food and Drug Administration known as VAERS. The program is an outgrowth of the 1986 National Childhood Vaccine Injury Act, which requires health care providers to report:

1. Any event listed by the vaccine manufacturer as a contraindication to subsequent doses of the vaccine.
2. Any event listed in the Reportable Events Table that occurs within the specified time period after vaccination. The data are stored electronically by the CDC in the Vaccine Safety Datalink.

VAERS is meant to act as a sort of 'early warning system'—a way for physicians and researchers to identify possible unforeseen reactions or side effects of vaccination for further study." – Wikipedia

1996 data from VAERS shows 872 serious events in children under age fourteen that received the hepatitis B vaccine. These children were either taken to an emergency room, had life-threatening health problems, were hospitalized, or were disabled following the vaccination. Of the 872 events, 214 had the hepatitis B vaccine alone while the rest had it in combination with other vaccines. Of the 872 events, 48 kids died from the vaccine reaction.

In 1996, only 279 cases of hepatitis B were reported in children under age fourteen. None of them died.

In 2007, there were 1,219 hepatitis B reactions reported to VAERS, about fifty percent more than in 1996!

So the current U.S. policy that requires every newborn to receive the hepatitis B vaccine kills forty-eight kids and injures another 824, with some of them permanently disabled. In those fortunate enough to escape vaccination, only 279 got hepatitis and none of them died.

So why are we forcing all our newborns to be exposed to this risk of death and disability with no benefit to anyone except Merck, which makes almost $1 billion per year from these vaccines? Economics vs. Science?

This is an example of why we spend twice the amount per capita as any other country in the world but still have the quality of health care on a par with Cuba!

The War on Cancer is a Failure

You will often hear that the success of some cancer therapy is fifty percent or eighty percent. What does that mean? It means that if the tumor shrinks at any time during the therapy, the system considers that patient "cured." It doesn't matter if they are dead one week later. They still are considered "cured."

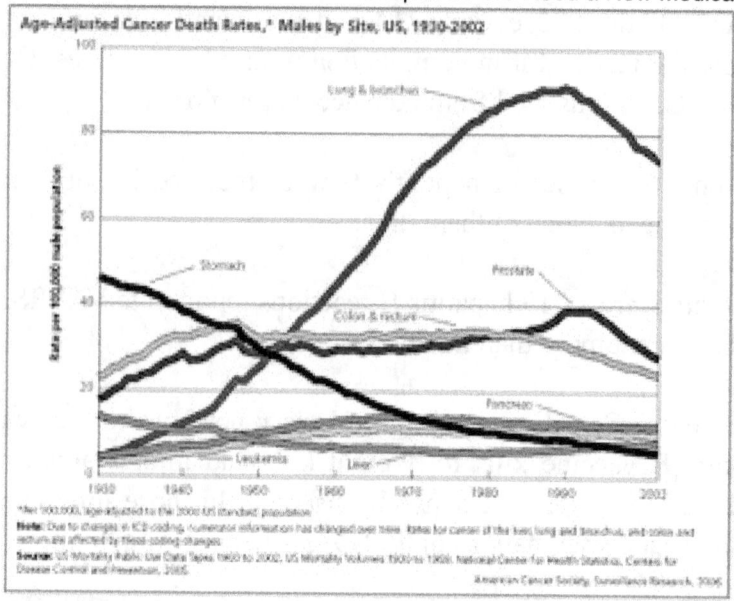

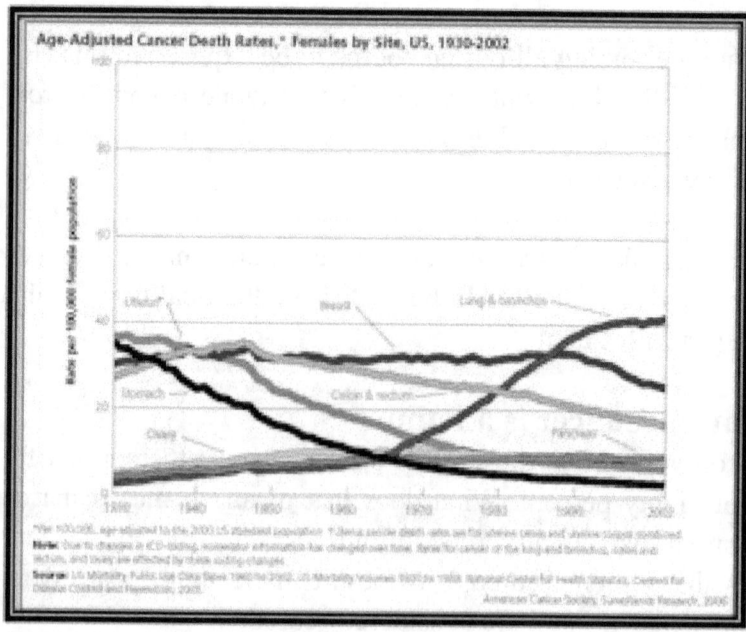

The American Cancer Society released the data shown in the chart in 2006. Note that in both men and women, the deaths from lung cancer increased dramatically. Deaths in both men and women decreased for stomach cancer, and deaths from uterine cancer also decreased. Deaths from other cancers are essentially unchanged from 1950 to 2002! The War on Cancer is a dismal failure. We need to re-examine the cancer paradigm because our current one isn't working.

This chart shows many of the chemotherapy agents approved by the FDA during the 1990s and early 2000s. What you see is that the mean time to death is 7.6 months! Few doctors tell their patients that the mean time to death from the drugs they are recommending is only 7.6 months and that much of this time will be spent in pain with vomiting and severe fatigue. Doctors are even turning to the courts to force patients to undergo this unsuccessful treatment of chemotherapy! Economics vs. Science?

The FDA requires that every drug approved be tested against a placebo—except for chemotherapy drugs. They will not allow chemotherapy drugs to be tested against a placebo. I can find only one study in the Medline database that compares chemotherapy with "supportive care." That is a Canadian study.

What you see is that the chemotherapy group lived an average of three months longer than the supportive care group, but the price they paid was that four of them died from bone marrow damage, forty percent had lung damage, and twenty-one percent had serious

Docetaxel Vs Supportive Rx	
J Clin Oncol 2000; 18:2095-103	
Docetaxel	7.5 months survival
Supportive Care	4.6 months survival
Side effects = cost for living three months longer	
Hair loss = 56 percent	
Bone marrow damage = four deaths	
Lung toxicity = 40 percent	
Serious lung damage = 21 percent	

lung damage. I don't believe many would consider living three months longer not being able to breathe is a good trade-off along with being sick from the chemotherapy for the seven months they lived. And this also ignores the cost of therapy.

A recent Australian study also looked at the science of treating cancer with chemotherapy:

> "The Contribution of Cytotoxic Chemotherapy to 5-year Survival in Adult Malignancies," Morgan G., Ward, R., and Barton, M., Department of Radiation Oncology, Sydney, NSW, Australia
>
> AIMS: The debate on the funding and availability of cytotoxic drugs raises questions about the contribution of curative or adjuvant cytotoxic chemotherapy to survival in adult cancer patients.
>
> MATERIALS AND METHODS: We undertook a literature search for randomized clinical trials reporting a 5-year survival benefit attributable solely to cytotoxic chemotherapy in adult malignancies. The total number of newly diagnosed cancer patients for 22 major adult malignancies was determined from cancer registry data in Australia and from the Surveillance Epidemiology and End Results data in the USA for 1998.
>
> For each malignancy, the absolute number to benefit was the product of (a) the total number of persons with that malignancy; (b) the proportion or subgroup(s) of that malignancy showing a benefit; and (c) the percentage increase in 5-year survival due solely to cytotoxic chemotherapy. The overall contribution was the sum total of the absolute numbers showing a 5-year survival benefit expressed as a percentage of the total number for the 22 malignancies.
>
> RESULTS: The overall contribution of curative and adjuvant cytotoxic chemotherapy to 5-year survival in adults was estimated to be 2.3% in Australia and 2.1% in the USA.

CONCLUSION: As the 5-year relative survival rate for cancer in Australia is now over 60%, it is clear that cytotoxic chemotherapy only makes a minor contribution to cancer survival. To justify the continued funding and availability of drugs used in cytotoxic chemotherapy, a rigorous evaluation of the cost effectiveness and impact on quality of life is urgently required.

If the mean time to death with chemotherapy drugs is 7.6 months and the contribution of these drugs to survival is only 2.1 percent, why are we forcing our population to have this horrible therapy? Economics vs. Science?

Obesity

Our population is becoming more obese.

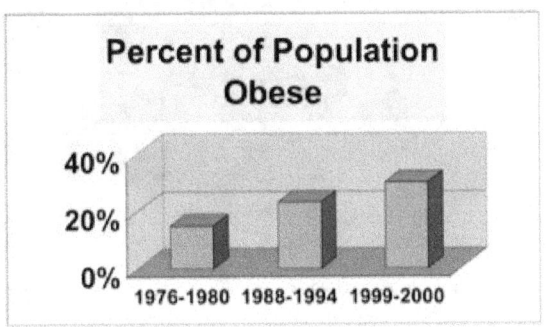

Obesity is defined as having a Body Mass Index (BMI) over 30. The formula to calculate your BMI is

$$BMI = \frac{(weight\ in\ pounds\ *\ 703)}{Height\ in\ inches^2}$$

You can find BMI calculators on the web so you don't have to do the math.

As we will discuss, fluoridation causes hypothyroidism.

Hypothyroidism causes obesity. The CDC data shows a correlation between the amount of fluoridation and the amount of obesity in states.

This graph shows the percentage of people in each state that are obese vs. the percentage of people in each state with fluoridated city water. In order to compare them, we did a trend analysis on the fluoridation and got the following graph:

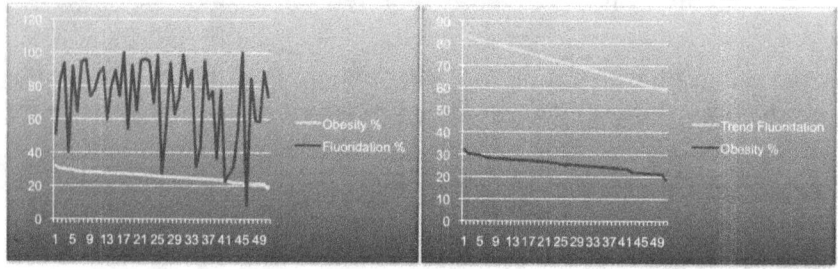

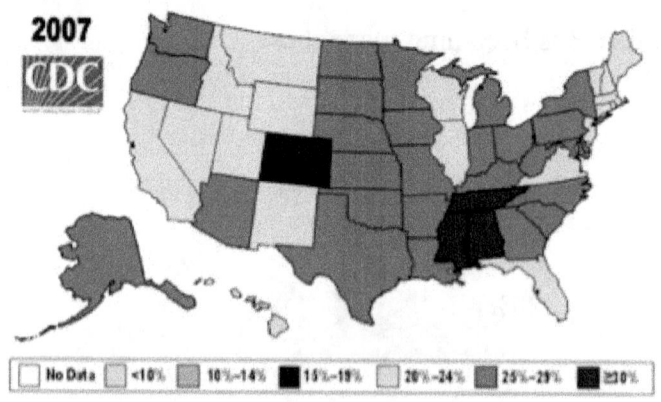

Thus we can see that the states with the most fluoridation tend to have the most obesity. Although not proof that fluoridation is causing our obesity epidemic, I think you will be convinced after reading the chapter on hypothyroidism.

Just recently on ABC News, they were discussing doing gastric bypass surgery on obese children. Are we going to do gastric bypass surgery on twenty-five percent of our population or simply take fluoride out of the water, toothpaste, and dental offices? Economics vs. Science?

Causes of Death in the United States

Anderson, R.N., "Deaths: Leading Causes for 2000," National Vital Statistics Reports 50(10), 2002

Cause of Death	Deaths
Heart Disease	710,760
Cancer	553,091
Medical Care	225,400
Stroke	167,661
Lung Disease	122,009
Accidents	97,900
Diabetes	69,301
Influenza and Pneumonia	65,313

Note that the third leading cause of death in the United States is medical errors in hospitals!

These are listed in the *Journal of the American Medical Association*: Starfield, B., "Is U.S. Health Care Really the Best in the World?" *JAMA* 284 (2000): 483–485.

Medication Errors	7,400
Unnecessary Surgery	12,000
Other Preventable Errors in Hospital	20,000
Hospital Borne Infections	80,000
Adverse Drug Effects	106,000
Total	225,400

In-Hospital Drug Reactions/Deaths

"Incidence of Adverse Drug Reactions in Hospitalized Patients: A Meta-analysis of Prospective Studies," Lazarou, J., Pomeranz, B.H., and Corey, P.N., Department of Zoology, University of Toronto, Ontario, Canada

OBJECTIVE: To estimate the incidence of serious and fatal adverse drug reactions (ADR) in hospital patients.

DATA SOURCES: Four electronic databases were searched from 1966 to 1996.

STUDY SELECTION: Of 153, we selected 39 prospective studies from U.S. hospitals.

DATA EXTRACTION: Data extracted independently by 2 investigators were analyzed by a random-effects model. To obtain the overall incidence of ADRs in hospitalized patients, we combined the incidence of ADRs occurring while in the hospital plus the incidence of ADRs causing admission to hospital. We excluded errors in drug administration, noncompliance, overdose, drug abuse, therapeutic failures, and possible ADRs. Serious ADRs were defined as those that required hospitalization, were permanently disabling, or resulted in death.

DATA SYNTHESIS: The overall incidence of serious ADRs was 6.7% (95% confidence interval [CI], 5.2%–8.2%) and of fatal ADRs was 0.32% (95% CI, 0.23%–0.41%) of hospitalized patients. We estimated that in 1994 overall 2,216,000 (1,721,000–2,711,000) hospitalized patients had serious ADRs and 106,000 (76,000–137,000) had fatal ADRs, making these reactions between the fourth and sixth leading cause of death.

CONCLUSIONS: The incidence of serious and fatal adverse drug reactions in U.S. hospitals was found to be extremely high. While our results must be viewed with circumspection because of heterogeneity among studies and small biases in the samples, these data nevertheless suggest that adverse drug reactions represent an important clinical issue.

As you can see, this study found that almost seven people out of a hundred who enter a hospital will have a serious drug reaction, and three out of a thousand will die from a drug reaction!

"Modern Health Care System is the Leading Cause of Death"

Null, Gary, PhD; Dean, Carolyn, MD ND; Feldman, Martin, MD; Rasio, Debora, MD; and Smith, Dorothy, PhD.

Null et al. added the hospital deaths to other drug-induced deaths and came to the conclusion that iatrogenic (caused by doctors) deaths are the leading cause of death in the U.S.

Our projected statistic of 7.8 million iatrogenic deaths is more than all the casualties from wars that America has fought in its entire history."

Thus if you add untoward hospital deaths to deaths from the side effects of drugs, the leading cause of death in the United States is health care! The approximately eight million Americans killed by health care is certainly more than the approximately 1.25 million killed in all the wars Americans have fought!

The table below shows the number of U.S. soldiers killed in battle beginning with the Revolutionary War.

41

Revolutionary	4,435
War of 1812	2,260
Mexican	13,283
Civil War	823,028
Spanish-American	2,446
WW I	116,708
WW II	407,316
Korean	36,914
Vietnam	58,169
Persian Gulf	269
Iraq	4,232
Total	1,469,060

The single drug Vioxx is now estimated to have killed approximately 130,000 people in the United States alone.

Myth: There is a Safe Dose of Chemicals that can be put Into the Human Body.

In 1927, J.W. Trevan attempted to find a way to estimate the relative poisoning potency of drugs and medicines used at that time. He developed the LD50 test because the use of death as a "target" allows for comparisons between chemicals that poison the body. "LD" stands for "Lethal Dose." LD50 is the amount of a material, given all at once, which causes the death of fifty percent (one half) of a group of test animals. The LD50 is one way to

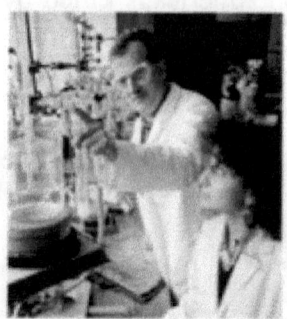

measure the short-term poisoning potential (acute toxicity) of a material.

To determine what dose of a drug to give, pharmaceutical companies determine how much of the drug is required to kill half of the mice or other animals it is given to. This is called the Lethal Dose 50% (LD50).

Then they determine how much drug must be given to humans to get an effect in fifty percent. This is called the Effective Dose 50% (ED50). Dividing the LD50/ED50 gives you the Therapeutic Index. If it takes 400/mg/ Kg of a drug to kill half of the mice and 100 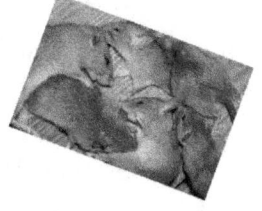 mg/Kg to get a result in people, the TI is 4. The closer the ED50 is to the LD50, the more toxic the drug.

Drugs are approved as "Safe and Effective" when the FDA determines the number of people who will die from the drug is acceptable "collateral damage." Patients (and often doctors) tend to believe that "Safe and Effective" means just that in all patients. They ignore the "acceptable collateral damage" implied by LD50/ ED50 that tells us that *all* drugs will kill or injure some of those who take them. Over time, the FDA seems to have allowed more toxic drugs to be called "Safe and Effective." Witness what has happened with Neurontin, Vioxx, Bextra, Avandia, Baycol, Propulsid, Posicor, Astemizole, Omniflox, Fen-Phen, and many OTC drugs that were declared "safe and effective" and then had to be removed from the market.

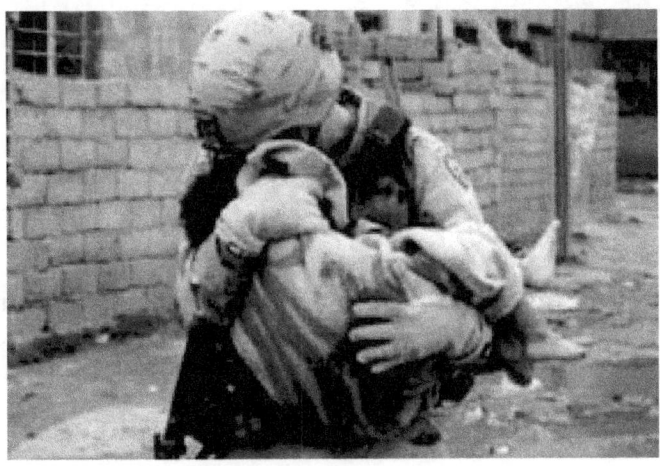

The diabetes drug Avandia increases the risk of fatal heart attack by sixty-four percent. The FDA has recently ruled that this is acceptable collateral damage and should remain on the market.

All chemicals (medicines) you put into your body have three effects:
1. Those you hope will happen.
2. Those you hope won't happen.
3. Those you don't know are happening.

Most pharmaceuticals and surgery speak to eliminating symptoms, but do not speak to healing. Absence of symptoms is not the same as healed and healthy. For example, taking aspirin or Tylenol may make you not know your joints are hurting, but they are still degenerating.

Myth: Most illness is genetic. We will find drugs to cure most disease by studying genes.

Proteins are the "gears" that make cells capable of doing their work. Every cell contains thousands of proteins. When a cell needs

to make some more proteins, it needs to read the gene's information on how to make the protein (reads the blueprint). DNA contains the genetic blueprints to make new proteins. Genes don't *do* anything. They are just blueprints. Genes are kept hidden like keeping blueprints in a drawer.
You can't see them until the drawer is opened.

The genes are covered with a protein sleeve. When the cell needs to make new proteins, an electronic signal causes the protein drawer (sleeve covering DNA) to open (move), revealing the necessary genes. The "drawers" concealing the genes are called "regulatory proteins."

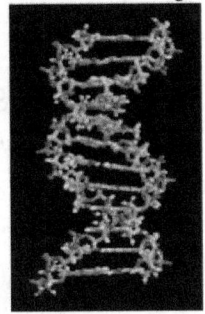

After accessing the DNA, the genetic information is imprinted onto a protein molecule called "messenger RNA." Messenger RNA is like a photocopy of the genes. The messenger RNA leaves the nucleus and enters the cytoplasm. It goes to a unit called the ribosome. Ribosomes are protein assembly factories that use the instruction set from the messenger RNA to build the protein from the blueprint carried by the messenger RNA. Once the protein is manufactured by the ribosome factory, it moves out into the cytoplasm of the cell to takes its place and begin to do its work.

The first correct description of DNA was by J. Watson and F. Crick in *Nature*, 1953:

"Molecular Structure of Nucleic Acids"; "A Structure for Deoxyribose Nucleic Acid," Watson, J. D., and Crick, F.H.C., *Nature* 171, 737–738 (1953), Macmillan Publishers Ltd., Medical Research Council Unit for the Study of Molecular Structure of Biological Systems, Cavendish Laboratory, Cambridge

There is no doubt that some genes are responsible for certain diseases. Examples are Huntington's chorea, beta thalassemia, and cystic fibrosis. However, only two percent of disorders are due to single gene defects! The thousands of people who sit and worry that they are destined to get cancer, diabetes, and other diseases because one of their relatives had it do so without good scientific basis.

The theory that genes control everything about us began to unravel with the publication of "The Origin of Mutants" by John Cairns et al. They took bacteria that lacked the gene to utilize lactose and placed them into an environment where the only nutrient was lactose. They were surprised to find that the bacteria lived instead of dying. This could only mean that the bacteria changed their genetic structure so that they could use lactose!

"The Origin of Mutants," Cairns, J., Overbaugh, J., and Miller, S., *Nature* (1988 Sep 8), 335 (6186): 142–5; Department Of Cancer Biology, Harvard School of Public Health, Boston, Massachusetts

Nucleic acids are replicated with conspicuous fidelity. Infrequently, however, they undergo changes in sequence, and this process of change (mutation) generates the variability that allows evolution. As the result of studies of bacterial variation, it is now widely believed that mutations arise continuously and without any consideration for their utility. In this paper, we briefly review the source of this idea and then describe some experiments suggesting that cells may have mechanisms for choosing which mutations will occur.

"Transposable Elements: Targets for Early Nutritional Effects on Epigenetic Gene Regulation," Waterland, R.A., and Jirtle, R.L., *Mol Cell Biol* (2003 Aug), 23(15): 5293–300 ISSN: 0270-7306

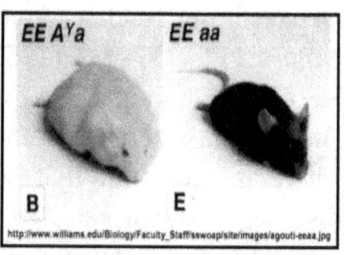

Another example of the ability of environment to change genes was described by Waterland et al. Usually yellow and fat, Agouti mice fed folic acid, vitamin B12, choline, and betaine changed their genes to have slender brown offspring. Thus we see that our genes can be changed by changing our diet.

Genome Project

One of the findings that is causing the genetic control myth to evaporate is the Genome Project. This project was the mapping of the genes of the human. It takes over 120,000 different proteins for the human body to work. It is still being taught that there is a specific gene present to make each protein. However, when the genes were all mapped, it was found that the human only has about 25,000 genes! Oops! There is obviously something wrong with the theory, isn't there?

In 1957, Howard Temin won the Nobel Prize for showing that the genes in DNA could be altered. RNA could go against the DNA/RNA concept and rewrite the DNA. We now know that the flow should be in both directions and is controlled by the environment:

Organism	Number of Genes
Human	25,000
Yeast Cell	6,000
Fruit fly	13,000
Worm	18,000
Plant	26,000

25,000 genes

26,000 genes

6,000 genes

13,000 genes

18,000 genes

"Environment Regulatory Proteins DNA RNA Proteins: From Heresy to Dogma in Accounts of Opposition to Howard Temin's DNA Provirus Hypothesis," Marcum, J.A., *Hist Philos Life Sci* (2002) 24(2): 165–92 ISSN: 0391-9714

Stem Cells

Primitive cells (totipotential cells, stem cells) have the entire genetic code of the organism. As cells differentiate into specialized cells such as liver, brain, heart, etc., the entire code is still present. However, the unused codes are switched off. Under the right conditions, these codes are switched back on, and the cell dedifferentiates back into a stem cell.

It has been found that the genes that we received from our parents can be altered by our environment. The study of this phenomenon has come to be called *epigenetics*. Not only can our genes change, these changes can be passed on to the next generation.

> "Reprogramming of Genome Function through Epigenetic Inheritance," Surani, M. Azim, *Nature*, Vol. 414, Issue 6859 (2001): 122–28.

> Most cells contain the same set of genes and yet they are extremely diverse in appearance and functions. It is the selective expression and repression of genes that determines the specific properties of individual cells. Nevertheless, even when fully differentiated, any cell can potentially be reprogrammed back to totipotency, which in turn results in re-differentiation of the full repertoire of adult cells from a single original cell of any kind. Mechanisms that regulate this exceptional genomic plasticity and the state of totipotency are being unraveled and will enhance our ability to manipulate stem cells for therapeutic purposes.

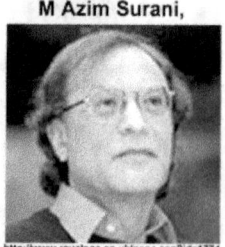

M Azim Surani,

http://www.royalsoc.ac.uk/page.asp?id=1774

We see that almost any of our cells can revert back to adult stem cells. There is no need, and perhaps no advantage, in using embryonic stem cells.

Evidence-based Medicine

Most doctors rely on "double-blind studies" published in peer-reviewed journals for information about how to treat patients. Actually many doctors rely on information from drug salespeople on how to treat patients.

> "Selective Publication of Antidepressant Trials and its Influence on Apparent Efficacy," Turner, E.H., Matthews, A.M., Linardatos, E., Tell, R.A., and Rosenthal, R.. *N Engl*

J Med (2008 Jan 17), 358(3): 252–60 ISSN: 1533-4406

Abstract:

BACKGROUND: Evidence-based medicine is valuable to the extent that the evidence base is complete and unbiased. Selective publication of clinical trials—and the outcomes within those trials—can lead to unrealistic estimates of drug effectiveness and alter the apparent risk-benefit ratio.

METHODS: We obtained reviews from the Food and Drug Administration (FDA) for studies of 12 antidepressant agents involving 12,564 patients. We conducted a systematic literature search to identify matching publications. For trials that were reported in the literature, we compared the published outcomes with the FDA outcomes. We also compared the effect size derived from the published reports with the effect size derived from the entire FDA data set.

RESULTS: Among 74 FDA-registered studies, 31%, accounting for 3,449 study participants, were not published. Whether and how the studies were published was associated with the study outcome. A total of 37 studies viewed by the FDA as having positive results were published; 1 study viewed as positive was not published.

Studies viewed by the FDA as having negative or questionable results were, with 3 exceptions, either not published (22 studies) or published in a way that, in our opinion, conveyed a positive outcome (11 studies). According to the published literature, it appeared that 94% of the trials conducted were positive. By contrast, the FDA analysis showed that 51% were positive. Separate meta-analyses of the FDA and journal data sets showed that the increase in effect size ranged from 11% to 69% for individual drugs and was 32% overall.

CONCLUSIONS: We cannot determine whether the bias observed resulted from a failure to submit manuscripts on the part of authors and sponsors, from decisions by journal editors and reviewers not to publish, or both. Selective reporting of clinical trial results may have adverse consequences for researchers, study participants, health care professionals, and patients.

Most doctors will say that they will not consider a treatment for their patients unless it has been approved by the FDA and results of double-blind, crossover studies have been published in peer reviewed journals. What is clearly demonstrated by the article above is that what is published in our journals is cherry-picked so that it appears that therapies work when indeed the totality of studies show just the opposite. This modification of the truth by drug companies and medical journals is criminal! The paradigm that doctors so fervently believe regarding published studies is like believing in the tooth fairy! This becomes even worse when you understand that many of the published studies were never even done!

"Guest Authorship and Ghostwriting in Publications Related to Rofecoxib: A Case Study of Industry Documents From Rofecoxib (Vioxx) Litigation," Ross, J.S., Hill, K.P., Egilman, D.S., and Krumholz, H.M., *JAMA* (2008 Apr 16), 299(15): 1800–12

Abstract:

CONTEXT: Authorship in biomedical publication provides recognition and establishes accountability and responsibility. Recent litigation related to rofecoxib (Vioxx) provided a unique opportunity to examine guest authorship and ghostwriting, practices that have been suspected in biomedical publication but for which there is little documentation.

OBJECTIVE: To characterize different types and the extent of guest authorship and ghostwriting in 1 case study.

DATA SOURCES: Court documents originally obtained during litigation related to rofecoxib (Vioxx) against Merck & Co. Inc. Documents were created predominantly between 1996 and 2004. In addition, publicly available articles related to rofecoxib identified via MEDLINE.

DATA EXTRACTION: All documents were reviewed by one author, with selected review by coauthors, using an iterative process of review, discussion, and re-review of documents to identify information related to guest authorship or ghostwriting.

DATA SYNTHESIS: Approximately 250 documents were relevant to our review. For the publication of clinical trials, documents were found describing Merck employees working either independently or in collaboration with medical publishing companies to prepare manuscripts and subsequently recruiting external, academically affiliated investigators to be authors. Recruited authors were frequently placed in the first and second positions of the authorship list.

For the publication of scientific review papers, documents were found describing Merck marketing employees developing plans for manuscripts, contracting with medical publishing companies to ghostwrite manuscripts, and recruiting external, academically affiliated investigators to be authors. Recruited authors were commonly the sole author on the manuscript and offered honoraria for their participation.

Among 96 relevant published articles, we found that 92% (22 of 24) of clinical trial articles published a disclosure of

51

Merck's financial support, but only 50% (36 of 72) of review articles published either a disclosure of Merck sponsorship or a disclosure of whether the author had received any financial compensation from the company.

CONCLUSIONS: This case-study review of industry documents demonstrates that clinical trial manuscripts related to rofecoxib (Vioxx) were authored by sponsor employees but often attributed first authorship to academically affiliated investigators who did not always disclose industry financial support. Review manuscripts were often prepared by unacknowledged authors and subsequently attributed authorship to academically affiliated investigators who often did not disclose industry financial support.

This report shows that Merck, the manufacturer of Vioxx, had its marketing department write up studies to show the safety of Vioxx. They then paid professors of medicine to say that they did the study when, in reality, no study was ever done. The professors names were placed on the study and it was submitted to journals and the FDA as if the study actually happened. It was all fraudulent and criminal. It resulted in the death of at least one hundred thousand Americans and many more in other countries. Merck paid a small fine in relation to the amount of money they made on the drug. I have not read that anyone went to jail.

The database of the National Library of Medicine is the MEDLINE computer database. This database is widely used by physicians to understand medical issues. Few physicians know that less than twenty percent of the world's medical studies are indexed here. They tend to refuse to index studies that do not support drug sales. They tend to refuse to publish studies that show that natural remedies work.

How can we doctors know what therapies to recommend to our

patients when only the positive studies get published and many of them never even happened? The paradigm must change. This ongoing criminal behavior makes medical care the leading cause of death in the United States!

Understanding Medical Studies

In addition to publishing only positive studies and hiding negative ones, publishing fake studies, and only indexing twenty percent of the studies, another deceit has come into prominence. It is the difference between absolute risk and relative risk.

A good explanation of this problem is the book entitled *The Illusion of Certainty: Health Benefits and Risks* by Ed Bouwer and Eric Rivkin from Johns Hopkins University.

Absolute risk is your risk of developing a disease over a specified period of time. Absolute risk reflects the number of people who will be harmed compared to the total number of people being considered.

If six out of one hundred get a disease and die, the AR is 6/100 or 0.06 or 6 percent.

"Absolute Risk Reduction" is the difference between two absolute risks in two groups. In the above example, if people take a drug and only four out of one hundred get the disease and die, the ARR is 6% - 4% = 2%. Two lives are saved out of one hundred.

ARR compares the number of people who will benefit from intervention to the total number of people being considered.

Relative risks are based on the ratio of two absolute risk numbers. When using relative risks, the absolute risk levels for the experimental and control groups are not known. If taking a new drug reduces the number of disease deaths from six out of one hundred (6%) to four out of one hundred (4%), then the relative risk difference is thirty-three percent, because four percent is thirty-three percent less than six percent. The absolute risk difference is two percent (6% - 4%). However, thirty-three percent sounds much better than two percent.

Let's say we looked at ten thousand people, five thousand of whom chewed bubble gum and five thousand that did not. If one of five thousand that chewed bubble gum had a heart attack and two out of the five thousand that did not chew bubble gum had a heart attack, we could report that only half as many people developed a heart attack when they chewed bubble gum. The FDA would then allow us to market bubble gum as preventing fifty percent of heart attacks because the relative risk is 0.5. This ignores the fact that 0.02 percent of those that chewed bubble gum had a heart attack while 0.04 percent of those that did chew gum did not have the same event. Certainly one case different between the two groups is not significant. However, it can be reported as a relative risk of fifty percent.

This is a significant problem in that almost all medical studies are now reported with relative risk instead of absolute risk. This sleight-of-hand reporting is the primary way that physicians are tricked into believing that drugs work.

This graph is from the MRFIT Study and shows deaths vs. cholesterol levels. It assumes a current benchmark of 200 mg/100 ml.

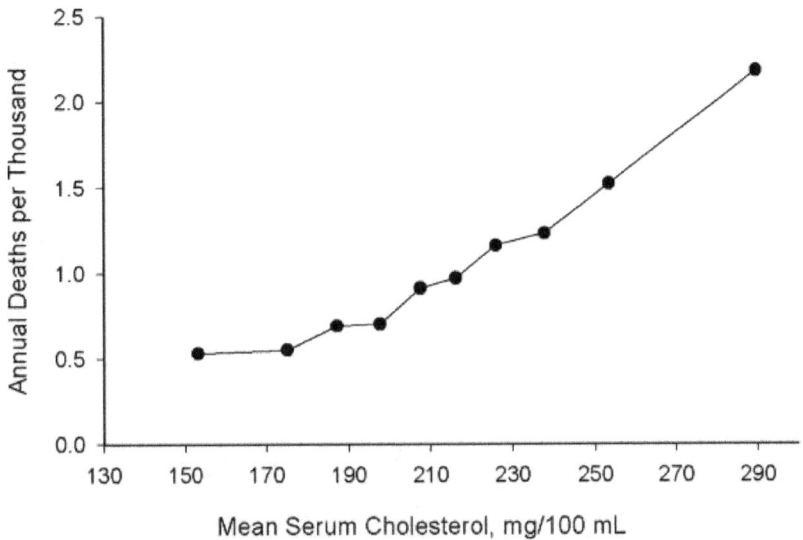

Mean Serum Cholesterol, mg/100 mL

"Is Relationship Between Serum Cholesterol and Risk of Premature Death From Coronary Heart Disease Continuous and Graded? Findings in 356,222 Primary Screenees of the Multiple Risk Factor Intervention Trial (MRFIT)," Stamler J., Wentworth, D., and Neaton, J.D., *JAMA* (1986 Nov 28), 256(20): 28238 ISSN: 0098-7484

Out of two thousand people with cholesterol over 200 mg/100 ml, there will be one additional death each year from CHD as compared to two thousand people with normal cholesterol. This means that 99.95 percent of the population would not benefit from efforts (diet and/or drugs) to reduce blood serum cholesterol levels.

Deaths per 1000

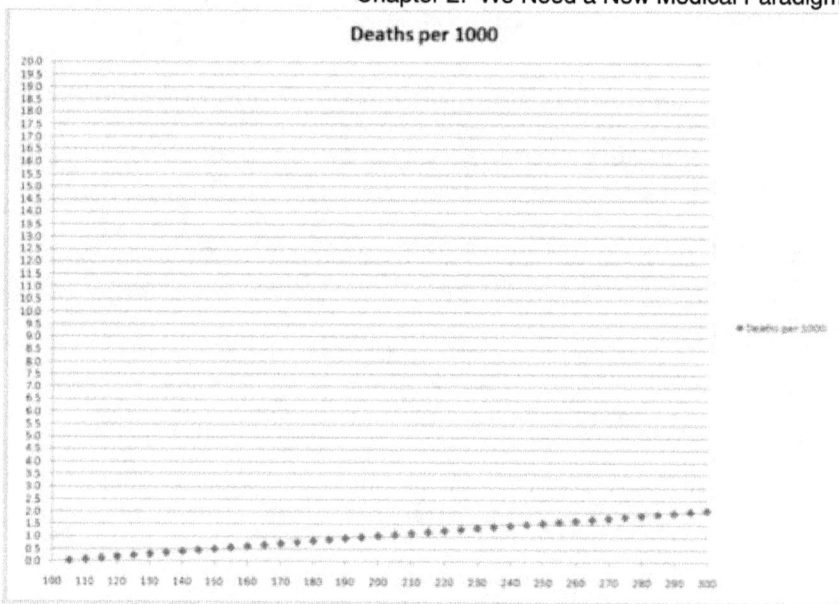

The graph above is the same data as above except the data line has been trended and the y-axis extended to make it more obvious visually how little difference cholesterol makes in deaths per thousand.

To put it another way, for 1,999 out of 2,000 individuals each year, it makes no difference whether they have elevated cholesterol or normal cholesterol in terms of whether or not they develop coronary heart disease!

I will discuss this in greater detail in the chapter on heart disease. It is clear that it doesn't make much sense to focus so much time and energy and money on the subject of cholesterol. Despite the science, the politics of medicine says that doctors should lose their license if they don't put patients with "elevated" cholesterol on statin drugs. The American Heart Association states that you are at high risk of coronary heart disease if your cholesterol level is above 240. However, the study showed that the cholesterol of 240 is only 0.5 percent more likely to have a heart attack than those with the cholesterol of 200. Economics vs. Science at work again!

Current guidelines suggest that anyone with a cholesterol level over 180 should be put on statin drugs. If you have a heart attack, you are put on statins no matter how low your cholesterol already is.

Statin drugs cost between $900 and $1,400 per year per person. This means that we waste about 12.5 billion dollars per year in therapies that are not supported by science for cholesterol treatment alone. Now expand this into all areas of medicine. It then becomes easy to see why Americans spend more money on health care than anyone in the world and yet have outcomes equivalent to Third World countries.

The Chemistry vs. Biophysics Paradigm

Myth: The human body is controlled primarily by chemistry.

Fact: the human body is controlled primarily by electronics (physics), not chemistry. Thus to really understand how the body works, we must understand something about physics and electronics.

Most physicians operate as if the body works like a clock. If a clock stops working, you take it apart to find the broken gear. You then replace that gear with a new one and the clock will work again. This concept is called *reductionism* and is a part of what is called Newtonian physics (after the theories of Isaac Newton).

The mathematics of reductionism is, at its most basic, the use of fractions, which holds that dividing and multiplying are opposites. The statement "four divided by two equals two" is the idea that dividing the system into two parts and then putting them back together restores the original system.

Simply put, reductionism is the idea that if you take a ten-pound bag of flour and put five pounds in one bucket, three pounds in another, and two pounds in another, you have ten pounds. Then if you put it all back into a sack, you will have the same ten pounds.

Isaac Newton lived from 1642 to 1727. Newton's book *Philosophiae Naturalis Principia Mathematica* demonstrated for the first time that celestial bodies follow the laws of dynamics and, formulating the law of universal gravitation, give mathematical solutions to most of the problems concerning motion. Newton created the mathematics called calculus. Newton's laws of motion became the basis for what we today call physics or Newtonian physics.

Modern medicine assumes that the body is Newtonian. We keep looking for the smallest particles of the body assuming that there we will find the answers to disease, for example, gene mapping. This is valid for systems where only the total mass of a system matters, such as for weights or collections of small, weakly interacting particles, like a pound of flour.

Later when people began to consider atoms instead, Newton's laws didn't work. *Newton's laws work for large objects but don't work for atoms or the human body while it lives.*

Atoms
(A short history of the knowledge of the atom)
Compiled by Jim Walker

The following history of the theories of atoms is reprinted here with the permission of Jim Walker, http://www.nobeliefs.com/atom.htm. I have taken the liberty of recreating some of the graphics since the copies from the website do not reproduce well. For Dr. Walker's original graphics, please see his website.

Atom n.: A unit of matter, the smallest unit of an element,

58

consisting of a dense, central, positively charged nucleus surrounded by a system of electrons, equal in number to the number of nuclear protons, the entire structure having an approximate diameter of 10^{-8} centimeter and characteristically remaining undivided in chemical reactions except for limited removal, transfer, or exchange of certain electrons.

The history of the study of the atomic nature of matter illustrates the thinking process that goes on in the philosophers' and scientists' heads. The models they use do not provide an absolute understanding of the atom but only a way of abstracting so that they can make useful predictions about them. The epistemological methods that scientists use provide us with the best known way of arriving at useful science and factual knowledge. No other method has yet proven as successful.

In the beginning

Actually, the thought about electricity came before atoms. In about 600 B.C. Thales of Miletus discovered that a piece of amber, after rubbing it with fur, attracted bits of hair and feathers and other light objects. He suggested that this mysterious force came from the amber. Thales, however, did not connect this force with any atomic particle.

Not until around 460 B.C. did a Greek philosopher, Democritus, develop the idea of atoms. He asked this question: If you break a piece of matter in half, and then break it in half again, how many breaks will you have to make before you can break it no further? Democritus thought that it ended at some point, a smallest possible bit of matter. He called these basic matter particles "atoms."

Unfortunately, the atomic ideas of Democritus had no lasting effects on other Greek philosophers, including Aristotle. In fact, Aristotle dismissed the atomic idea as worthless. People considered Aristotle's opinions very important, and if Aristotle thought the atomic idea had no merit, then most other people thought the same also. (Primates have great mimicking ability.)

For more than 2,000 years nobody did anything to continue the explorations that the Greeks had started into the nature of matter. Not until the early 1800s did people begin again to question the structure of matter.

In the 1800s, English chemist John Dalton performed experiments with various chemicals that showed that matter, indeed, seem to consist of elementary lumpy particles (atoms). Although he did not know about their structure, he knew that the evidence pointed to something fundamental.

Thomson's "Raisin in the Pudding" Model Of The Atom

(Plum pudding originated as a mixture of minced meat, suet, oatmeal, and dried plums thickened with bread crumbs seasoned with spices, and bound together

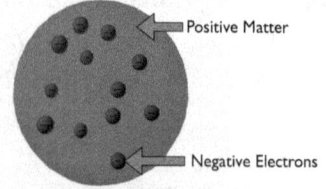

with eggs. This mixture would have either been eaten as a kind of thick soup or stuffed into animal stomachs and boiled in cauldrons over open fire.)

In 1897, the English physicist J.J. Thomson discovered the electron and proposed a model for the structure of the atom. Thomson knew that electrons had a negative charge and thought that matter must have a positive charge. His model looked like raisins stuck on the surface of a lump of pudding.

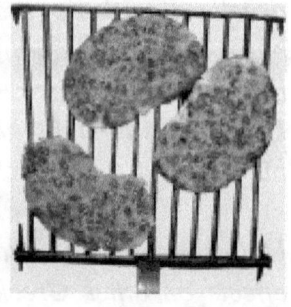

In 1900, Max Planck, a professor of theoretical physics in Berlin,

showed that when you vibrate atoms strong enough, such as when you heat an object until it glows, you can measure the energy only in discrete units. He called these energy packets "quanta."

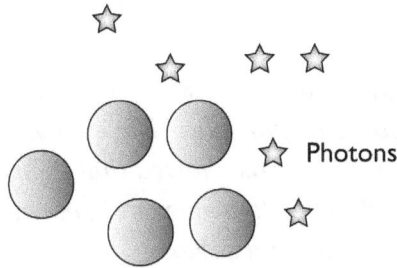

Physicists at the time thought that light consisted of waves but, according to Albert Einstein, the quanta behaved like discrete particles. Physicists call Einstein's discrete light particle a "photon."*

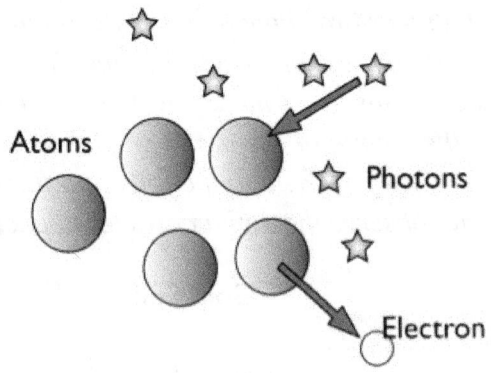

* Note: I anachronistically use the word "photon" here. Actually physicists did not refer to light quanta as photons until after Gilbert N. Lewis proposed the name in an article in *Nature*, Vol. 118, Pt. 2, December 18, 1926.

Photoelectric effect

Atoms not only emit photons, but they can also absorb them. In 1905, Albert Einstein wrote a ground-breaking paper that explained that light absorption can release electrons from atoms, a phenomenon called the "photoelectric effect." Einstein received his only Nobel Prize for physics in 1921 for his work on the photoelectric effect.

A heated controversy occurred for many years on deciding whether light consisted of waves or particles. The evidence appeared strong for both cases. Later, physicists showed that light appears as either wave-like or particle-like (but never both at the same time) depending on the experimental setup.

Other particles discovered around this time were called alpha rays. These particles had a positive charge and physicists thought that they consisted of the positive parts of the Thompson atom (now known as the nucleus of atoms).

In 1911, Ernest Rutherford thought it would prove interesting to bombard atoms with these alpha rays, figuring that this experiment could investigate the inside of the atom (sort of like a probe). He used radium as the source of the alpha particles and shined them onto the atoms in gold foil. Behind the foil sat a fluorescent screen for which he could observe the alpha particles impact.

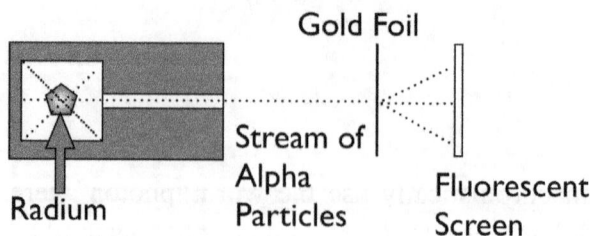

The results of the experiments were unexpected. Most of the alpha particles went smoothly through the foil. Only an occasional alpha veered sharply from its original path, sometimes bouncing straight back from the foil!

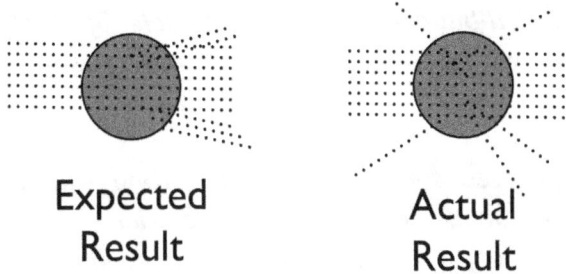

**Expected
Result**

**Actual
Result**

Rutherford reasoned that they must get scattered by tiny bits of positively charged matter. Most of the space around these positive centers had nothing in them. He thought that the electrons must exist somewhere within this empty space.

Rutherford thought that the negative electrons orbited a positive center in a manner like the solar system where the planets orbit the sun.

Rutherford's Atom

Rutherford knew that atoms consist of a compact, positively charged nucleus, around which circulate negative electrons at a relatively large distance. The nucleus occupies less than one thousand million millionth of the atomic volume, but contains almost all of the atom's mass. If an atom had the size of the earth, the nucleus would have the size of a football stadium.

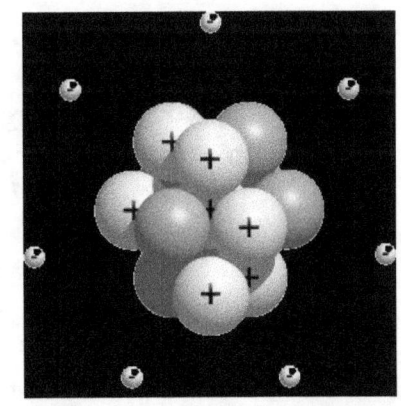

Not until 1919 did Rutherford finally identify the particles of the nucleus as discrete positive charges of matter. Using alpha particles as bullets, Rutherford knocked hydrogen nuclei out of atoms of six elements: boron,

fluorine, sodium, aluminum, phosphorus, and nitrogen. He named them "protons," from the Greek for "first," for they consisted of the first identified building blocks of the nuclei of all elements. He found the protons mass was 1,836 times as great as the mass of the electron.

But there appeared something terribly wrong with Rutherford's model of the atom. The theory of electricity and magnetism predicted that opposite charges attract each other and the electrons should gradually lose energy and spiral inward. Moreover, physicists reasoned that the atoms should give off a rainbow of colors as they did so. But no experiment could verify this rainbow.

In 1912, a Danish physicist, Niels Bohr, came up with a theory that said the electrons do not spiral into the nucleus and came up with some rules for what does happen. (This began a new approach to science because for the first time rules had to fit the observation regardless of how they conflicted with the theories of the time.)

Bohr said, "Here's some rules that seem impossible, but they describe the way atoms operate, so let's pretend they're correct and use them." Bohr came up with two rules that agreed with his experiments:

RULE 1: Electrons can orbit only at certain allowed distances from the nucleus.
RULE 2: Atoms radiate energy when an electron jumps from a higher-energy orbit to a lower-energy orbit. Also, an atom absorbs energy when an electron gets boosted from a low-energy orbit to a high-energy orbit.

Bohr's Atom for Hydrogen

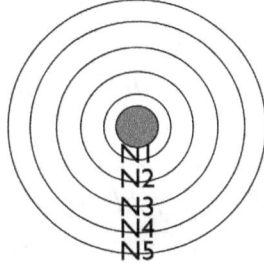

Orbit N	Distance from Nucleus
I	0.529A
2	2.116A
3	4.761A
4	8.464A
5	13.225A

The red line in the atomic spectrum occurs from electrons dropping from the 3rd orbit to the 2nd orbit.

The electron can exist in only one of the orbits. (The diagram shows only five orbits, but any number of orbits can theoretically exist.)

Light (photons) is emitted whenever an electron jumps from one orbit to another. The jumps seem to happen instantaneously without moving through a trajectory. (The example above shows only one possibility from Rule 2.)

By the 1920s, further experiments showed that Bohr's model of the atom had some troubles. Bohr's atom seemed too simple to describe the heavier elements. In fact it only worked roughly in these cases. The spectral lines did not appear correct when a strong magnetic field influenced the atoms.

65

Bohr- Sommerfeld Model of the Atom

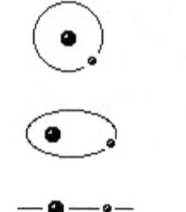

Direction of magnetic field

Bohr and a German physicist, Arnold Sommerfeld, expanded the original Bohr model to explain these variations. According to the Bohr-Sommerfeld model, not only do electrons travel in certain orbits but the orbits have different shapes and the orbits could tilt in the presence of a magnetic field. Orbits can appear circular or elliptical, and they can even swing back and forth through the nucleus in a straight line.

The orbit shapes and various angles to the magnetic field could only have certain shapes, similar to an electron in a certain orbit. As an example, the fourth orbit in a hydrogen atom can have only three possible shapes and seven possible traits. These added states allowed more possibilities for different spectral lines to appear. This brought the model of the atom into closer agreement with experimental data.

The conditions of the state of the orbit got assigned quantum

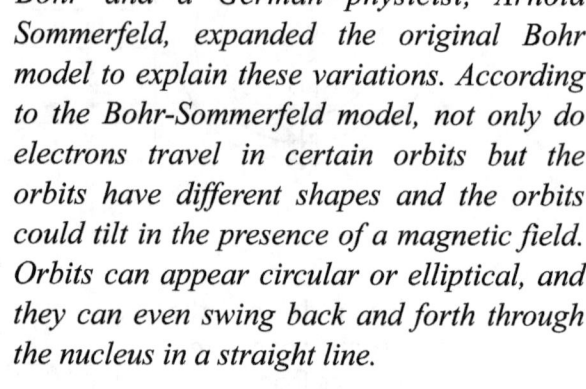

Helium
atom

numbers. The three states discussed so far consist of: orbit number (n), orbit shape (l) and orbit tilt (m).
In 1924, an Austrian physicist, Wolfgang Pauli, predicted that an electron should spin (kind of like a top) while it orbits around the nucleus. The electron can spin in either of two directions. This spin consisted of a fourth quantum number: electron spin (s).

Pauli's Exclusion Principle

Pauli gave a rule governing the behavior of electrons within the atom that agreed with experiments. If an electron has a certain set of quantum numbers, then no other electron in that atom can have the same set of quantum numbers. Physicists call this "Pauli's Exclusion Principle." It provides an important principle to this day and has even outlived the Bohr-Sommerfeld model that Pauli designed it for.

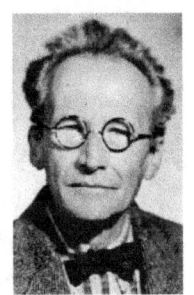

In 1924, a Frenchman named Louis de Broglie thought about particles of matter. He thought that if light can exist as both particles and waves, why couldn't atom particles also behave like waves? In a few equations derived from Einstein's famous equation ($E=mc^2$), he showed what matter waves would behave like if they existed at all. (Experiments later proved him correct.)

In 1926, the Austrian physicist Erwin Schrödinger had an interesting idea: Why not go all the way with particle waves and try to form a model of the atom on that basis? His theory worked kind of like harmonic theory for a violin string except that the vibrations traveled in circles.

The world of the atom, indeed, began to appear very strange. It proved difficult to form an accurate picture of an atom because nothing in our world really compares with it.

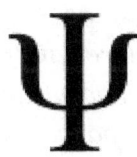

Schrödinger's wave mechanics did not question the makeup of the waves, but he had to call it something so he gave it a symbol seen here. The "psi" symbol of Schrödinger's wave came from the Greek lettering system.

In 1926, German physicist Max Born had an idea about "psi." Born thought they resembled waves of chance. These ripples moved along waves of chance, made up of places where particles may occur and places where no particles occurred. The waves of chance ripple around in circles when the particle appears like an electron in an atomic orbit, and they ripple back and forth when the electron orbit goes straight through the nucleus, and they ripple along in straight lines when a free particle moves through interatomic space. You can think of them as waves when traveling through space and as particles whenever they travel in circles.

However, they cannot exist as both waves and particles at the same time.

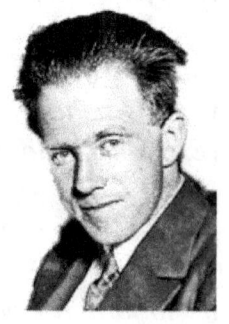

Just before Schrödinger proposed his theory, German physicist Werner Heisenberg, in 1925, had a theory of his own called matrix mechanics that also explained the behavior of atoms. The two theories seemed to have an entirely different set of assumptions yet they both worked. Heisenberg based his theory on mathematical quantities called matrices that fit with the conception of electrons as particles whereas Schrödinger based his theory on waves. Actually, the results of both theories appeared mathematically the same.

In 1927, Heisenberg formulated an idea, which agreed with tests, that no experiment can measure the position and momentum of a quantum particle simultaneously. Scientists call this the "Heisenberg Uncertainty Principle." This implies that as one measures the certainty of the position of a particle, the uncertainty in the momentum gets correspondingly larger. Or, with an accurate momentum measurement, the knowledge about the particle's position gets correspondingly less.

The visual concept of the atom now *appeared as an electron "cloud" that* *surrounds a nucleus. The cloud consists of* *a probability distribution map, which* *determines the most probable location of* *an electron. For example, if one could* *take a snapshot of the location of the* *electron at different times and then* 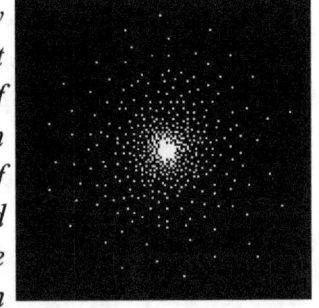 *superimpose all of the shots into one photo, then it might look* *something like the view here.*

Note: Just as no map can equal a territory, no concept of an atom *can possibly equal its nature. These models of the atom simply* *served as a way of thinking about them, albeit they contained* *limitations (all models do).*

Although the mathematical concept of the atom got better, the *visual concept of the atom got worse. Regardless, even simplistic* *visual models can still prove useful. Chemists usually describe the* *atom as a simple solar system model similar to Bohr's model but* *without the different orbit shapes. The important emphasis for* *chemistry attempts to show the groupings of electrons in orbital* *shells.*

Chemical behavior of the elements form together to create *molecules. Molecules may share electrons as the hydrogen and* *oxygen in water molecules. (Atoms that share electrons have the* *name "ions.") The outer electron shell of an atom actually does* *the sharing and bonding of the atoms. This in turn allows chemists* *to describe the interactions of chemistry. **Even though the orbit*** ***model of the atom does not provide an accurate model, it works*** ***well for describing chemistry.***

A mystery of the nature of the nucleus remained unsolved. The *nucleus contains most of the atom's mass as well as the positive* *charge. The protons supposedly accounted for this mass. **However,*** *a nucleus with twice the charge of another should have twice the number of protons and twice the mass. But this did not prove correct.* Rutherford speculated in 1920 that there existed electrically neutral particles with the protons that make up the missing mass, but no one accepted his idea at the time.

Not until 1932 did the English physicist James Chadwick finally discover the neutron. He found it to measure slightly heavier than the proton with a mass of 1,840 electrons and with no charge (neutral). The proton-neutron together received the name "nucleon."

Isotopes of Hydrogen

Although scientists knew that atoms of a particular element have the same number of protons, they discovered that some of these atoms have slightly different masses. They concluded that the variations in mass result, more or less, from the number of neutrons in the nucleus of the atom. Atoms of an element having the same atomic number but different atomic masses are called "isotopes" of that element.

Antimatter

In 1928, Paul Dirac produced equations that predicted an unthinkable thing at the time—a positive charged electron. He did not accept his own theory at the time. In 1932, in experiments with cosmic rays, Carl Anderson discovered the anti-electron, which proved Dirac's equations. Physicists call it the "positron."

For each variety of matter there should exist a corresponding "opposite," or antimatter. Physicists now know that antimatter exists. However, because matter and antimatter annihilates whenever they come in contact, it does not stay around for very long. (By the way, an unsolved problem remains as to why the universe consists of mostly regular matter and not an equal *amount of antimatter. Physicists call this "symmetry breaking.")*

There exists not only anti-electrons, but in 1955, physicists found the anti-proto, and later the anti-neutron. This allows the existence for anti-atoms, a true form of antimatter.

When scientists found out about the atomic nucleus, they questioned why the positively charged protons should remain so close without repelling. The scientists realized that there must exist new forces at work and the secrets must lie within the nucleus. They knew that the force which holds the protons together must occur much stronger than the electromagnetic force and that the force must act over very small distances (otherwise they would have noticed this force in interactions between the nucleus and the outer electrons).

In 1932, Werner Heisenberg concluded that charged particles bounce photons of light back and forth between them. This exchange of photons provides a way for the electromagnetic forces to act between the particles. The theory says that a proton shoots a photon at the electron, and the electron shoots a photon back at the proton. These photon exchanges go on all the time, very rapidly. However, because no one can see them (measure them), Heisenberg called these exchange particles "virtual photons" (virtual meaning not exactly "real").

In 1935, a Japanese physicist, Hideki Yukawa, suggested that exchange forces might also describe the strong force between nucleons. However, virtual photons did not have enough strength for this force, so he thought that there must exist a new kind of virtual particle. Yukawa used Heisenberg's uncertainty principle to explain that a virtual particle could exist for an extremely small fraction of a second. Since its time of existence occurs nearly exactly, there would occur a great uncertainty in the energy of the virtual particle. This uncertainty allows the particles to exist very strongly only at certain times, and the particles could slip in and

71

out of existence. He also calculated that these particles should be about 250 times as heavy as an electron. Later, in 1947, the physicist Cecil F. Powell detected this particle and called it the "pion."

Although the pions describe the transmitters of the strong force, they do not get classed with the other force-transmitting particles, such as the photon or the W and Z particles. Pions now appear not as elementary particles but rather composites made up of "quarks." The strong force gets transmitted by the pions only at relatively larger nuclear levels.

Physicists presently think that all the forces in the universe get carried by some kind of quantum particle. This theory started in 1928 with Paul Dirac stating that photons transmit the electromagnetic force. The theory called "quantum electrodynamics," or QED, developed from work by Richard Feynman, Julian Schwinger, and Sin-Itiro in the late 1940s.

From the time of the ancient Greeks until today, the visual concept of the atom has proved elusive and obscure, yet the mathematical concepts have grown stronger. Although nothing has yet proven absolute, humans can now predict the behavior of atoms with great accuracy. But the world of the atom, the quanta of particles, appears so strange that we can no longer visualize what we think and talk about. The particles have a quality of complete random existence and non-existence about them; and yet the methods of quantum electrodynamics (QED), quantum chromodynamics (QCD), and the whole of quantum mechanics provide such precise, useful, and powerful tools that it encompasses all of the classical physical laws.

The predictions of quantum mechanics have verified themselves many times and to a precision of better than one part in a billion. No predictive method has yet come as close. Even the unproven psychics, soothsayers, and prophets can only dream about such powers of prediction.

Review and a New Theory

H 1																	He 2
Li 3	Be 4											B 5	C 6	N 7	O 8	F 9	Ne 10
Na 11	Mg 12											Al 13	Si 14	P 15	S 16	Cl 17	Ar 18
K 19	Ca 20	Sc 21	Ti 22	V 23	Cr 24	Mn 25	Fe 26	Co 27	Ni 28	Cu 29	Zn 30	Ga 31	Ge 32	As 33	Se 34	Br 35	Kr 36
Rb 37	Sr 38	Y 39	Zr 40	Nb 41	Mo 42	Tc 43	Ru 44	Rh 45	Pd 46	Ag 47	Cd 48	In 49	Sn 50	Sb 51	Te 52	I 53	Xe 54
Cs 55	Ba 56	57-70	Lu 71	Hf 72	Ta 73	W 74	Re 75	Os 76	Ir 77	Pt 78	Au 79	Hg 80	Tl 81	Pb 82	Bi 83	Po 84	At 85	Rn 86
Fr 87	Ra 88	89-102	Lr 103	Rf 104	Db 105	Sg 106	Bh 107	Hs 108	Mt 109	Uun 110	Uuu 111	Uub 112		Uuq 114				

*Lanthanide series	La 57	Ce 58	Pr 59	Nd 60	Pm 61	Sm 62	Eu 63	Gd 64	Tb 65	Dy 66	Ho 67	Er 68	Tm 69	Yb 70
**Actinide series	Ac 89	Th 90	Pa 91	U 92	Np 93	Pu 94	Am 95	Cm 96	Bk 97	Cf 98	Es 99	Fm 100	Md 101	No 102

In 1869, a Russian chemist named Dmitri Mendeleev came up with a way of organizing the elements that were known at the time. He set them out in order of atomic weight and grouped them into rows and columns based on their chemical and physical properties.

In 1897, J.J. Thomson stated that atoms have a negative charge and there must therefore also be a positive particle. His model was like raisins in pudding.

In the early part of the twentieth century, scientists finally derived a model of the atom. In this model, an atom was supposed to consist of various protons, neutrons, and electrons. The atom had a nucleus of heavy particles, and these were either protons or a combination of protons and neutrons. Orbiting around the nucleus were electrons that were much smaller than either protons or neutrons (approximately 1,800 times smaller). Each proton was considered to have a fixed electric charge of +1, the neutron had no charge, and the electron had a fixed electrical charge of -1. Units of the charge didn't matter for this explanation. The idea was that all stable atoms had to be electrically neutral overall.

Each different type of atom was one distinct element on the chemical periodic table. So the simplest atom, which consisted of just one proton and one electron and usually no neutrons, was hydrogen. The next one, helium, had two protons, two neutrons, and two electrons, the second element in the periodic table, and so on.

Photoelectric Effect

Atoms not only emit photons, but they can also absorb them. In 1905, Albert Einstein wrote a ground-breaking paper that explained that light absorption can release electrons from atoms, a phenomenon called the "photoelectric effect." Einstein received his only Nobel Prize for physics in 1921 for his work on the photoelectric effect.

If you heat up atoms of any particular element, they will start to emit light, and the light has specific colors. Sodium would give intense yellow, strontium would give bright red, and copper would give blue-green, and so on. Some property of the atom somehow makes these colors.

In 1905, Albert Einstein came up with a new theory. He found that elements also responded to certain colors of light, and that by shining light on metals he could cause a voltage to appear across the metal. This was called the photoelectric effect. It was the thing that made Einstein famous and won him the Nobel Prize. The colors of the light that caused the electrons to move in any particular element were the same as the colors emitted when that element was heated to incandescence. Einstein managed to prove that the different colors of light had different energies, and so it followed that electrons were bound to atoms by certain amounts of energy. In different atoms the electrons have different energy levels.

A Dutch scientist named Niels Bohr worked out that the electron was rather like a ball tied to a string that was whirled around the atom. It was easy to see that the string was in fact the electrical force between the positive proton and the negative electron. But Bohr had a problem. For many years scientists have known that if you accelerated a charged object, the object would start to emit radiation. He suddenly realized that his electron whirling around the atom was a charged particle, 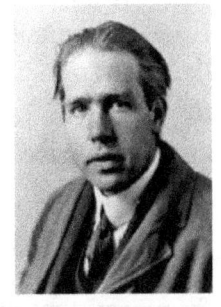 and that it was accelerating. Yet if the atoms were consistently emitting radiation they would constantly lose energy. The only place that energy could come from was within the matter of the atom itself. If this were true, all atoms would get lighter and eventually fade away.

Bohr proposed that maybe there were special fixed energy states in an atom (remember that these energy states are just different orbits of electrons) and that as long as the electron was only in one of these special orbits it would not emit radiation. Scientists found that electrons usually behave like small charged particles of matter. But in some cases they found electrons could also behave like waves! This was very confusing. It was impossible to determine if the electron was a particle or a wave, and to explain the results they had, it had to be both at the same time.

They discovered this was true of all subatomic particles, and it was equally valid to think of them as either particles or waves. Equations were worked out that let the scientists calculate the wavelength of particles. For the electron this became known as its "Compton wavelength." The wave/particle duality was described by de Broglie.

Bohr knew about this, and it gave him another clue. If the electron was a wave instead of a particle, he figured that any orbit around any atom must have a total circumference that was exactly equal to a whole number of wavelengths of the Compton wavelength of the electron. The theory was that an electron could only exist in one of a specific number of fixed energy levels (for example orbits that Bohr had calculated to be exact electron wavelength multiples). If that were true, then adding energy to an electron would not cause it to change its orbit unless the amount of energy was exactly the amount needed to move the electron from one permitted orbit to another permitted orbit.

Light that was absorbed by an atom had to be of an exact frequency that contained just the right amount of energy to move the electron from one permitted orbit to another. If the electron fell from a higher energy orbit to a lower one, it would also emit light of exactly that same frequency.

The most important departure from conventional physics was this idea that only certain energy states were permissible. It implied that at the atomic level, all energy interacted in steps, not continuous amounts. These discrete steps were given a name. They were called "quanta." The whole theory that energy was always stepped became known as "quantum theory."

However, there was a problem! When Bohr tried to work out the energy levels of the second simplest atom, helium, he got stuck. Because helium has two electrons, not one (and two protons and two neutrons), the calculation not only had to work out the permitted energy levels of the two electrons, it had to take into account interactions between the electrons themselves. If he assumed the energy level of one electron to be fixed, then it would alter the energy level of the second electron. And the moment that the energy of the second electron changed, it would affect the energy level of the first electron, and so on. So it was impossible to solve! The problem only got worse with all the higher elements.

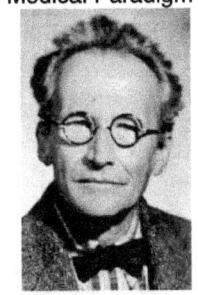

Around 1923, another scientist named Schrödinger came up with a new way of working out the hydrogen solution using only waves and not considering particles at all. He came up with a master equation that should solve any energy level in anything. It looked promising. He worked out hydrogen, but his equation decomposed in exactly the same way as Bohr's equation.

Nobody has ever come up with an acceptable *exact* solution to the Schrödinger Equation for multiple particle atoms. However, the Schrödinger Equation did have some promise. If it were squared (mathematically) it could be approximated (although not solved exactly) and the approximation to the square gave something called a probability density function for the energy levels of the atoms.

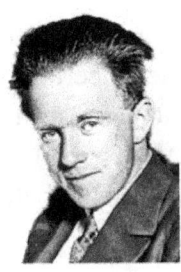

Another scientist, Werner Heisenberg, had derived another aspect of quantum theory. He proposed that it was impossible to know exactly *where* an electron was at any time *and* its exact energy. You could know one or the other, but never both at the same time. This is called Heisenberg's Uncertainty Principle. He also theorized that the mere effort to measure the electron changed it.

Putting together the Heisenberg Uncertainty Principle and the probability function of the Schrödinger Equation, it was obvious that one could never know where the electron was at any time with one hundred percent certainty or probability. So the usefulness of the probability function was not to tell you exactly where the electron was, but to estimate with ninety percent predictability where it *should* be. From an analysis of the geometry of these probability functions for various atoms, scientists were able to work out that electrons move in complicated geometrical shapes around atoms.

There are two important things to remember from all the above:

1. All energy is quantized; i.e., all energy interactions (or state changes) occur in definite discrete steps called quanta.
2. No quantum function can ever be solved exactly; the best you can do is estimate the probability of something happening.

The science of playing about with quantum functions later became broadly known as quantum mechanics. Quantum mechanics is based on clever mathematical manipulations of things like the Schrödinger Equation. If anyone could solve the Schrödinger Equation exactly, the mathematics would actually be easier. Because it can't be solved, mathematicians have to resort to all kinds of complicated tricks to do anything useful with it all.

The second reason is that quantum mechanics is *not* an exact science (because of that unsolvable equation and the uncertainty principle). So we can never say that this equals that because it's impossible to prove. The best we can do is to say "There is a ninety percent probability that this is equal to that...most of the time!"

The equations are so complicated that they usually have more than one answer even for the probability! So in quantum mechanics you often get a ridiculous situation where two absolutely contradictory things are both probably equally true at the same time! The first rule of quantum mechanics is that anything is possible and true but some things are more probable than others. The second rule of quantum mechanics is that it is impossible to solve anything exactly or prove anything with absolute certainty.

Be cautious when someone tells you that a device works with quantum physics. That can be true, but it can also be a means to confuse the unknowledgeable about the relationship of quantum mechanics in the human body.

Remember that Newton's laws apply to the things you can see but don't work well for small things. Quantum physics laws apply to small things you can't see, like atoms. The energy exchange between atoms occurs before chemical reactions occur.

The universe appears to have a Newtonian component superimposed on a quantic component. The body is the same. The body is controlled by quantum laws until it dies. It then becomes Newtonian. Much of medicine treats the body as if it were Newtonian. At the moment the body loses its magnetic field, the body dies.

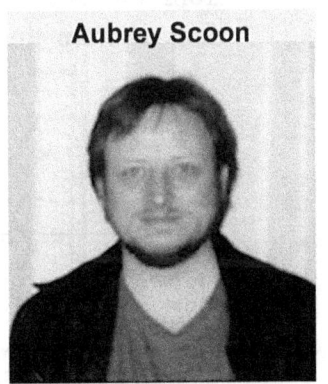

Aubrey Scoon

I wish to give special acknowledgment to the brilliant Scottish scientist Aubrey Scoon, who taught me the things I have discussed above about quantum physics.

Are Electrons Waves or Particles?

Physicists take a position that is unique in science. They can't figure out if an electron is a wave or matter, so they decided they would claim whichever one is needed at any moment to support the theory they are using! This clearly suggests that the basic theory is wrong when you have to change the rules to make sense of your experiment.

This dilemma is clearly demonstrated by the classical "Two-Slit Experiment."

In quantum mechanics the double-slit experiment

demonstrates the inseparability of the wave and particle natures of light and other quantum particles (wave–particle duality). The setup used by Young, and by Newton, differs from the modern version; they passed a beam of light over a thin object, such as a slip of card (in Young's case) or a hair (in Newton's case).

More recently a point light source illuminates a thin plate with two parallel slits, and the light passing through the slits strikes a screen behind them. The beams emerging from the two slits are coherent, in phase, as they are derived from the same source. The wave nature of light

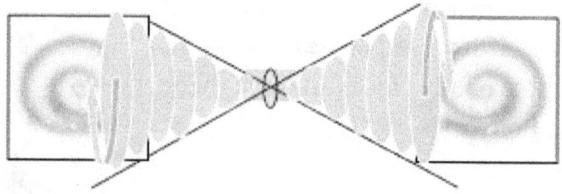

causes the coherent light waves passing through the two slits to interfere, creating a pattern of bright and dark bands on the screen. (However, at the screen the light is always found to be absorbed as though it were composed of discrete particles, photons.) – Wikipedia

Tennant Theory of Atoms

- One can solve the riddle of whether electrons are particles or waves by assuming the nucleus is not a proton but rather a capacitor. The capacitor of each atom is different. It can store/emit different frequencies of light (electrons) depending on whether it is, say, hydrogen or helium.
- There is no such thing as a proton.
- Each electron is a vortex of energy radiating away from or toward the central capacitor.
- Each atom has specific frequencies of light that

characterize it. You can find those in the *Handbook of Chemistry and Physics*. Hydrogen has about 100 frequencies. Oxygen has about 400. However, each atom has dominant frequencies.

- Light is simply the vortex of energy known as electrons. Since we cannot measure where it is now because it is moving in a vortex, Heisenberg found he could not figure out where it was at any moment.
- The two-slit experiment that confused the issue about whether an electron is a particle or wave can be understood when acknowledging that an electron is a moving vortex of light.
- The frequency of each light vortex (electron) is the distance between the arcs of the vortex.
- Two atoms join when the frequency of each atom is in phase with the other. It is not necessary to theorize that one atom is positive and one is negative. This can be explained by whether the direction of the vortex is clockwise or counter-clockwise, expanding or contracting as it moves.

This is a theory modified from the ideas of Robert James. James described his theories to me by drawing a vertical line where the vortices intersect. He did not have a description of what he thought this line was in our discussions. It occurred to me that the line he suggested was indeed acting as a capacitor and represented matter. However, his theories of vortices suggested a logical explanation of why clouds levitate, etc.

A similar theory has been proposed by Dr. Nuno Nina of Portugal. He believes that matter is simply a holographic illusion created by intersecting waves. What I have described as a capacitor he would say is the hologram. Thus a primary difference between our theories is that I have suggested each atom has matter that is unique in that it receives and emits unique frequencies that create each atom's characteristics. Nina suggests that matter only exists as an illusion and can be thought to be real only if there is an observer to detect the hologram thought to be matter. I have not researched whether this theory is original to Nina.

To understand this theory and the following one, you must understand fractals and holograms.

Fractals

Cats, canaries, or kangaroos are similar if they are alike in some way. In geometry, though, *self-similar* means something very specific. Geometric figures are similar if they have the same shape. I don't mean two rectangles or two triangles, but really the same shape.

http://math.rice.edu/~lanius/fractals/

If the corresponding sides are in proportion (and the corresponding angles are also of equal measure), the figures are the same shape and are similar.

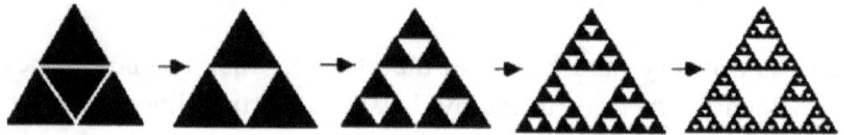

Consider similarity in another way. In order for one figure to be similar to another, you must be able to magnify the length of the small figure by the scale factor, and it will become exactly the same size as the larger figure. In the image above, you start with four equilateral triangles of the same size and assemble them into one larger triangle. Cut out the center triangle. Now make an equilateral triangle inside each of the remaining triangles. Repeat this step over and over an infinite number of times. Note that each triangle is self-similar to any one of the original triangles; it is just proportionally smaller. This is called a "fractal," a name given to this system by Benoit Mandelbrot, a German scientist working at IBM.

All livings things are fractal!

Winter Theory and the Golden Mean

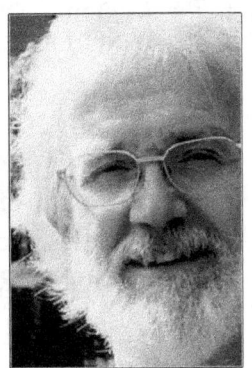

After I published the above in the first edition of this book, I became aware of the writings of Dan Winter. It became obvious that his understanding of how atoms work was far superior to mine. I visited him in France and learned the following. There is obviously much I don't understand, but I feel that his explanation is more complete than mine.

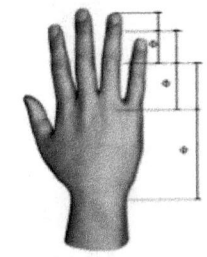

First one must understand the term "Golden Mean" or "Golden Ratio." Golden mean is based on what is called the Fibonacci number set. The Fibonacci number set appears to have first been introduced in Indian mathematics from 400 AD to 1200 AD. However, they are usually credited to Filius Bonacci or Leonardo of Pisa, generally known as Fibonacci or "son of Bonacci."

The Fibonacci number set starts by taking the numbers zero and one and adding successive numbers. So $0 + 1 = 1$. Now add the last two numbers: $1 + 1 = 2$. Then $2 + 1 = 3$. Then $3 + 2 = 5$. Then $5 + 3 = 8$. Then $8 + 5 = 13$. Keep adding the last two numbers of the sequences.

0,1,1,2,3,5,8,13,21,34,55, etc.

Now divide each number by the previous number. You will get 1.618 each time.

Everything that is alive has this ratio. If you measure a leaf that is inserted inside a box, the length will be 1.618 times the width. The first branch of a tree exits the trunk 1.618 times the diameter of the trunk.

If you look at your hand, the second bone in your finger is 1.618 times the length of the bone at the end of your finger. The next bone is 1.618 times the length of the middle bone, etc. This is called the Golden Ratio or the Golden Mean.

Holograms

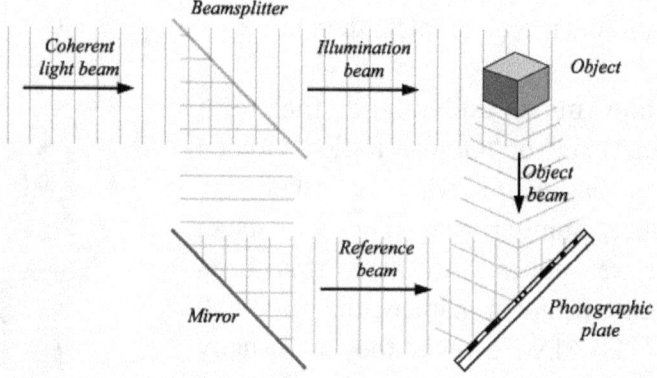

Holography is a method that uses the wave character of light, which depicts an exact description that goes beyond the options of classic photography. In contrast to photography, holography not only records the intensity of light, but also its difference of phase. All pieces of information reflected by the object are recorded. For

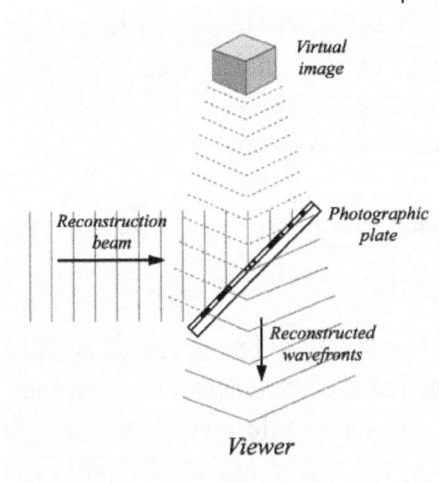

a hologram you need a laser beam, which gets enlarged by a dispersing lens and goes through a semi-penetrable mirror. Only a piece of this laser beam goes through the mirror. Then this beam becomes the reference wave that is recorded on the film. The other piece of the laser beam will be reflected on the mirror and runs as the so-called exposure wave at the object. The object reflects this wave on the film.

The process of creating a hologram is nearly identical to photography through diverse chemicals. To look at a hologram just recorded, you have to light the film with the reference wave. These waves are reflected on the film (hologram) and create (within the proper angle of sight) a virtual picture of the recorded object. http://simple.wikipedia.org/wiki/Holography

To review, if you shine a regular light onto an object, such as a person, and the light is reflected onto film, you get a photo. If you tear the photo in half, you can only see half the person.

If you shine a laser (one frequency) light onto a person and it reflects onto the film while at the same time you shine the same light onto the film, the two beams will interfere with each other in front of the film. This process contains the entire three-dimensional information of the person.

Now remove the person and simply shine the same frequency of light onto the film and you will see a three-dimensional image of the person. Now if you tear that photo in half, you still see the whole person, just smaller. If you keep tearing pieces off the hologram photo, you continue to see the whole person in smaller and smaller images. Thus the hologram is fractal.

Winter's Golden Mean Model of Atoms

The following discussion is from the book *Implosion* by Dan Winter.

Everything in the universe is made of waves. The universe is filled with a medium or ether that becomes electrons, atoms, photons, molecules, people, galaxies, etc. Only sharable waves that can get into phase survive. The universe is organized as 3D sine waves in the shape of donuts.

Wherever waves meet they interfere with each other. Charge waves in a pine cone, your heart, your pineal gland, or the earth and you make *gravity.*

Implosion: the correct geometry that allows waves to charge compression into *acceleration.* It is the "Golden Mean."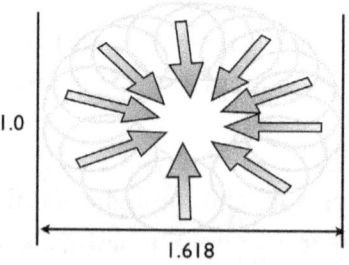

1.0

1.618

Waves must both add and multiply to produce constructive interference. The "Golden Mean Spiral" is the only way for waves to nest without interfering because it is the only ratio sequence that both adds and multiplies:

$0.618 + 1.0 = 1.618$
$1.618 \times 1.0 = 1.618$
$1.618 \times 1.618 = 2.618$, etc.

Waves always spin in such a way that when they reach the other side of the donut, they don't cancel out. This is called *symmetry.* Think of a slinky in a coil where the ends of the slinky are touching. The circular wires of the slinky are the waves. The donut created by the circular slinky creates an implosion of energy into the center of the donut.

The implosion from the top and bottom of the donut creates a tornado with the wide part at the outside of the donut hole and the pointed part at the center of the donut hole. As the wave becomes a

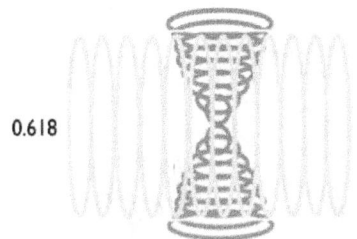

0.618

donut its movement creates a centripetal force to the donut hole. This creates a "tornado" from the top and another from the bottom. These are "electrons." The pointed portions of each tornado touch each other nose-to-nose in the center of the donut hole. The only shape that allows the donut to be stable is the "Golden Mean."

The most stable form is when multiple donuts combine to form *atoms*. The forms that allow for stability are called *platonic solids*. A platonic solid is a 3D shape where each face is the same regular polygon and the same number of polygons meet at each vertex (corner). There are only five platonic solids:

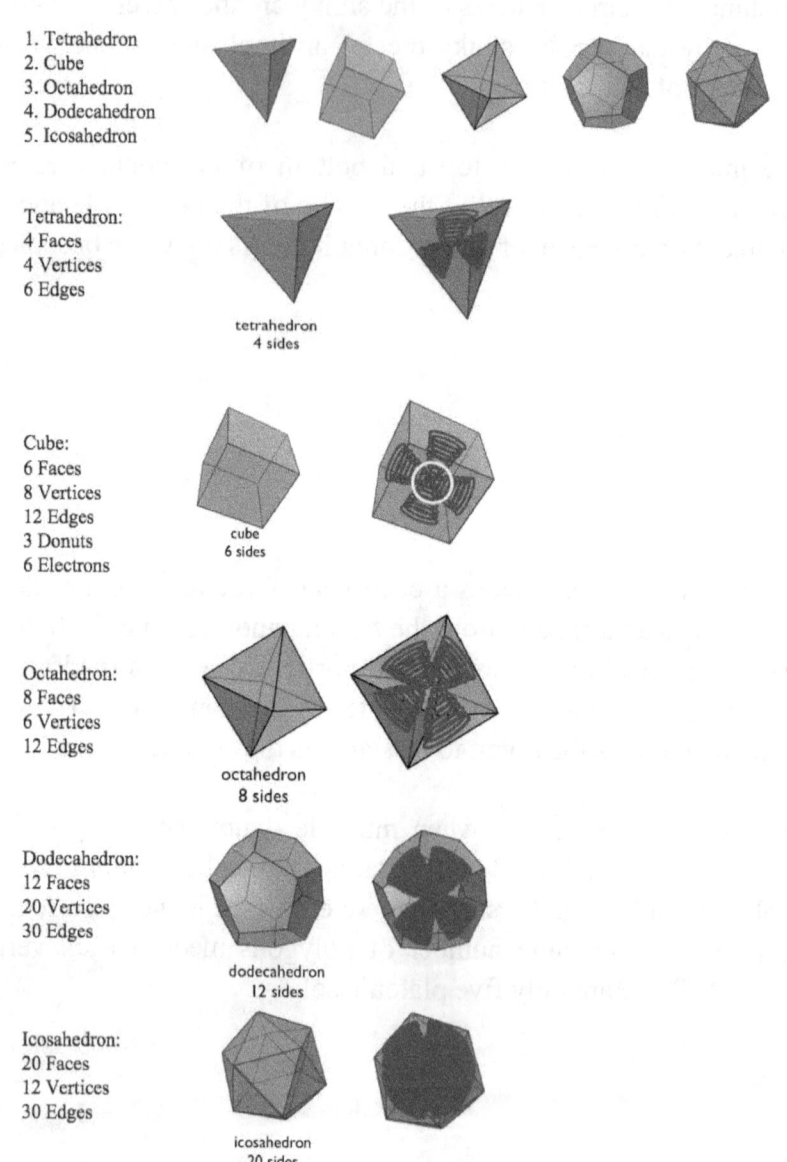

1. Tetrahedron
2. Cube
3. Octahedron
4. Dodecahedron
5. Icosahedron

Tetrahedron:
4 Faces
4 Vertices
6 Edges

tetrahedron
4 sides

Cube:
6 Faces
8 Vertices
12 Edges
3 Donuts
6 Electrons

cube
6 sides

Octahedron:
8 Faces
6 Vertices
12 Edges

octahedron
8 sides

Dodecahedron:
12 Faces
20 Vertices
30 Edges

dodecahedron
12 sides

Icosahedron:
20 Faces
12 Vertices
30 Edges

icosahedron
20 sides

The nucleus of each atom is self-similar to the electron vortices making each atom a fractal hologram in the shape of a platonic solid. The details of this theory are beyond the scope of this book as well as beyond my understanding. You can read more about it at http://goldenmean.info/creation

3 Healing is Voltage

You will recall that I began my journey toward getting well by recognizing that cells are designed to run between a pH of 7.35 and 7.45. I also began my journey with the idea that if I could figure out how to make one cell work I could make them all work.

The following chart shows the requirements for a cell to work properly.

Requirement	Range for Cell	Abnormally High	Abnormally Low
Glucose	80-110 mg/dl	Diabetes	Hypoglycemia
Temperature	98.6-100° F.	Fever	Hypothyroidism
Blood Pressure	120-140/80-90	Hypertension	Hypotension (Dizziness)
pH	7.35-7.45	Throbbing Pain	Chronic Pain
Oxygen	paO2 >95%	Doesn't Occur	Anaerobic Metabolism –>Lactic Acid –>Lowered pH

We doctors are trained to pay particular attention to things that are abnormally high. For example, we watch carefully for a high blood sugar (diabetes); however, we rarely think about hypoglycemia unless a patient is dizzy or faint. We watch carefully for high temperature indicating fever, but we are not trained that a low temperature indicates hypothyroidism. We watch carefully for high blood pressure and are insensitive to the fact that low pressures due to over-exuberant prescription of medication is causing our patients to be dizzy. We rarely look at pH levels or oxygen levels unless the patient is in intensive care.

I want to focus on the importance of pH. When I was trying to figure out how to get well, I couldn't remember a lot about pH. I remembered that it was something about acid/base balance but I knew little more than that. So I began to read about pH. What I discovered is that pH (shorthand for "potential hydrogen") is really a measurement of voltage.

When electrons are running through a conductor such as a copper wire, they are there or not. If the switch is on, you have an electron donor. If the switch is off, there are no electrons.

However, a solution provides a different situation. The solution may be an electron donor or an electron stealer. One measures the voltage of the solution with a sophisticated voltmeter. By convention, if the solution is an electron donor, one puts a minus sign in front of the voltage. If, however, the solution is an electron stealer, one puts a plus sign in front of the voltage.

For example, if your pH voltmeter measures +150 millivolts, it means that the solution is an electron stealer with 150 millivolts of stealing power. If your pH voltmeter measures -200 millivolts, it means that the solution is an electron donor with 200 millivolts of donating power.

After measuring the voltage of the solution, one can convert that to a logarithmic scale called pH. A voltage of +400 mV is the same as a pH of zero. A voltage of -400 mV is the same as a pH of 14. A solution that is neither an electron donor nor electron stealer is called a pH of seven.

With this understanding, one can see that a pH of 7.35 is the same as a voltage of -20 mV. A pH of 7.45 is the same as a voltage of -25 mV. Thus we see that all cellular biology texts tell us that cells are designed to run between -20 and -25 millivolts of electron donor status!

pH	0	7	14
Voltage	+400 mV	0mV	-400mV

The following chart begins to help us understand the difference between electron donors and electron stealers as it relates to the human body.

Electron Stealer	Electron Donor
Causes damage	Can Do Work
pH 0–6.9	pH 7.1–14
Acidic	Alkaline
Free Radical	Antioxidant
Positive Pole	Negative Pole
Destructive	Constructive
Spins Left	Spins Right

Electron stealers cause damage, are a pH from 0 to 6.9, are acidic, are free radicals, are the positive pole, are destructive, and at the atomic level spin left.

You will hear statements such as "all disease occurs when you are acidic." What this is really saying is that all disease occurs when your voltage is low or in an electronic stealer state.

You will hear statements such as "alkalize or die." What this means is that you must have electrons available to do work or your cells will die.

A free radical is a molecule that is missing electrons. It is like a mugger looking for someone's purse to steal. When a free radical steals electrons from the cell, it damages the cell.

An antioxidant is a molecule capable of giving away electrons. Thus when your mother says "eat your vegetables" she is saying that the vegetables contain electrons that are good for you.

We maintain our health and heal primarily by making new cells. To make a new cell requires a voltage of -50 mV.

Cell Voltage	Cell pH	
-50	7.88	Make New Cells
-45	7.79	
-40	7.70	
-35	7.61	Normal for kids
-30	7.53	
-25	7.44	Normal for adults
-20	7.35	
-15	7.26	Tired
-10	7.18	Sick
-5	7.09	
0	7.00	Change polarity
+5	6.91	
+10	6.83	
+20	6.65	
+30	6.48	Cancer occurs

Salivary and urinary pH are about 0.8 pH units less than cell pH. Salivary pH is a rough indicator of cellular voltage. Urinary pH is a rough indicator of the voltage in the fluids around cells. When normal, both should be 6.5. If you add 0.8 to 6.5, you get a pH of 7.3. This equates to -20 millivolts.

Now let's consider my thumb. My thumb is running at a voltage of -25 mV. It is pink, feels fine, and works well. Now I hit it with a hammer. The thumb is red, swollen, hot, and has a pulsing pain. It has automatically gone to -50 mV. This is necessary to make new cells needed to replace the ones I damaged with a hammer. At -50 mV, blood vessels dilate and dump raw materials such as proteins, carbohydrates, fats, vitamins, minerals, etc. into the neighborhood. I need these raw materials to build new cells. I also need -50 mV to have the energy to turn these raw materials into new cells.

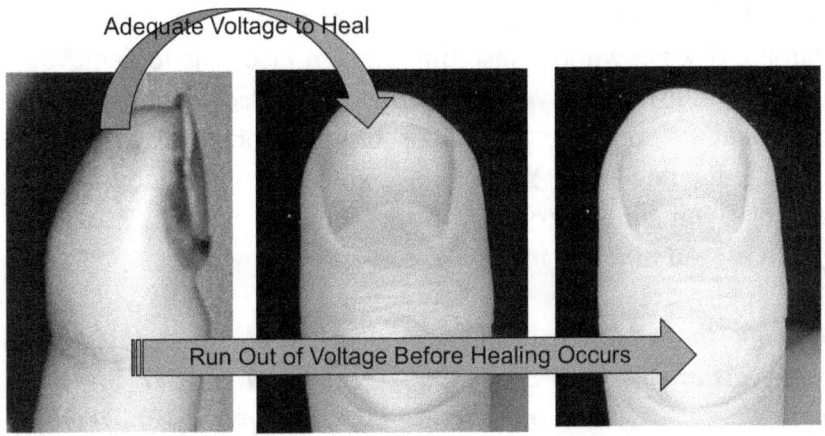

Adequate Voltage to Heal

Run Out of Voltage Before Healing Occurs

Pain and Healing Voltage -50 mV	Normal Voltage -20 mV	Pain and Degeneration Voltage <-20 mV

As soon as I finish making enough cells to replace those I damaged with the hammer, my thumb goes back to -25 mV. It is normal and I am happy.

Now let's assume that I ran out of voltage before I was able to make enough new cells to replace those I injured with a hammer. My voltage dropped to -10 millivolts. Now I am stuck in chronic disease. I cannot heal unless I can make new cells. I cannot make new cells unless I have -50 mV and all the raw materials I need to make new cells. In chronic disease, my thumb hurts all the time, it is white, and it doesn't work very well.

Thus we see that chronic

Any cellular biology book will tell you that the normal pH of body tissue is 7.35 (-20 millivolts) to 7.45 (-25 millivolts). However, if you measure the gradient across a cell membrane the voltage is up to -90 millivolts. Don't be confused: -20 to -25 is the operating environment; -90 is the gradient.

Even if you wanted to say that the "normal" voltage of cells is -90 millivolts, the same logic and understanding applies to making new cells to heal. You must simply define whether you are measuring across a membrane in a petri dish or via the acupuncture system with an ohmmeter.

93

disease is always defined by having low voltage. One cannot cure chronic disease without inserting enough electrons to achieve -50 mV. One must also have the raw materials necessary to make new cells and to eliminate the toxins or infections present that will damage the new cells. You can take all of the medications you like and do as much surgery as you like, but you will not heal unless you have -50 mV, raw materials, and lack of toxins.

Without the ability to achieve -50 mV and the necessary raw materials to make new cells, you cannot maintain your health, and you will suffer aging and chronic disease. You also are unable to repair injuries, so they can also lead to chronic disease. You don't need drugs to heal. You need to make new cells that work to heal. To make good cells, you need voltage and a good diet. You also need to remove toxins from your body that damage cells and make you obese.

Once you begin to understand that chronic disease and healing are controlled by voltage, you must ask the following questions:

1. How do cells normally get voltage?
2. How do cells store voltage?
3. Why did my voltage drop enough to allow me to get sick?
4. How do I measure the voltage of organs?
5. What do I do when I find the voltage is low?

Several bad things happen when voltage drops. The obvious one is that organs simply don't have enough horsepower to do their job. Another is that they don't have the energy to get rid of toxic waste, which begins to accumulate.

Remember that at -50 mV, there is a pulsing pain. When you have low voltage, it simply hurts all the time. Thus pain is simply a symptom of abnormal voltage. You correct it by correcting the voltage.

If you put a tube into a glass of water and began bubbling oxygen into the water, the amount of oxygen that will dissolve in the water is dictated by the voltage of the water. As voltage is raised, more oxygen will dissolve in water. However, as voltage drops, oxygen comes out of solution and leaves the water.

Our cells are seventy percent water. Thus as voltage begins to drop in us, oxygen leaves the cells. This has serious consequences.

Our cells contain a process for turning fatty acids into glucose. They are processed through a series of chemical reactions called the Krebs cycle. The end result is a rechargeable battery called ATP. As ATP provides electrons to keep the cell functioning, it becomes a discharged, rechargeable battery called ADP.

When oxygen is available, for every unit of fatty acids run through the Krebs cycle, we create thirty-eight molecules of ATP. However, if oxygen is unavailable, only two molecules of ATP are created for every unit of fatty acids. Thus as voltage drops and oxygen levels drop, our metabolism goes from "thirty-eight miles per gallon to two miles per gallon." Thus it is very difficult for cells to have enough energy to function with such inefficient metabolism.

Another problem of decreased oxygen is infections. Our bodies contain perhaps 1 trillion microorganisms. However, most of these are inactive as long as oxygen is present. However, when oxygen levels drop, these bugs wake up. The first thing they want to do is have lunch. And they want to have you for lunch.

Since these bugs don't have teeth, they must put out digestive enzymes to dissolve you so that they can acquire the nutrients from the cells.

One of the problems has to do with these digestive enzymes. Let's assume that you have a Streptococcus bacteria having lunch on your tonsil. You, of course, recognize this as a sore, painful throat.

95

We all know, however, that the digestive enzymes produced by these Streptococcus bacteria can enter our bloodstream and cause damage to our heart valves. They can also damage our joints.

The same process can happen anywhere in the body. Let's assume you have low voltage in your gallbladder. This means that your gallbladder will hurt, have decreased oxygen and inefficient metabolism, and have bugs having lunch on the gallbladder. The toxins produced by these bugs can enter the bloodstream and cause brain damage. You may have infections in your large intestine, in your sinuses, or other places causing damage an autoimmune problem. However, it is simply bugs having lunch because your voltage and thus your oxygen levels are low.

I have seen a number of patients with a diagnosis of lupus. A blood test called the ANA test is used to make the diagnosis of lupus. If you correct the voltages in such patients, their symptoms go away and their ANA test goes back to normal.

As voltage continues to drop, it will go from an electron donor to electron stealer status. This is known as a change in polarity. When voltage drops to +30 mV, you have cancer.

It is generally taught in western medicine that the blood is sterile. This is because placing blood into a Petri dish does not normally show growth. Generally speaking, only bacteria that have cell membranes reproduce in Petri dishes. However, if you look at blood under a high-powered microscope without the blood stains or other chemicals, you will easily identify many microorganisms. These microorganisms do not have cell membranes. As voltage and oxygen levels drop and as toxins build up in the system, you will see these organisms change from spherical to rod-shaped to yeast-like and finally fungus with hyphae.

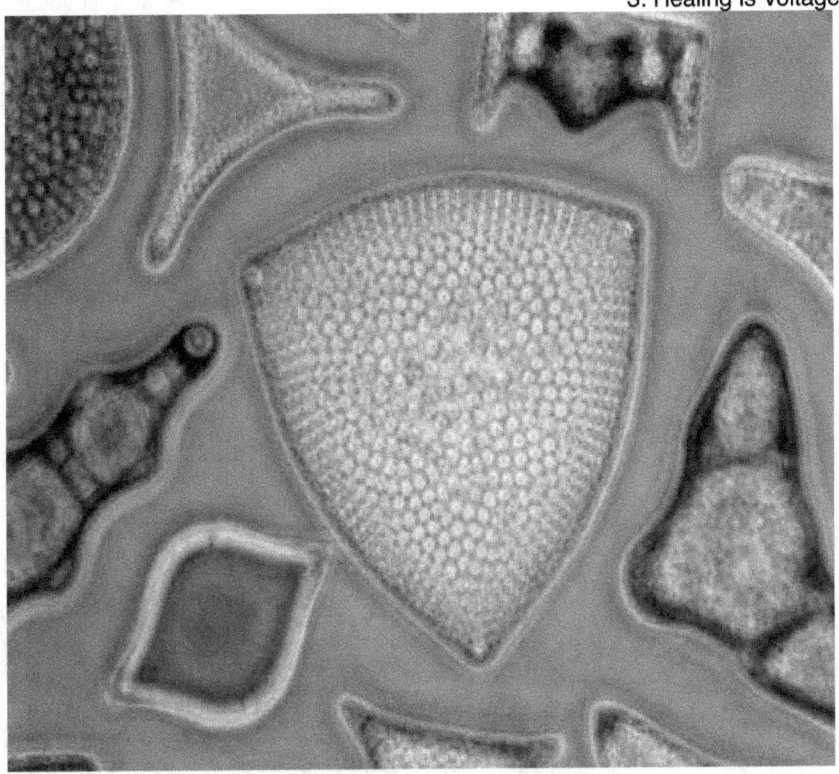

The association of finding fungal-like forms in the blood with the development of tumors was reported as long ago as 1840 and has continued to be reported ever since. Although the existence of these forms has generally been denied by most microbiologists and oncologists, the development of the German microscope known as the Ergonom makes these denials no longer credible. This microscope is capable of 15,000 to 40,000 power and allows one to see even viruses in their live state.

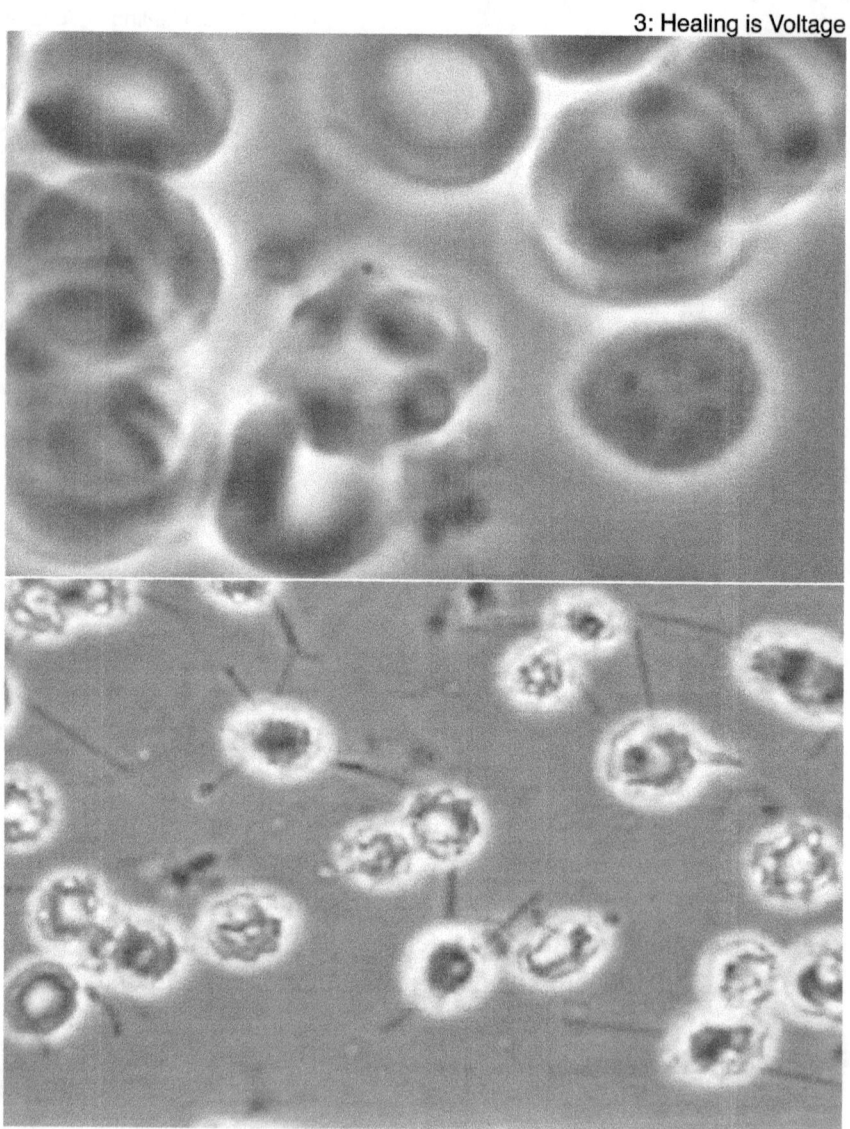

Please look at the videos at www.grayfieldoptical.com.

How do Cells Normally Get Voltage?

There are many ways that the body is intended to get electrons. However, our modern culture has tended to eliminate most of these sources.

Ion	Volts
Fluoride	+2.85
Peroxide	+1.77
Chloride	+1.36
Ferric	+0.76
Copper +	+0.52
Copper ++	+0.34
Hydrogen	0
Chromium	-0.41
Ferrous	-0.44
Zinc	-0.76
Aluminum	-2.23
Magnesium	-2.71
Sodium	-2.87
Calcium	-2.89
Barium	-2.92
Potassium	-2.99
Cesium	-3.02
Lithium	-3.04

Earth is a large electromagnet. If you take the electrodes of a voltmeter and stick them into the dirt, you will measure voltage. An area of high voltage always causes electrons to flow to an area of low voltage. If your body has lower voltage than the earth, walking barefoot on the dirt or grass will cause electrons to flow from the earth into your body, recharging you. However, if you walk with shoes, this cannot occur.

Water from the ground contains electrons. We call this "alkaline water." However, when chlorine and fluoride are placed in the water, it turns into an electron stealer. Thus every time we drink such water, it steals electrons from us. The water we should be drinking should contain electrons and be clean and free from toxins. Again, you can test your water to see if it is an electron donor or electron stealer by simply placing the electrodes of the voltmeter into the water. If the voltmeter shows minus voltage, the water is an electron donor. If the voltmeter shows plus voltage, the water is an electron stealer.

If you stick a voltmeter into a raw potato, you will measure voltage. However, if you bake a potato or freeze the potato and then insert the voltmeter, most of the voltage will be gone. Unprocessed food contains voltage. Once we process food, most of the voltage disappears. We are designed to eat unprocessed food so that it brings its own electrons with it. When you eat food that has been processed, your body must provide electrons from other sources to digest it. You can actually tell the quality of food such as vegetables by simply using a voltmeter to compare the voltage in one product versus another.

Remember that voltage always moves from an area of higher voltage to an area of lower voltage. When my wife and I hug each other, there is obviously an emotional element. However, there is also an issue of pure physics. The one of us with the lower voltage will get a donation of electrons from the other one. As we continue to hug, soon we will be the same voltage.

This process continues when any two living things touch. For example, if I hold a dog or cat and I am lower voltage than the dog or cat, the animal will donate electrons to me. Then it will run outside, recharge itself, and bring me some more voltage. If I lean against a tree, the tree will donate voltage to me.

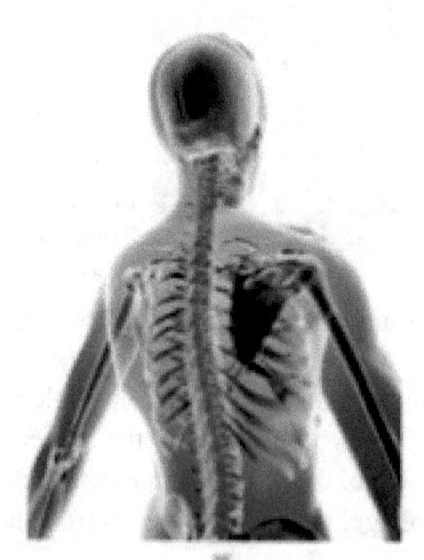

Moving water is always an electron donor. Still water is an electron stealer. Thus taking a shower will energize me whereas taking a bath will make me tired. Swimming in the ocean will give you electrons, but swimming in a chlorinated pool will steal voltage from you.

Moving air is an electron stealer. Thus people often feel tired if they sleep under a fan. Riding in a convertible is great fun, but you are always tired when you get to your destination.

If you take a voltmeter that measures in millivolts and hold it in the air inside your home, you will measure a small amount of voltage. Now take it outside. You will find there is much more voltage out

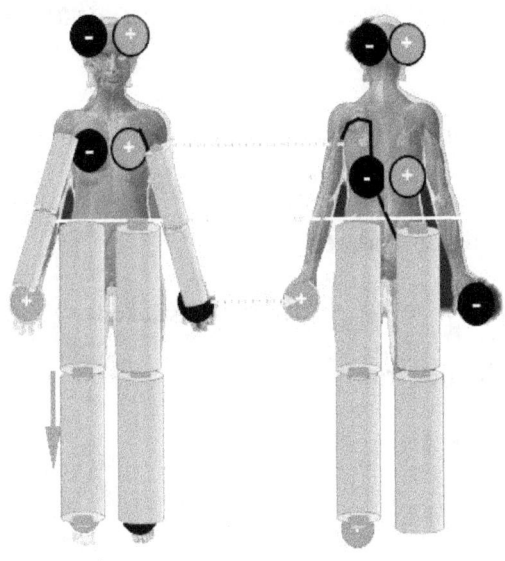

in the sun.

If you take a quartz crystal and squeeze it with a pair of pliers, it will emit electrons. This is called the *piezoelectric effect*. Our muscles are piezoelectric crystals. Thus when we exercise, our muscles create electrons. The muscles are also rechargeable batteries. Thus the movement of our muscles re-charges our muscle batteries. Exercise is a major way the body acquires electrons.

There is a pump within the skull and down the spine called the *craniosacral pump*. Each time this pump activates, it sends a surge of electrons through the body.

Thus you can see that the human is designed to get voltage primarily the way our grandparents got it. They worked out in the sun, drank water from a well, ate unprocessed foods, weren't afraid to touch the earth with their hands or feet, hugged their family, leaned against a tree or stood in moving water while they were fishing, and weren't afraid to stand in the rain.

Common Ways Electrons are Taken from the Human Body

1. Acidic water (tap water, chlorinated water, fluoride, most bottled water)

2. Carbonated beverages

3. Caffeinated beverages (pop, coffee, tea)

4. Alcoholic beverages

5. Cooked food

6. Processed food

7. Healer/doctors who touch their patients lose electrons to the patient

8. Hugs transfer electrons form one person to another

9. Parent holding sick child: child gets well quicker and parent left tired

10. Moving air: wind, air conditioning, fans, convertibles, and hair dryers

How Do Cells Store Electrons?

Cell membranes are made up of opposing layers of fats called phospholipids. This unusual fat is made up of a ball with two legs. The ball is an electron conductor. The legs are insulators.

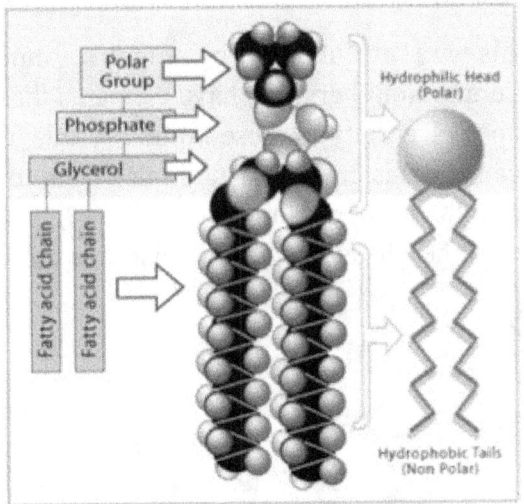

Anytime two conductors are separated by an insulator, you have an electronic device called a capacitor. Capacitors are designed to store electrons. Thus cell membranes serve as "battery packs" for the cells.

Cell Membrane With Opposing Molecules of Phospholipids

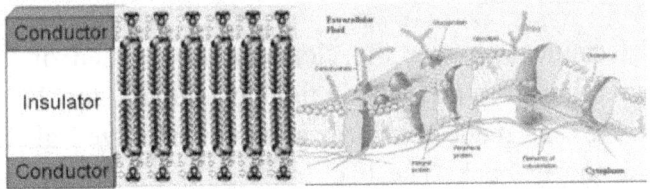

Two Conductors Separated by an Insulator Creates a Capacitor

Liquid Crystals

Dr. Bruce Lipton recently discovered that the cell membrane also serves as a liquid crystal. The molecules in solid things stay in one location. An example of a solid is a crystal. However, in liquids, the molecules move about. In some substances called liquid crystals, the molecules can move about but act like solids. This means that liquid crystals are neither a solid nor a liquid. Thus the name seems strange in that we are calling a solid a liquid when we say "liquid crystal." We are basically saying "liquid solid."

Liquid crystals are influenced by electric current and/or temperature. Certain liquid crystals have elements that are twisted. When one applies electricity to these liquid crystals, they begin to unwind. One can use this characteristic to use them to either block the passage of light through them or allow the light to pass This depends upon whether the elements are twisted or untwisted.

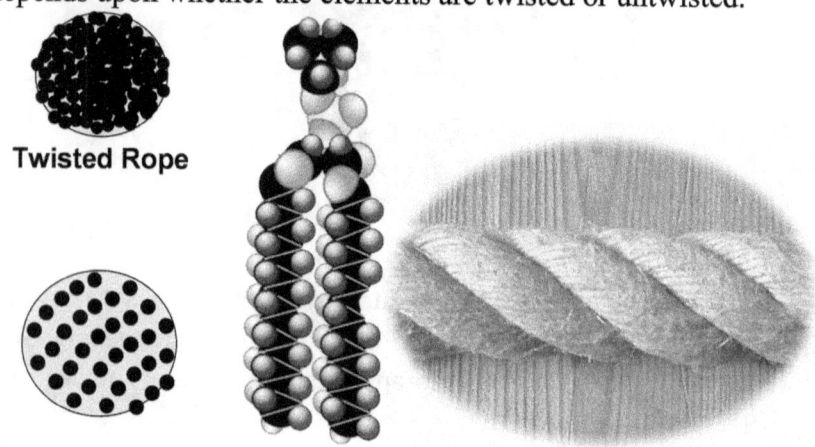

Twisted Rope

Untwisted Rope

What determines whether the elements are twisted or untwisted can be anything from a magnetic field to a surface that has grooves in it. An LCD is made with two plates of polarized glass, one in front and one in back. The back one is polarized ninety degrees from the front one. In between these two plates are filters coated with liquid crystals. The orientation of the crystals is aligned with or opposed to the passage of light depending upon the voltage applied. It is like having a rope with its fibers twisted tightly so light cannot pass down its length, or a rope with its fibers untwisted so that there are spaces between the fibers that allow light to pass down its length. The function is very much like a rotating diaphragm that opens or closes depending upon whether voltage is present or not.

The phospholipids that make up a cell membrane have legs that can twist or untwist to permit light or water or other molecules to be blocked or pass through the cell membrane. They open and close depending upon the voltage applied.

Semiconductors

The elements carbon, silicon, and germanium are called semiconductors. Each has four electrons in their outer shell. This allows each atom to attach the four other atoms in a nice crystalline structure called a lattice. The carbon lattice is called a diamond.

Carbon, silicon, and germanium in their crystal state are electronic insulators. Because they do not have free electrons (all are bonded to each other), they insulate rather than conduct electricity. However, one can turn these insulators into what are called "semiconductors" by adding impurities to the crystals. This process is called "doping."

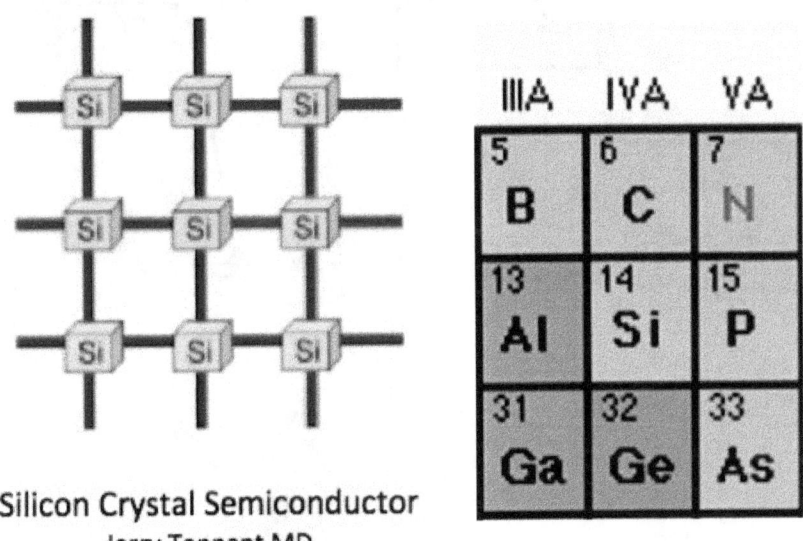

Silicon Crystal Semiconductor
Jerry Tennant MD

As you can see in the graphic of a portion of the periodic table, carbon, silicon, and germanium are in a column. The column next to them has nitrogen, phosphorous, and arsenic. To the left, the column contains boron, aluminum, and gallium.

Arsenic and phosphorous each has five outer shell electrons. When you place one of them into a lattice of carbon, silicon, or germanium (each of them has four electrons), there is an extra electron per set of four atoms. This extra electron can move from place to place turning the insulating crystal into a "semiconductor" that allows some electric current to flow through it. Since this semiconductor has a negative charge, it is called an "N-type." If you add boron or gallium to a crystal of carbon, silicon, or germanium, you have a different kind of semiconductor.

Since boron and gallium each have only three electrons in the outer shell, binding them to carbon, silicon, or gallium (each has four electrons) creates a hole in the latticework. This hole searches for electrons and accepts electrons that wander by. This creates a positive charged semiconductor called a P-type semiconductor.

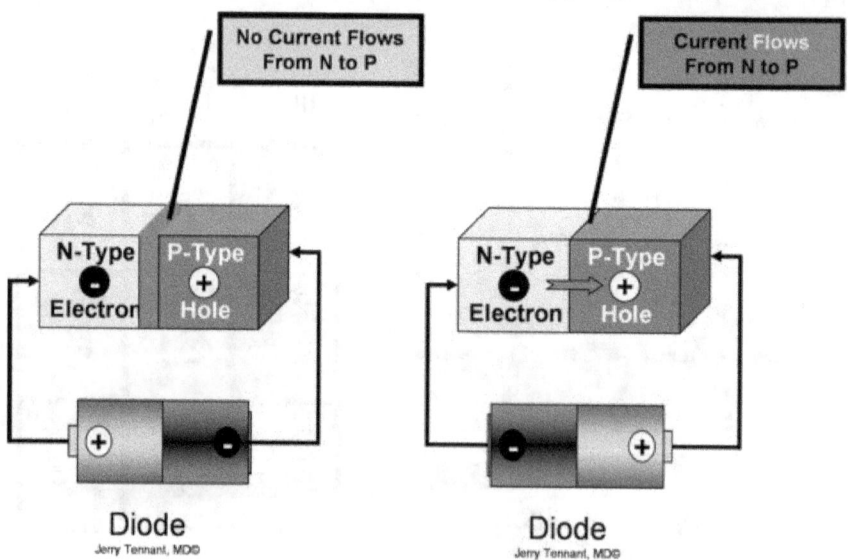

Diode
Jerry Tennant, MD©

Diode
Jerry Tennant, MD©

Diodes

When you place a negative and a positive semiconductor against each other, you have what is called a *diode*. What is unique about a diode is that it allows electric current to flow in one direction but not the other. It is a one-way street for electric current whereas conductors like copper allow the electric current to flow in either direction.

When you use a voltage source like a battery, as seen in the left part of the graphic, the plus part of the battery attracts and hold the electrons from the negative N-type semiconductor, and the minus pole of the battery attracts and holds the holes in the positive P-type semiconductor. The result is that no current flows through the semiconductors.

If you change the battery to the configuration you see in the right side of the graphic, electrons flow from the battery into the N-type semiconductor and then into the holes of the P-type semiconductor with the net effect that current flows through the diode.

Transistors

If you use three elements instead of two, you have a *transistor.* You can use two N-types with a P-type in the middle or two P-types with an N-type in the middle. The most commonly used type is two N-types and one P-type as it is easiest to use this format in a silicon sheet to make a chip.

A transistor normally blocks the flow of electricity through it, acting as a switch. However, when you apply voltage to the center layer, a large amount of voltage can move though the transistor, which makes it act as an amplifier. A small current can turn a larger current on and off.

N-P-N Transistor Can Function
As a Switch or Amplifier

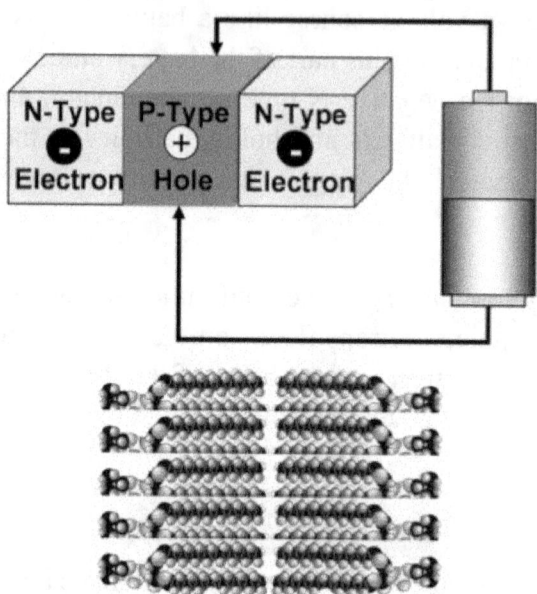

Phospholipids of Cell Membrane
Form N-P-N Transistors → Microprocessor Chip

As you can see, the phospholipids of the cell membrane act like a transistor and a microprocessor. A piece of silicon that can hold thousands of transistors is called a silicon chip. With transistors acting as switches, you can create Boolean gates, and with Boolean gates you can create microprocessor chips.

For an excellent discussion of LCDs and transistors, see http://www.howstuffworks.com/lcd1.htm.

Tesla Resonating Circuits

The Peripheral Cytoskeleton and Tesla's Resonating Circuits

In 1895, Nikola Tesla invented the "tuned circuit" or "resonating circuit." This is a capacitor and a coil wired in parallel. "Wired in parallel" means that the components are on a square, as can be seen in the diagram. Capacitors (abbreviated as "C") store electrons. Coils provide inductance (abbreviated as "L"). This is known as an "LC" circuit.

Parallel tuned circuits are used in radio and other electronics to couple resonant energy from one circuit to another in transmitters and receivers. This is the system used by the cell membrane and peripheral cytoskeleton to couple energy from to cell and into the cell. As you will recall, the cell membrane is made of two opposing layers of fat molecules that create a capacitor. Just under the cell membrane is a maze of protein called the *peripheral cytoskeleton*. These two are wired together in parallel in what is known as an RC circuit = resistor/capacitor circuit.

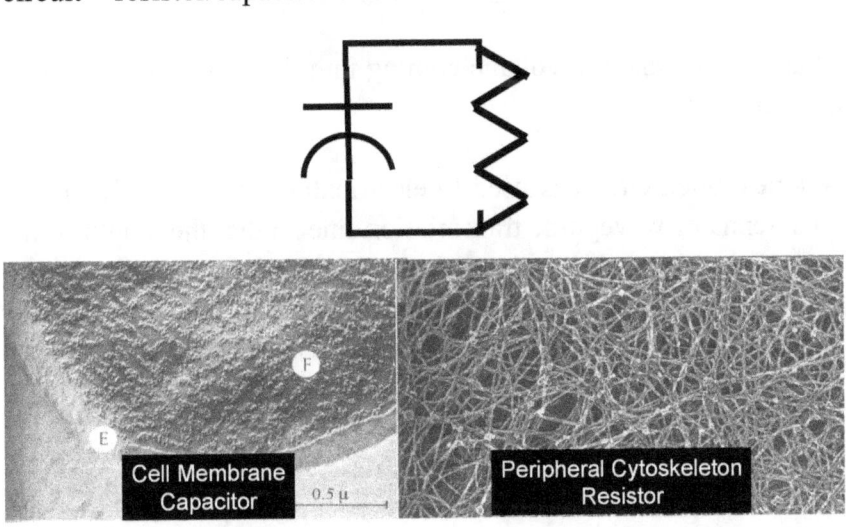

RC circuits work much like your checking account and savings account. In the photo, assume cash is coming into the top of the circuit and that the resistor is your checkbook and the capacitor is your savings account. As the cash comes in, it flows through your checking account to pay your bills. Any cash left over is transferred into your savings account. During months in which there isn't enough cash coming in to pay your bills, you take some out of savings and transfer it into your checking account to keep things going. So it is with an RC circuit. Electrons come into the circuit and flow through the resistor (peripheral cytoskeleton of the cell) to keep energy flowing into the cell so it can do its work.

When more electrons are being delivered by the perineural system —the acupuncture system, water, ionic transfer, etc.—than are needed to supply the requirements of the cell, the excess is stored in the capacitor (cell membrane). When the cell is inflamed, delivery of more electrons is reduced because the cell becomes somewhat isolated from the delivery systems by the edema. Thus the cell must operate on the electrons stored in the cell membrane. This is the same as "running on battery power."

Thus you see that the voltage coming into the cell is controlled by a Tesla RC circuit.

A series-tuned circuit is used to electrically "stretch" or "shorten" an antenna or waveguide transmission line so that the length of the antenna or waveguide will match the length of the incoming wave. For example, radio stations each put out a different frequency or wavelength. If you have a wire that is exactly the same length, the energy from the radio signal will be absorbed and you will hear that station on your radio.

Thus to hear all the radio stations in your area, you would need a separate wire for each station to match the wire lengths and wavelengths. However, if you attach your wire to the series coil above and make the capacitor variable in power, it changes the effective length of the wire. That is the tuning knob on your radio. In the body, extracellular fluid (impedance) and organs (capacitance) are wired in series as a series-tuned circuit.

We now see that the cell membrane is the *brain* of the cell. It is a *capacitor* that stores voltage for the cell to use. It is a *microprocessor* that controls the functions of the cell by interacting with the environment around the cell. It is a *liquid crystal* that can open and close to allow things to enter the cell or keep them out and also allow things to exit the cell or keep them in. It is part of a *Tesla resonating circuit* that allows it to communicate with other cells.

Remember that every cell is designed to run at about a negative 20–25 millivolts. When cells need to repair themselves, the voltage is increased to 50 millivolts. This is controlled by the cell membrane/peripheral cytoskeleton resonating circuit. Since the electrons necessary to allow this to happen are stored in the fat of the cell membrane, the fat is critical to the cell being able to do its work at -20 mV and to repair itself at -50 mV. Without an adequate amount of good fat, the cell membranes can't function and thus the cell can't function.

Remember that cells also replace themselves frequently. If you don't give the cell new building materials, including adequate amounts of good fat, it will have to make a new cell with materials from the worn-out cell it is replacing. Building new things using worn-out parts creates a new thing that doesn't work much better than the old one did.

As you can see, cell membranes must be made with good phospholipids (fats) for them to work. Making them with plastic fats prevents the process from working correctly. Since all of the brain and nervous system, the liver, and every cell membrane are made of fat, you must eat lots of good fat to keep making good cells. A normal person is about twenty to twenty-five percent fat. That means you need to eat about twenty to twenty-five percent of your normal body weight in fat every eight months because your body completely replaces itself every eight months.

Trans Fats ("Plastic Fats")

In the 1920s, food merchants were concerned about the amount of money being lost due to spoilage. They wanted to find ways to keep food from spoiling. They found that if they put certain chemicals like nitrates into the food, it was less likely to spoil. The problem is these chemicals preserve cells in your body as well as the food so they stop working. Cells that don't work are what we call "disease."

Next, food manufacturers found that if they cook fats at about 350 degrees for about five hours, the fats turned into something similar to plastic. Fats processed in this way are called "partially hydrogenated fats" or "trans fats" or "plastic fats." If you look in your pantry, you will find that about forty percent of what is there contains partially hydrogenated fats. When you eat these plastic fats, your cell membranes become made of plastic. Cell membranes made of plastic won't hold voltage. Without voltage, your cells can't work.

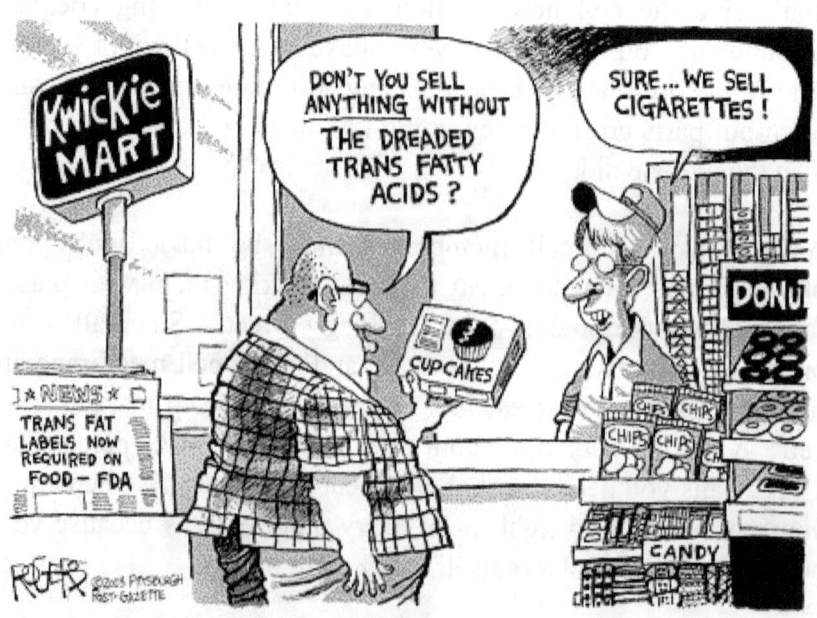

Think of a cell with a plastic membrane. It is like wrapping the cell in cellophane. The cell sends out signals that it is hungry. In response, the body sends glucose and insulin to the cell. However, they can't get through the plastic membrane. The cell continues to signal that it is hungry and the body continues to send insulin and glucose. Soon the cell is surrounded by insulin and glucose, but the cell is still hungry. This is known as insulin resistance and type II diabetes. The cell membrane becomes so saturated with glucose that it begins to off-load it into fat cells. Thus people who continue to eat plastic fats get fatter and fatter.

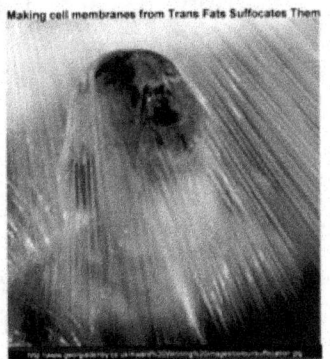

Making cell membranes from Trans Fats Suffocates Them

Guess what happens to a brain made of plastic? It doesn't work well and then becomes prone to depression, chronic fatigue, attention deficient, brain fog, etc.

Guess what happens to a liver that is made of plastic? It can't clean toxins out of your system and the toxins build up, causing things like fibromyalgia. Without a functional liver, your immune system fails and you get all sorts of chronic infections.

Another type of toxic fat is *canola oil*. Here is a summary of a few facts regarding canola oil:

1. It is genetically engineered rapeseed.
2. Rapeseed is lubricating oil used by small industry. It has never been meant for human consumption.
3. It is derived from the mustard family and is considered a toxic and poisonous weed, which when processed becomes rancid very quickly.
4. It has been shown to cause lung cancer.
5. It is very inexpensive to grow and harvest. Insects won't eat it.
6. Some typical and possible side effects include loss of vision, disruption of the central nervous system,

respiratory illness, anemia, constipation, increased incidence of heart disease and cancer, low birth weights in infants, and irritability.

Here is a review article about canola oil (rapeseed oil) and its toxic effects from a Swedish medical journal:

"Physiopathological Effects of Rapeseed Oil: A Review," Borg, K., *Acta Med Scand Suppl* (1975), 585: 5–13 ISSN: 0365-463X

Rapeseed oil has a growth retarding effect in animals. Some investigators claim that the high content of erucic acid in rapeseed oil alone causes this effect, while others consider the low ratio saturated/monounsaturated fatty acids in rapeseed oil to be a contributory factor. Normally erucic acid is not found or occurs in traces in body fat, but when the diet contains rapeseed oil, erucic acid is found in depot fat, organ fat, and milk fat. Erucic acid is metabolized in vivo to oleic acid.

The effects of rapeseed oil on reproduction and adrenals, testes, ovaries, liver, spleen, kidneys, blood, heart, and skeletal muscles have been investigated. Fatty infiltration in the heart muscle cells has been observed in the species investigated. In long-term experiments in rats erucic acid produces fibrosis of the myocardium. Erucic acid lowers the respiratory capacity of the heart mitochondria. The reduction of respiratory capacity is roughly proportional to the content of erucic acid in the diet, and diminishes on continued administration of erucic acid. The lifespan of rats is the same on corn oil, soybean oil, coconut oil, whale oil, and rapeseed oil diet. Rats fed a diet with erucic acid or other docosenoic acids showed a lowered tolerance to cold stress (+ 4 degrees C). In Sweden erucic acid constituted 3–4% of the average intake of calories up to 1970 compared

114

with about 0.4% at present.

What this study showed was that eating rapeseed oil (canola oil) causes the following damage:
1. Growth retardation
2. Damage to heart muscle
3. Lowered lung capacity
4. Lowered tolerance to cold temperatures

Generally rapeseed has a cumulative effect, taking almost ten years before symptoms begin to manifest. It has a tendency to inhibit proper metabolism of foods and prohibits normal enzyme function. Canola is four percent trans fatty acid, which has shown to have a direct link to cancer. These trans fatty acids are labeled as hydrogenated or partially hydrogenated oils. Avoid all of them!

According to John Thomas' book *Young Again*, twelve years ago in England and Europe, rapeseed was fed to cows, pigs, and sheep that later went blind and began attacking people. There were no further attacks after the rapeseed was eliminated from their diet. Source: David Dancu, ND, http://www.karinya.com/canola.htm

"Alkaline Heating of Canola and Rapeseed Meals Reduces Toxicity for Chicks," Barrett, J.E., Klopfenstein, C.F., and Leipold, H.W., *Plant Foods Hum Nutr* (1998), 52(1): 9–15 ISSN: 0921-9668, Department of Biology, Kansas State University, Manhattan, Kansas

Published Abstract:
A simple method for improving the nutritive quality of canola and high glucosinolate rapeseed meals for monogastric animals (chicks) was developed; the meals were mixed with $NaHCO_3$ and NH_4HCO_3 then heated in a conventional oven. Chicks fed untreated canola or rapeseed meals gained less weight than those fed a soybean meal

diet, whereas chicks fed the alkaline heated meals had weight gains not significantly different than those fed the soybean diet.

The antithyroid effect of the untreated rapeseed meal was reduced by alkaline treatment of the meals, as shown by improved T4 and free T4 levels in chicks fed the processed products. In chicks fed untreated or alkaline-treated canola or alkaline heated rapeseed meal, all thyroid hormone levels were similar to those of birds fed the soybean meal diet. However, heart tissue of chicks fed diets containing rapeseed or canola meals showed muscle fiber degeneration, although relative heart weights were the same in all groups.

Liver tissue from most of the chicks in all dietary groups appeared normal or only slightly abnormal. The nutritive value of both rapeseed and canola meals was improved by this simple processing technique.

This study shows that eating canola oil depressed weight gain in the young, depressed thyroid function, and damaged heart muscle.

"Effect of Dietary Cysteine Supplements on Canola Meal Toxicity and Altered Hepatic Glutathione Metabolism in the Rat," Smith, T.K., and Bray, T.M., *J Anim Sci* (1992 Aug), 70(8): 2510–5 ISSN: 0021-8812, Department of Nutritional Sciences, University of Guelph, Ontario, Canada

Published Abstract:
Experiments were conducted to determine the effects of feeding canola meal (Brassica campestris and Brassica napus) on the rat hepatic glutathione detoxification system and whether dietary cysteine supplements might modify

such effects. Rats were fed test diets for 14 d. Body weight change, feed consumption, hepatic glutathione concentration, and hepatic glutathione-Stransferase (GSHS-T) activities were determined. Weight gain was decreased when canola meal was fed, whereas hepatic glutathione concentrations increased, as did hepatic GSH-S-T activity. All effects correlated with total glucosinolate concentration in the canola meal.

Dietary cysteine supplements, however, did not influence the growth reduction and increased hepatic glutathione concentrations caused by feeding canola meal. Supplemental cysteine prevented the elevation in hepatic GSH-S- T activity. The elevation in hepatic glutathione concentration caused by canola meals was not an overcompensation caused by an initial depletion and therefore reflected a general hepatotoxicity.

Feeding supplemental cysteine increased hepatic glutathione levels at early time intervals and delayed the induction of GSH-S-T caused by canola meal toxicity. There was no beneficial effect of supplemental dietary cysteine in overcoming the toxicity of high levels of canola meal, but supplemental cysteine did modify the canola meal-induced changes in hepatic glutathione metabolism.

This study shows that eating canola oil causes liver damage. It prevents the liver from detoxifying harmful things from the body.

"Numerical Density of Cardiac Myocytes in Aged Rats fed a Cholesterol-rich Diet and a Canola Oil Diet (n-3 fatty acid rich)," Aguila, M.B., and Mandarim-de-Lacerda, C.A., *Virchows Arch* (1999 May), 434(5): 451-3 ISSN: 0945-6317, Laboratory of Morphometry and Cardiovascular Morphology State University of Rio de Janeiro, Brazil

Published Abstract:
We studied the myocardium of 45 aged rats fed from 21 days after birth until 15 months of age with a standard rat diet (A) a cholesterol- rich diet (CHO) or canola oil (O). We analyzed the cardiac weight (CW) and, using unbiased stereological estimates, studied isotropic, uniform, random sections of the free left ventricular wall to determine the numerical density of the myocytes (NV[myocyte]). The CW was not statistically different between groups A and CHO: it was smallest in animals in group O (21.2% smaller in group O than in group A and 15.3% smaller in group O than in group CHO).

NV[myocyte] was statistically different in all three groups and was greatest in animals in group O. By comparison with rats in group A, group CHO rats had an NV[myocyte] that was 51.3% smaller and group O, 33.3% greater. Aged rats fed with canola oil diet have a well-vascularized myocardium, which is probably associated with preservation of NV [myocyte] in the myocardium of these animals.

This study compared the size of hearts in rats fed one of three diets, a standard rat diet, a diet high in cholesterol, and a diet high in canola oil. Those fed the canola oil had the smallest hearts, supporting the previous study showing that canola oil damages heart muscles.

Eating Fat and Obesity

The next issue is the belief that eating fat will make you fat. The truth is that eating *plastic fat* (trans fats, canola oil) makes you fat. If you make cell membranes from plastic fats, you will keep eating because your cells are starving even while they are coated with glucose that can't get into the cell. Also, eating plastic fats makes a liver that won't work leading to inability to manage your metabolism. Eating plastic fats makes a brain that can't control your endocrine system causing your thyroid, adrenals, pancreas, and gonads to malfunction. The paradox is that eating more good fat and stopping plastic fats causes you to become your normal weight.

To digest fat, you must have bile. The liver normally makes one and one-half quarts of bile per day. Because it makes so much, it needs a storage tank. That is the function of the gall bladder.

When you eat a fatty meal, the gall bladder must empty bile into the intestine to digest it. If you don't have enough bile, eating fat makes you nauseated. If your liver can't work well because it is made of plastic or is full of toxins, it can't make enough bile. If you have a gall bladder that is full of muddy debris because it rarely gets emptied or if your gall bladder is missing, you will not have enough bile to digest the fats you eat.

As you can see, this becomes a vicious cycle. You can't repair your liver without eating and absorbing enough fat (about 0.1 to 0.2 pounds per day). You can't eat enough fat if you don't have enough bile because a lack of bile means you will be nauseated when you try to eat fat, and even if you keep it down, you can't absorb it.

The secret is to take bile supplements with each meal until your liver is repaired enough to make bile normally. You can get "Ox Bile" at most health food stores. If you don't have a gall bladder, you must take bile supplements with every meal the rest of your life or you won't be able to make normal cells. That means you will be sick.

Measuring Cell Membranes

We can measure the function of cell membranes using a device called the Biological Impedance

Biological Impedance Analysis (BIA)

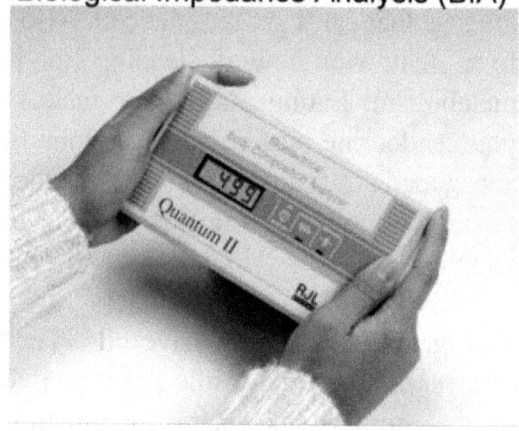

Analysis device (BIA). This device is in widespread use in every physiology department in the world. It gives us a measurement called "phase angle" that can suggest to us if you are made of plastic fat.

ATP/ADP

We have been discussing the storage of electrons by the cells. We have discussed how cell membranes are primary capacitors to store electrons for use by the cells. This voltage is used primarily to control the electronic circuitry of the cell membrane since it functions as a semi-conductor, a diode, a transistor, and a microprocessor.

Inside the cell, we have another electron storage system known as ATP/ADP. This rechargeable battery system is used to make many of the cell's chemical functions work.

Remember that when oxygen is available, we make thirty-eight molecules of ATP from one unit of fatty acids, but when oxygen is unavailable, we only make two! This inability to provide electrons for critical chemical pathways of the cell is part of chronic illness.

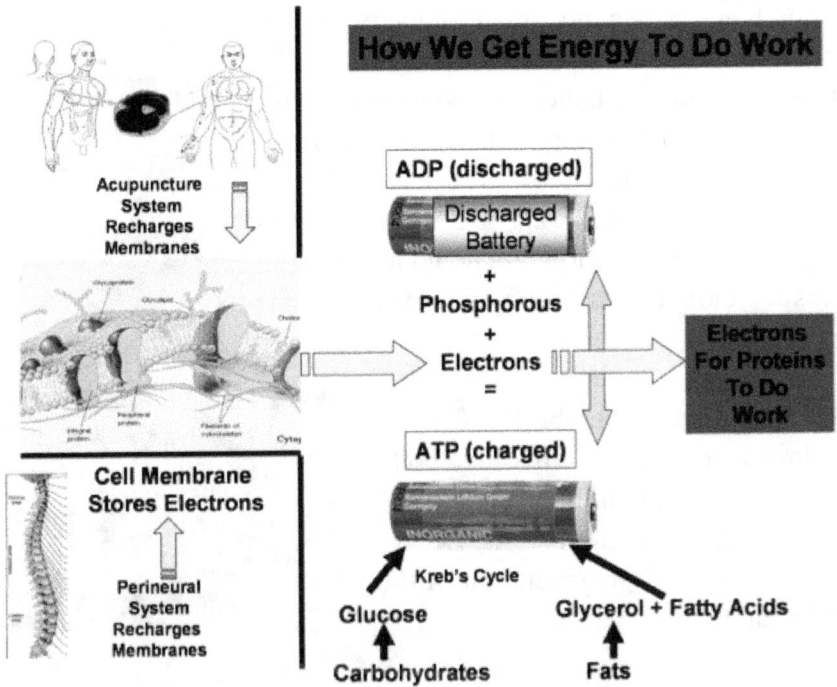

How are Electrons Moved From Place to Place in the Body?

Fibrous tissue has the least impedance or resistance to the flow of electrons of any tissue in the body. Therefore, wherever you find fibrous tissue in the body, it is serving two functions. One is structural, providing support for the adjacent tissue. The second function is to move electrons from place to place.

The human body has two wiring systems. Both are made of fibrous tissue. One is the fibrous encasement of nerves that Robert Becker named the *analog perineural nervous system*. The other is the acupuncture system.

Analog Perineural Nervous System

Robert Becker was an orthopedic surgeon. His classic book, *The*

Body Electric, is a must-read for everyone interested in healing. He

became interested in the fact that if a human loses a piece of bone, his body will make more bone. If you lose a piece of any other tissue, it is replaced by scar tissue. In the human, it was believed that only bone is capable of regeneration. We now know that all tissue can regenerate with the proper conditions.

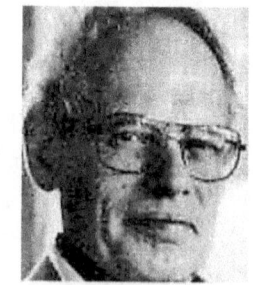

Regeneration is the ability of lower animals to replace missing body parts. It is particularly evident in the salamander. For this reason, Becker decided to study regeneration in the salamander.

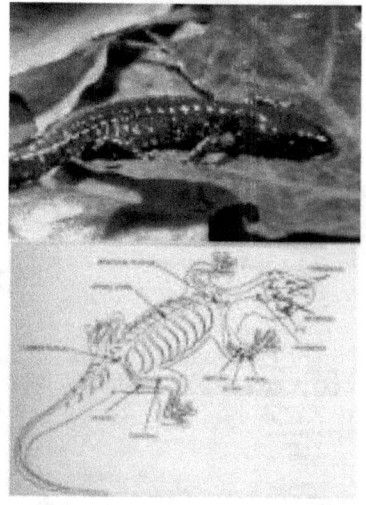

The salamander has essentially the same anatomy as the human, meaning the same number of bones, muscles, and nerves in the same arrangement.

The salamander is capable of growing an exact replacement of an arm, leg, eye, ear, up to one-third of its brain, almost all of its digestive tract, and up to half of its heart. If you poke out a salamander's eye, he simply grows a new one. If you cut off his

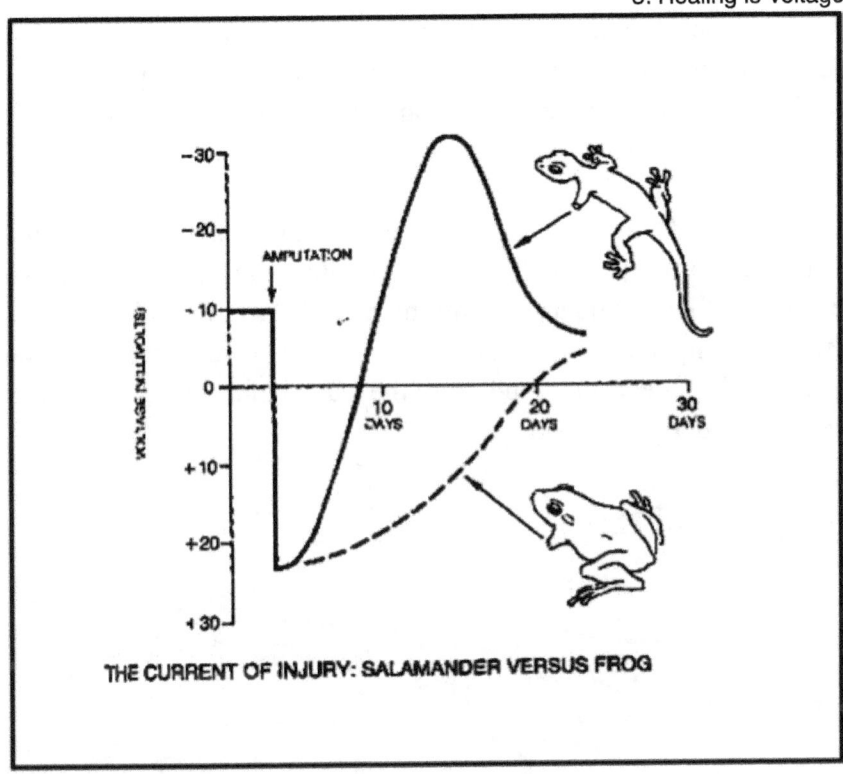

THE CURRENT OF INJURY: SALAMANDER VERSUS FROG

arm, he simply grows another one. The question is, "Why can the salamander grow new parts when we can't?"

The salamander is so efficient at regeneration that it does not get cancer! The regeneration of the salamander cannot be explained by the chemical-mechanistic views of traditional medicine.

To study regeneration, Becker would amputate the arm of the salamander. He found that the stump would become electropositive (electron stealer) of about +25 mV, and he called this the "current of injury." The skin would grow over the stump. The cut ends of nerves in the stump would connect with each skin cell called neuroepithelial junction (NEJ).

As soon as the NEJ forms, the reversed polarity changes normal cells to adult stem cells, a process that was named "blastema" by Thomas Hunt Morgan. This mass of primitive cells that appears between the cut end of the stump and the NEJ (blastema or stem cells) are primitive cells from bone, muscle, etc. that have de-differentiated back to the embryonic state. As soon as they form, the voltage goes to -30 mV (electron donor).

Becker found that if he removed and re-implanted the blastema before ten days, it grew a duplicate of the organ it was near. For example, if he amputated an arm, made a slit near the salamander's tail and implanted it, a new second tail would grow. If he implanted it near the hind leg, the salamander would grow a second hind leg.

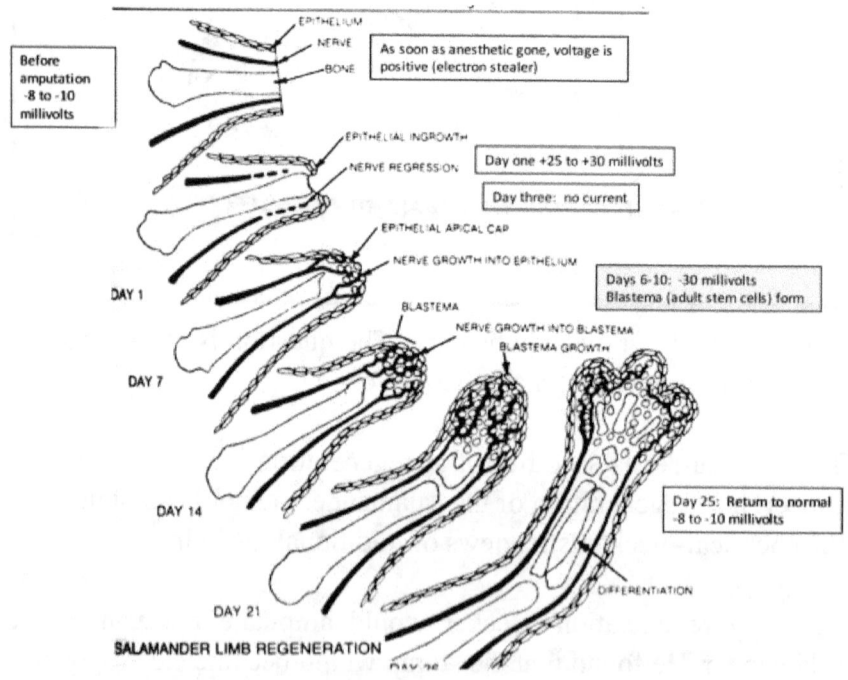

EPITHELIUM
NERVE
BONE

Before amputation -8 to -10 millivolts

As soon as anesthetic gone, voltage is positive (electron stealer)

EPITHELIAL INGROWTH
NERVE REGRESSION

Day one +25 to +30 millivolts

Day three: no current

EPITHELIAL APICAL CAP
NERVE GROWTH INTO EPITHELIUM

DAY 1

BLASTEMA

Days 6-10: -30 millivolts
Blastema (adult stem cells) form

NERVE GROWTH INTO BLASTEMA
BLASTEMA GROWTH

DAY 7

DAY 14

Day 25: Return to normal -8 to -10 millivolts

DIFFERENTIATION

DAY 21

SALAMANDER LIMB REGENERATION

Then he found something else unusual. If he removed and re-implanted the blastema after ten days, it grew a duplicate of the organ it was from. For example, if he amputated an arm but waited more than ten days after the blastema formed to remove and implant it near the tail, it grew an arm out of the tail area instead of another tail. Thus the blastema was being programmed what it was to become during the first ten days.

Becker wondered how the blastema was being programmed and assumed it was the nervous system. He then cut the nerves going to the arm and then amputated the arm. To his surprise, nothing changed. Harvesting and re-implanting the blastema before ten days grew a local organ and after ten days grew the same organ (or limb) that was amputated. He couldn't figure out how it was being programmed.

He then made one-millimeter sections of the area and found that the nerves were not growing back into the stem cells but that the fibrous tissue around the nerves were quickly growing into the stem cells (blastema). These fibrous cells were carrying the information to program the blastema.

Becker went on to discover that we have an entire second nervous system made of fibrous tissue surrounding our nerves.

He named this the *analog perineural nervous system.*"The nerve-impulse nerves of the brain and body are digital. That means that information is in discrete steps of on/off. It is sensitive to the frequency of the signal. It controls the conscious mind and the autonomic nervous system (automatic control of blood pressure, breathing, etc.).

The second nervous system of the body is the perineural system of glial cells and Schwann cells, etc., that surround the other nerves. It is an analog system, meaning continuously variable strength of signal, direction of flow, and waves of strength. It controls growth, healing, and biological cycles.

Where it was always thought that the fibrous tissue of the body serves only as structural support, Becker and Nördenstrom showed that fibrous tissue in the body also serves to conduct electrons, much like copper wire in our homes.

It seems that Becker never realized that the fibrous sheath called the perineural nervous system was actually bringing in electrons to change the voltage from operating voltage to healing voltage.

The analog perineural system:

1. Delivers information to the blastema about how to grow a new body part (regeneration). Nerves have nothing to do with it.
2. Senses injury and controls repair
3. Controls local environments.
4. Is the primary system in the brain
5. Regulates our consciousness
6. Regulates decision making

Most scientists do not believe that cells can dedifferentiate from normal cells back to adult stem cells. It is believed that once cells differentiate into functional cells, they cannot go back the other way. For example, once a stem cell becomes a liver cell, it can never be anything except a liver cell. Becker showed that isn't true. Frog red blood cells have a nucleus. Becker exposed them to small electron-stealer currents (in billionths of amperes). They became stem cells.

When cells differentiate into cells in organs, genes that are not needed are turned off. However, they are still present. With the proper voltage, these genes can be switched back on as the cell de-differentiates back into adult stem cells.

The easiest way to access the perineural nervous system is at the spine. In the chart, you can see where each autonomic nerve exits the spine and which organs are connected to each nerve. One can use an electronic device such as the Tennant BioModulator to tap into any of these wires to measure the voltage of the connected organ or to send electrons to that organ.

Vertebra	Areas Supplied by Nerves	Possible Effects or Conditions
C1	Blood supply to the head, pituitary, scalp, bones of the face, brain, inner and middle ear, sympathetic nervous system	Headache, nervousness, insomnia, head colds, high blood pressure, migraines, mental conditions, nervous breakdowns, amnesia, epilepsy, chronic tiredness
C2	Eyes, optic nerve, auditory nerve, sinuses, mastoid bones, tongue, forehead	Sinus trouble, allergies, crossed eyes, deafness, eye trouble, earache, fainting spells, blindness
C3	Cheeks, outer ear, facial bones, teeth, facial nerve	Neuralgia, tinnitus, acne, eczema
C4	Nose, lips, mouth, Eustachian tubes, mucous membranes	Hay fever, hearing loss, post-nasal drip.
C5	Vocal cords, neck lymph glands, pharynx	Laryngitis, hoarseness, sore throat
C6	Neck muscles, shoulders, tonsils	Stiff neck, pain in upper arm, tonsillitis, whooping cough, croup
C7	Thyroid gland, bursae in shoulders, elbows	Bursitis, colds, thyroid conditions, goiter, tennis elbow, tendonitis
T1	Arms from elbows down, hands, wrists, fingers, esophagus, trachea	Asthma, cough, difficult breathing, shortness of breath, pain in lower arms and hands, carpal tunnel syndrome.
T2	Heart, pericardium, valves, arteries	Heart conditions, angina
T3	Lungs, bronchial tubes, pleura, chest, breast, nipples	Bronchitis, pleuritis, pneumonia, congestion, influenza, grip
T4	Gall bladder and common duct	Gall bladder pain, jaundice, shingles
T5	Liver, solar plexus, blood	Liver conditions, low blood pressure, anemia, poor circulation, arthritis
T6	Stomach	Indigestion, heartburn, dyspepsia
T7	Pancreas, Islets of Langerhans, duodenum	Diabetes, ulcers, gastritis, hypoglycemia
T8	Spleen, diaphragm	Weakened immune system, acute and chronic infections, hiccoughs
T9	Adrenals	Allergies, hives, hypertension, anemia, hypoglycemia, obesity, hair loss

T10	Kidneys	Kidney stones, arteriosclerosis, chronic fatigue, nephritis, kidney infections
T11	Kidneys, ureters	Skin conditions like acne or pimples, boils, autoimmune diseases
T12	Small intestine, fallopian tubes, lymph, circulation	Joint pain, gas pain, bloating
L1	Large intestine, inguinal rings	Constipation, colitis, dysentery, diarrhea, hernias
L2	Appendix, abdomen, upper leg	Appendicitis, cramps, acidosis, varicose veins
L3	Sex organs, ovaries, testicles, uterus, bladder, knee	Bladder troubles, menstrual trouble, miscarriages, bed wetting, incontinence, menopausal symptoms, knee pain
L4	Prostate gland, low back muscles, sciatic nerve	Sciatica, low back pain, painful & frequent urination, backaches
L5	Lower legs, ankle, feet, toes, arteries	Poor circulation in legs, swollen ankles, cold feet, weakness in legs, leg cramps

The Acupuncture System

One of the body's wiring systems is the analog perineural nervous system. The other is the acupuncture system. Remember that both wiring systems are made of fibrous tissue.

A sheath or cable made of fibrous tissue is called *fascia*. Fascia interpenetrates and surrounds muscles, bones, organs, nerves, blood vessels, and other structures. Fascia is an uninterrupted, three-dimensional web of tissue that extends from head to toe, from front to back, from interior to exterior.

I encourage you to go back and read the section about semiconductors, diodes, transistors, and microprocessors.

The fascias of the body are semiconductors, diodes, transistors, and microprocessors. These connect with and communicate with the cells of each organ.

Remember that one of the characteristics of semiconductors is that electrons move in only one direction. This becomes important when considering how acupuncture meridians work.

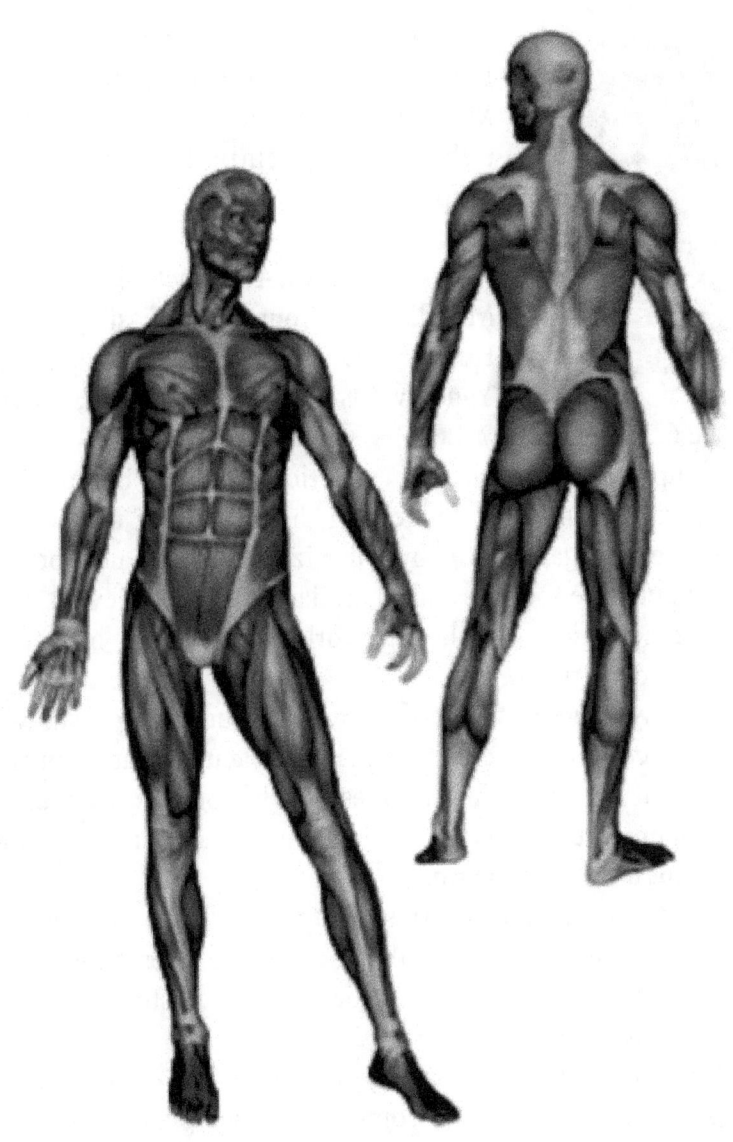

In the images you will notice that fascia surround each muscle, connect with a fascial sheath that surrounds each organ, and then small fibers connect the sheets around each organ down to each little cluster of cells. In this way, each cell of the body is wired to the common wire that goes up the center of the back and down the center of the front of the body. This is the acupuncture system.

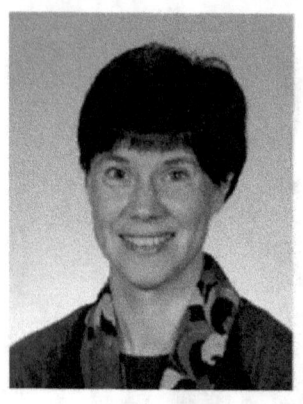

Helene Langevin, MD, is a research assistant professor of neurology at the University of Vermont School of Medicine. She and her colleagues published a seminal article about acupuncture meridians:

"Relationship of Acupuncture Points and Meridians to Connective Tissue Planes", Helene M. Langevin, and Jason A. Yandow, *The Anatomical Record*, Volume 269, Issue 6, 2002, pp. 257–265.

1. Acupuncture meridians traditionally are believed to constitute channels connecting the surface of the body to internal organs. We hypothesize that the network of acupuncture points and meridians can be viewed as a representation of the network formed by interstitial connective tissue.

2. This hypothesis is supported by ultrasound images showing connective tissue cleavage planes at acupuncture points in normal human subjects. To test this hypothesis, we mapped acupuncture points in serial gross anatomical sections through the human arm.

3. We found an 80% correspondence between the sites of acupuncture points and the location of inter-muscular or intramuscular connective tissue planes in postmortem tissue sections.

4. We propose that the anatomical relationship of acupuncture points and meridians to connective tissue planes is relevant to acupuncture's mechanism of action and suggests a potentially important integrative role for interstitial

connective tissue.

Thus Langevin and her colleagues have shown us that the acupuncture system is essentially the fascial planes of the body.

Remember that the fascia are made of fibrous tissue. Remember also that fibrous tissue has the least resistance to the flow of electrons through the body. Remember also that this tissue is an electronic semiconductor, diode, etc.

In the graphic you can see the cross section of an arm. You can also see the classical drawings for the lung and large intestine meridians. You can see in the cross-section the fascial wires in the arm that are at the fibrous wires known as the lung and large intestine meridians.

Lung and
Large Intestine Meridians

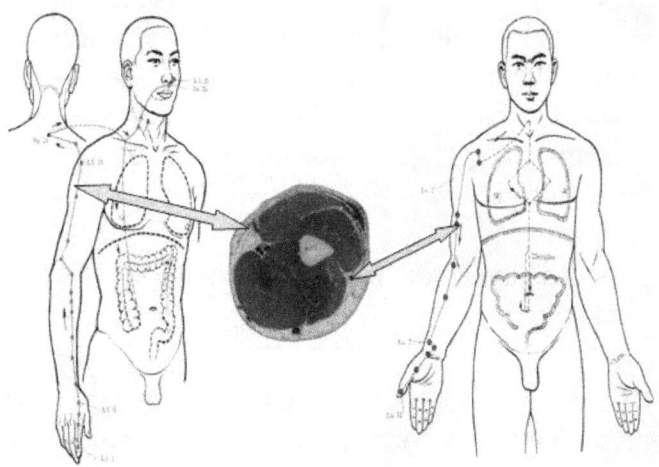

Ionic Transfer of Electrons

Besides the two wiring systems of the body (the perineural system and the acupuncture system) there is an additional means of moving electrons from place to place: an ionic transfer within the blood plasma. This was eloquently described by Björn Nördenstrom in his classical book *Biologically Closed Electric Circuits.*

In summary, there are three ways in which electrons are moved from place to place. One is by way of the wiring system known as the perineural nervous system. The second is by way of the wiring system known as the acupuncture meridian system. The third is ionically within the blood plasma.

How Do We Measure the Voltage in Organs?

It is difficult to use a voltmeter to measure the voltage in organs via the perineural nervous system or the acupuncture system. Voltage in the body pulses. Thus when you use a voltmeter, it will give a wide range of readings. It usually starts high and then, over a few minutes, it settles down to a more constant reading. Therefore it is common to use an ohmmeter to measure the voltage and then convert that to volts using Ohm's Law, which says that voltage = ohms x amps. If one assumes that amperage is constant, then ohms = voltage.

One can also use the assess mode of the Tennant BioModulator to estimate the voltage.

Measuring the Voltage of Organs Using the Perineural Nervous System or Acupuncture System

If you want to use the perineural system, refer to the chart displayed above to know what organ corresponds to which

132

vertebra.

The acupuncture system is more difficult for most to understand. Its origins are over five thousand years old—long before there was a clear understanding of anatomy and physiology. For example, there is no brain or nervous system in acupuncture theory.

Another system that is over five thousand years old is the Vedas and the concept of chakras. In this system it is believed that there are energy spheres in the body that connect to the universe. Disease results when these energy spheres, called chakras, spin incorrectly.

Chakras, as described above, are energy centers along the spine located at major branchings of the human nervous system, beginning at the base of the spinal column and moving upward to the top of the skull.

Chakras are considered to be a point or nexus of biophysical energy or *prana* of the human body. Shumsky states that "prana is the basic component of your subtle body, your energy field, and the entire chakra system...the key to life and source of energy in the universe."

The following seven primary chakras are commonly described:
1. Muladhara (Sanskrit: Mūlādhāra) Base or Root Chakra (last bone in spinal cord *coccyx*)
2. Swadhisthana (Sanskrit: Svādhiṣthāna) Sacral Chakra (ovaries/prostate)
3. Manipura (Sanskrit: Maṇipūra) Solar Plexus Chakra (navel area)

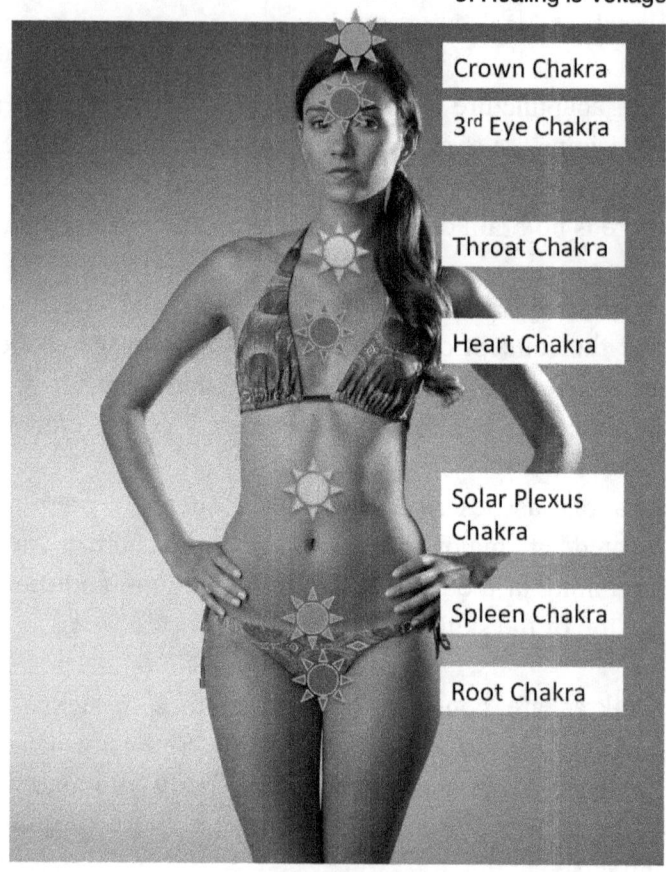

4.

Anahata (Sanskrit: Anāhata) Heart Chakra (heart area)

5. Vishuddha (Sanskrit: Viśuddha) Throat Chakra (throat and neck area)
6. Ajna (Sanskrit: Ājñā) Brow or Third Eye Chakra (pineal gland or third eye)
7. Sahasrara (Sanskrit: Sahasrāra) Crown Chakra (Top of the head; 'Soft spot' of a newborn) – Wikipedia

Another system of energy distribution was developed by Master Jiro Murai, a Japanese gentleman about to die in 1912. It is said that he went into a deep sleep and awoke well with the knowledge of how to balance energy in the body. Others report that he remembered a technique he was taught as a child and applied this to himself and was cured in one week.

134

The system is called *Jin Shin* or *Jin Shin Jyutsu*. The system consists of the therapist placing both hands on certain spots in a series of protocols to correct the flow of energy.

It is said that Jiro Murai taught Haruki Kato, MD, this method. Apparently Kato and Murai taught Mary Mariko Iino-Burmeister the techniques. Mary, a Japanese American, returned to California and began teaching the techniques there and later in Arizona.

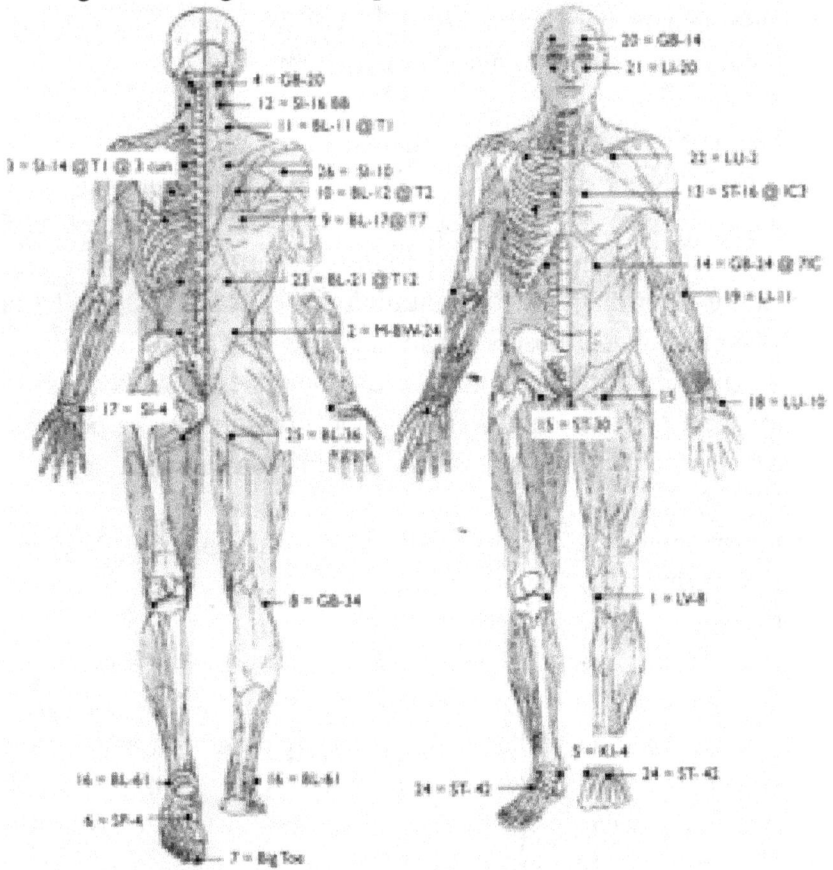

This graphic depicts the points used by Burmeister in her teachings and their acupuncture correspondences. In the Murai technique, the points are listed as a number. For example, you might use your hands to connect right #4 with right #20. This would be the same as connecting GB-20 and GB-14 in acupuncture terminology.

In the 1990s, Glenn King, PhD, of Dallas, Texas, sought to learn and understand Murai's system. He studied the methods taught by Mary Burmeister and eventually was given copies of Murai's drawings originally given to Mary Burmeister. His interpretation of the system differed from Burmeister's. He eventually developed a system called "The King Method" or TKM. Although I have been trained by him in his system, he strongly enforces his copyrights to the material. Since it is difficult to know what material is Murai's or more ancient and not covered by copyright and what King's version is, it is difficult to discuss his system.

I found it difficult to believe that the body contained different systems that were not working together. As I continued to study various acupuncture texts, it became apparent to me that there were spots on the primary acupuncture circuits (governor and conception meridians) where multiple meridians crossed. These points corresponded closely to the locations described for many of the chakras. Understanding that the acupuncture system is the same as the fascia system, I noted that the location of crossing points of the fascia were the same as some of the Jin Shin/Murai points.

Further examination of these facts led to the understanding that there is a primary cable that carries voltage up the back and down the front of the body. Also, there is a central terminal for each region of the body on that cable that sends voltage to every organ in that region. For example, there are points on the front and back of the skull that send voltage first to the right and left of the skull and then to each organ in the skull. The central terminal corresponds to what is classically called the third eye chakra. The lateral terminals correspond to what the Jin Shin/Murai system calls energy spheres #20 and acupuncture calls gall bladder 14 (GB-14).

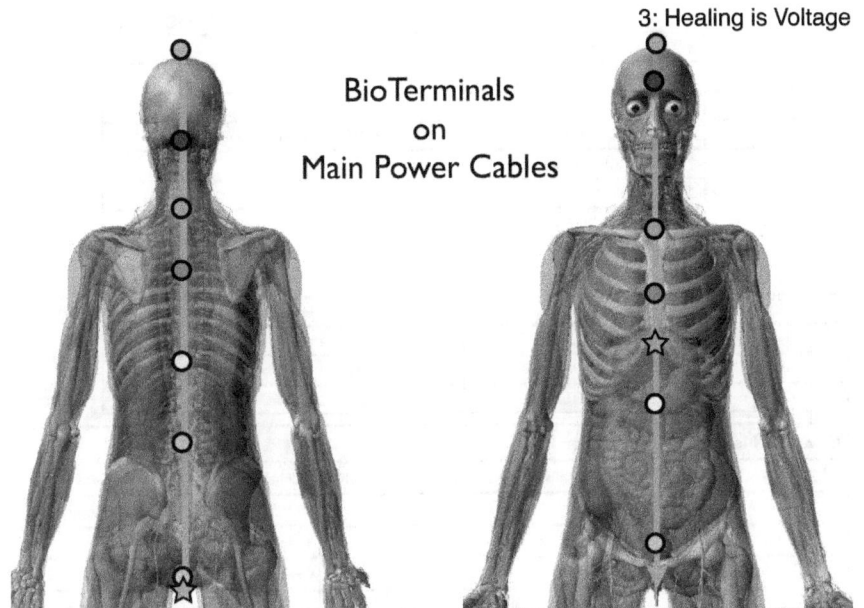

BioTerminals
on
Main Power Cables

I began to call these switching points on the primary meridians "Switching Terminals" or "**BioTerminals®**." I felt they needed a different name because they are close to, but not the same as, chakra positions.

The lateral BioTerminals are shown in the graphic. Notice that we have a central and right and left lateral BioTerminals for the head, neck/upper chest, chest, abdomen, and pelvis. Note they are basically the same as the "Energy Spheres" described in Jin Shin as shown on the right.

Look at the similarities between the BioTerminals and the bands of fascia in the graphic.

Now we have an easy way to determine the voltages of the organs in each region of the body. Let's say that you have pneumonia. You will certainly have low voltage in the chest BioTerminal®. It may be front or back or both. If you have stomach ulcers, you will have low voltage in the abdomen BioTerminal®. It can be on the left or the right or both.

Conception Meridian	Terminals	Switching Terminals
CV-1	CV, GV, and Penetrating	PRIMARY TERMINAL =Root Chakra
CV-2	CV, LV	
CV-3	CV, SP, LV, KI	PELVIS TERMINAL = Sacral Chakra
CV-4	CV, SP, LV, KI	
CV-7	CV, KI	
CV-10	CV, SP	
CV-12	CV, SI, TB, ST	ABDOMEN TERMINAL = Solar Plexus Chakra
CV-13	CV, ST, SI	
CV-15	Luo Point	xiphoid
CV-17	CV, SP, KI, SI, TB	CHEST TERMINAL = Mid-sternum; Heart Chakra
CV-22	CV, Yin Linking	THROAT TERMINAL = Supra-sternal notch; Throat Chakra
CV-24	CV, GV, LI, ST	Chin

Governor Meridian	Location	Terminals	BioTerminals
GV-1	Coccyx to Anus	Luo Point; GV, CV, GB, KI	PRIMARY TERMINAL = Root Chakra
GV-4	L-2/KI		PELVIS TERMINAL = L-2; Sacral Chakra
GV-6	T-11/SP		T-11; Solar Plexus Chakra
GV-11	T-5/HT		CHEST TERMINAL = T-5, Heart Chakra
GV-13	T-1	GV, BL	THROAT TERMINAL = C-7, T-1; Throat Chakra
GV-14	C-7	GV, Six Yang Channels	THROAT TERMINAL = C-7; Throat Chakra
GV-15	C-2	GV, Yang Linking Vessel	BRAIN TERMINAL = C-2; Brow Chakra
GV-16	C-1	GV, Yang Linking Vessel,	BRAIN TERMINAL = C-1; Brow Chakra
GV-17		GV, BL	
GV-20		GV, BL, GB, TB, LV	CROWN TERMINAL = Crown Chakra
GV-24		GV, BL, ST	
GV-26		GV, LI, ST	Upper Lip

The locations of these BioTerminals are noted above. The head BioTerminal® is between the brows on the front and

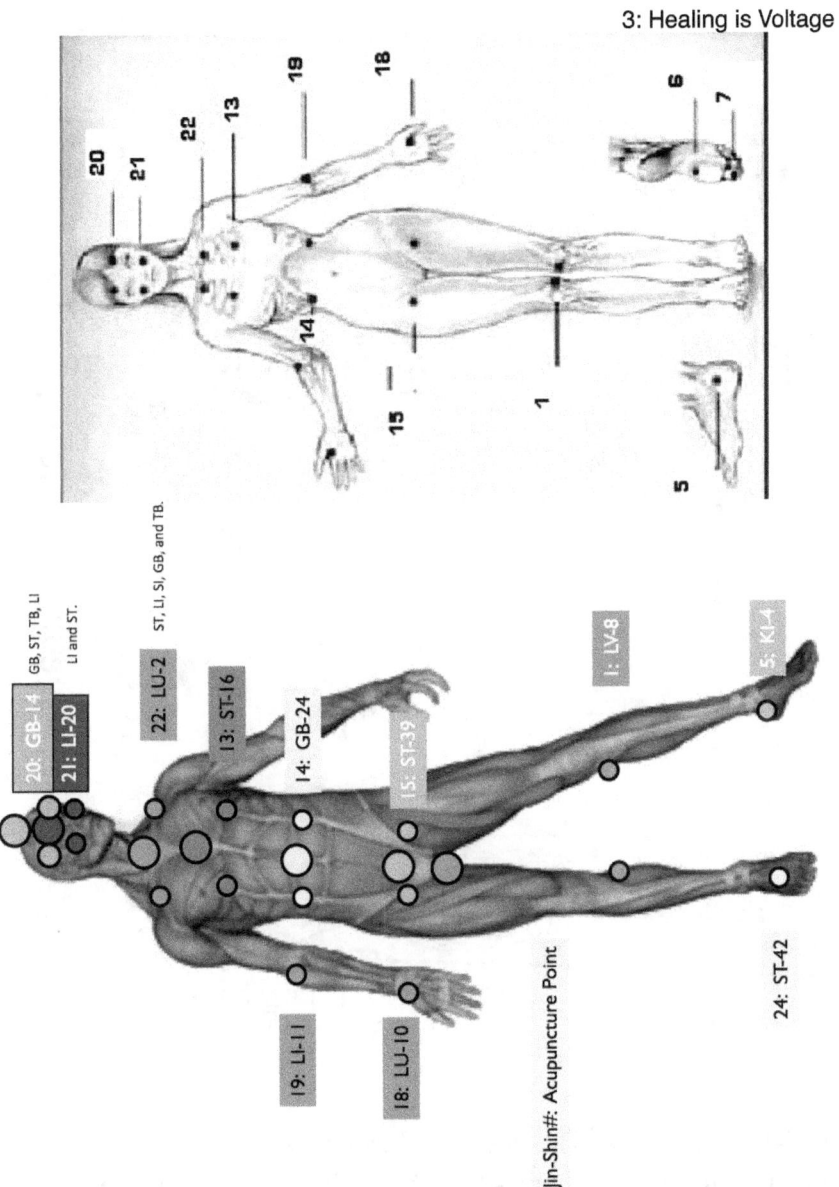

20: GB-14   GB, ST, TB, LI
21: LI-20   LI and ST.
22: LU-2   ST, LI, SI, GB, and TB.
13: ST-16
14: GB-24
15: ST-39
19: LI-11
18: LU-10
1: LV-8
5: KI-4
24: ST-42
Jin-Shin##: Acupuncture Point

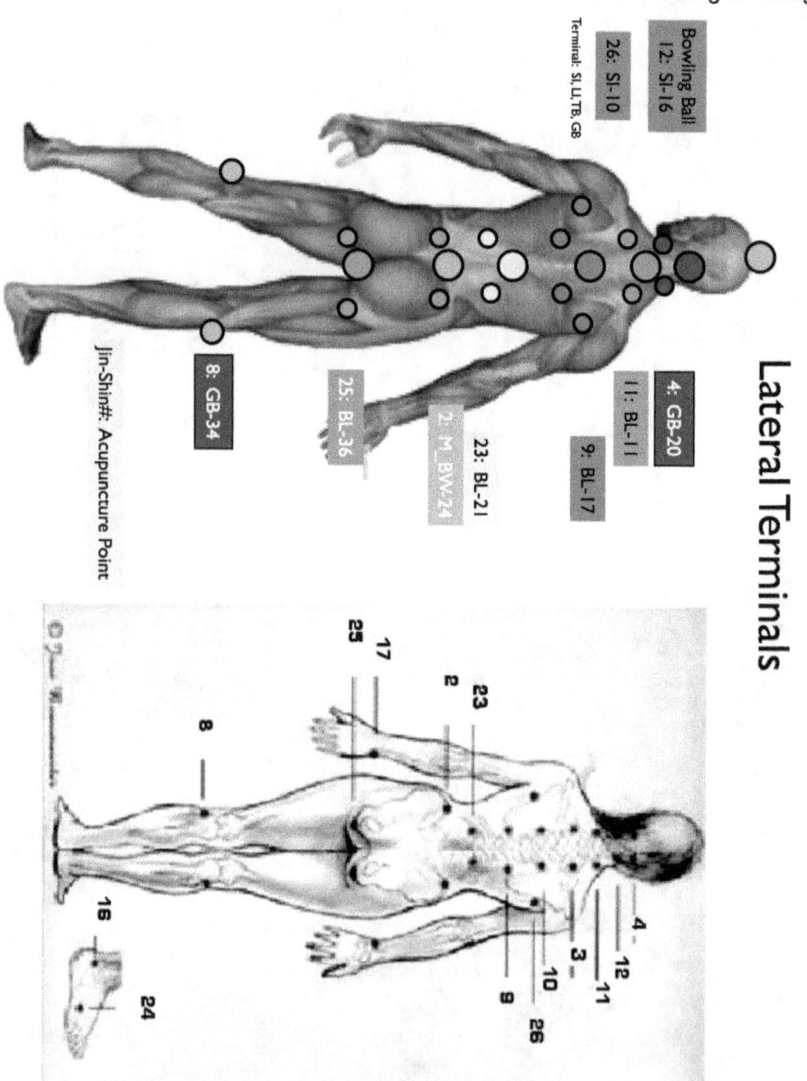

Lateral Terminals

Bowling Ball
12: SI-16

26: SI-10

Terminal: SI, LI,TB, GB

4: GB-20

11: BL-11

9: BL-17

23: BL-21

2: M_BW-24

25: BL-36

8: GB-34

Jin-Shin#: Acupuncture Point

at C-1 on the back. The neck BioTerminal® is at the supra-sternal notch in the front and at C-7 on the back. The chest BioTerminal® is at the mid-sternum in the front and at T-5 in the back. The abdomen BioTerminal® is halfway between the bottom of the sternum and the umbilicus on the front and at T-11 on the back. The pelvic BioTerminal® is just above the pubic bone on the front and at L-2 on the back.

There is also a BioTerminal® on the top of the skull and in the perineum. It can be measured over the coccyx.

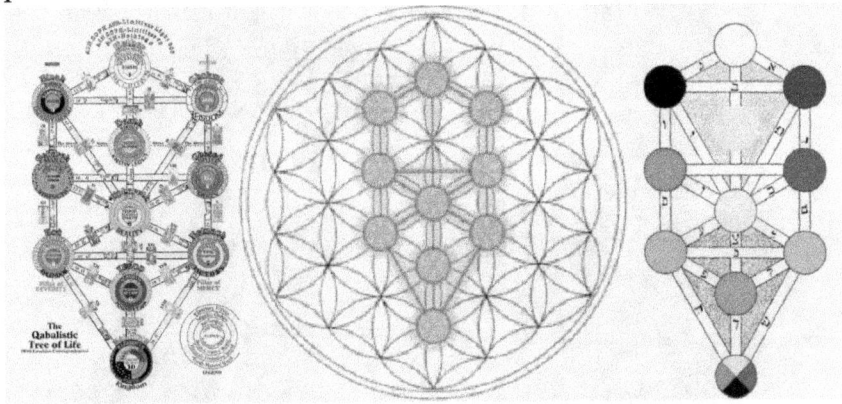

Note that the BioTerminal System has some similarities to the Kabbalah's Tree of Life. It also describes energetic pathways.

There is a safety circuit that connects the main cables in case one gets shorted out. It runs from the bottom of the sternum (xiphoid) to the coccyx. It is shown as a star in the graphic. This safety circuit often is necessary after abdominal surgery creates a scar that shorts out the normal flow of electrons through the main cables. You can see how the electrons normally flow up the back and down the front. Now imagine a scar on your abdomen from

141

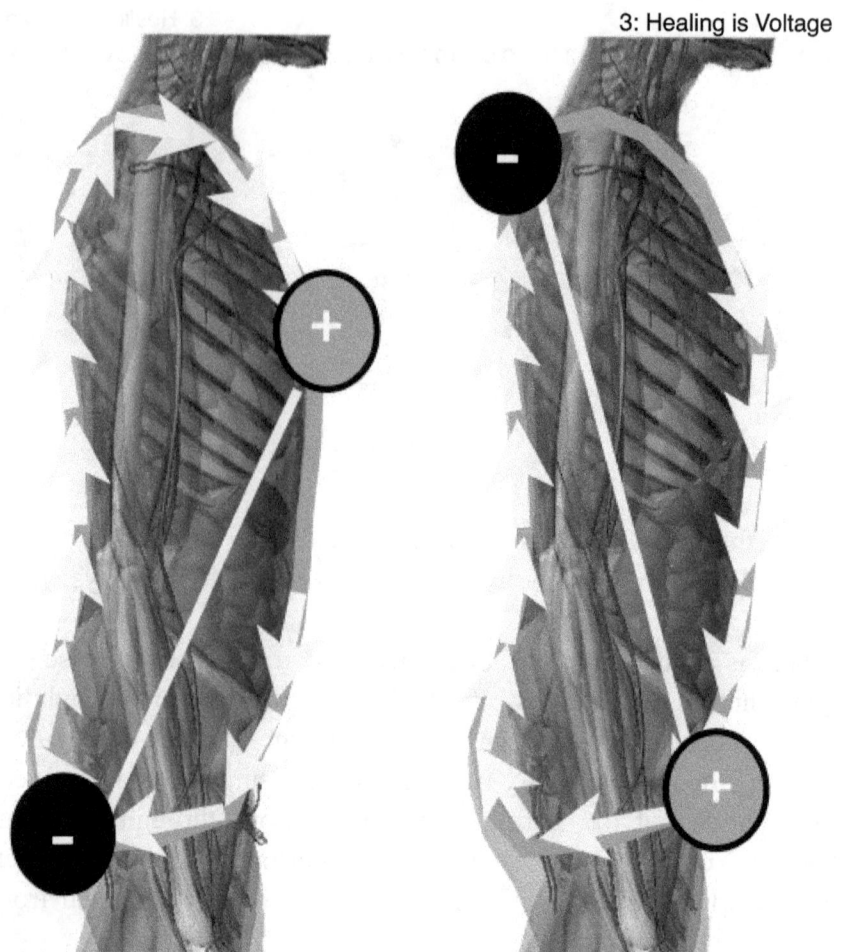

surgery or an injury. It would short out the circuit.

The body's defense against this is to use the "detour" from the xiphoid (bottom of sternum) to the coccyx. This protects the vital brain and heart, but it leaves the pelvis organs with reduced voltage, resulting in pelvic disorders. To overcome this, there is another "detour" from C-7 to the supra-pubic BioTerminal®. This allows some electrons to flow from C-7 to the pelvis to overcome blockages.

It is unfortunate that surgeons know nothing about the serious side effects of scars on the normal flow of electrons to organs via the acupuncture system of fascia.

One should treat scars with the Tennant Soreness Essential Oil Blend and the Tennant BioTransducer to reduce their shorting effect on the flow of electrons.

The Organs of the Body are Wired Together as Tesla Circuits

The father of electricity was Nikola Tesla. He had a much more dramatic influence on electronic devices and the delivery of electricity than Thomas Edison.

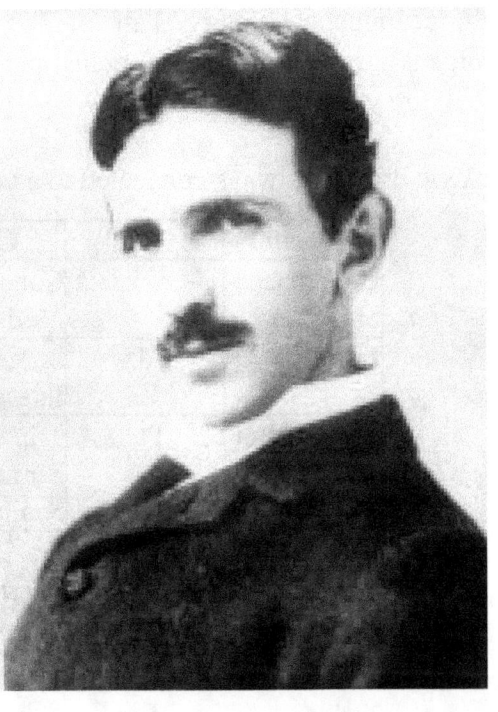

Nikola Tesla (10 July 1856–7 January 1943) was an inventor and a mechanical and electrical engineer. He was one of the most important contributors to the birth of commercial electricity and is best known for his many revolutionary developments in the field of electromagnetism in the late 19th and early 20th centuries. Tesla's patents and theoretical work formed the basis of modern alternating current (AC) electrical power systems, including the polyphase system of electrical distribution and the AC motor, with which he helped usher in the Second Industrial Revolution. – Wikipedia

In 1895, Tesla invented the tuned circuit, or resonating circuit. It consists of a coil wired to a capacitor. When they are wired on a box-shaped circuit, it is called "wired in parallel." Parallel tuned circuits are used in radio and other electronics to couple resonating energy from one circuit to another in transmitters and receivers.

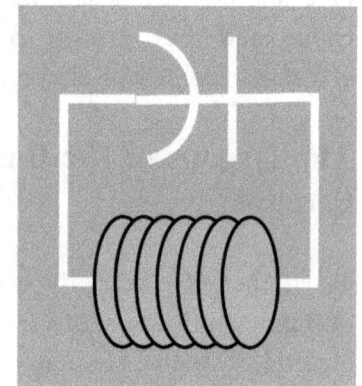

In acupuncture theory, half of the organs are said to be yin organs and half are yang organs.

A yin organ is always connected to a yang organ.

Capacitors	Yin	Coils	Yang
Governor Meridian	GV	Conception Meridian	CV
Lung	LU	Large Intestine	LI
Pericardium	PC	Triple Burner or Sanjiao	TB
Heart	HI	Small Intestine	SI
Liver	LV	Gall Bladder	GB

It became apparent to me that the yin organs are capacitors and the yang organs are hollow organs that serve as coils. They are wired together through connecting meridians to form Tesla resonating circuits.

The yin organs (capacitors; solid organs) are all wired to the main cable that runs up the back. The yang organs (coils; hollow organs) are all wired to the main cable that runs down the front of the body.

Point	Connected Meridians
LU-6	Lung Meridian
LU-7	Large Intestine Meridian
PC-8	Triple Burner (Sanjiao)
TB-5	Pericardium Meridian
Point	Connected Meridians
SI-7	Heart Meridian
HT-5	Small Intestine Meridian
BL-58	Kidney Meridian
KI-4	Bladder Meridian
GB-37	Liver Meridian
LV-5	Gall Bladder
ST-40	Spleen Meridian
SP-4	Stomach Meridian

What is confusing at first is that the wires that form the Tesla resonating circuits with each organ pain make a loop through either an arm or a leg. The loop also passes through a BioTerminal®. The loops connect in the arms or legs at what are called the "Luo Points" in acupuncture theory.

One circuit that is unique is the liver/gall bladder circuit. It controls the entire main cable system and is thus critical in the function of the entire system.

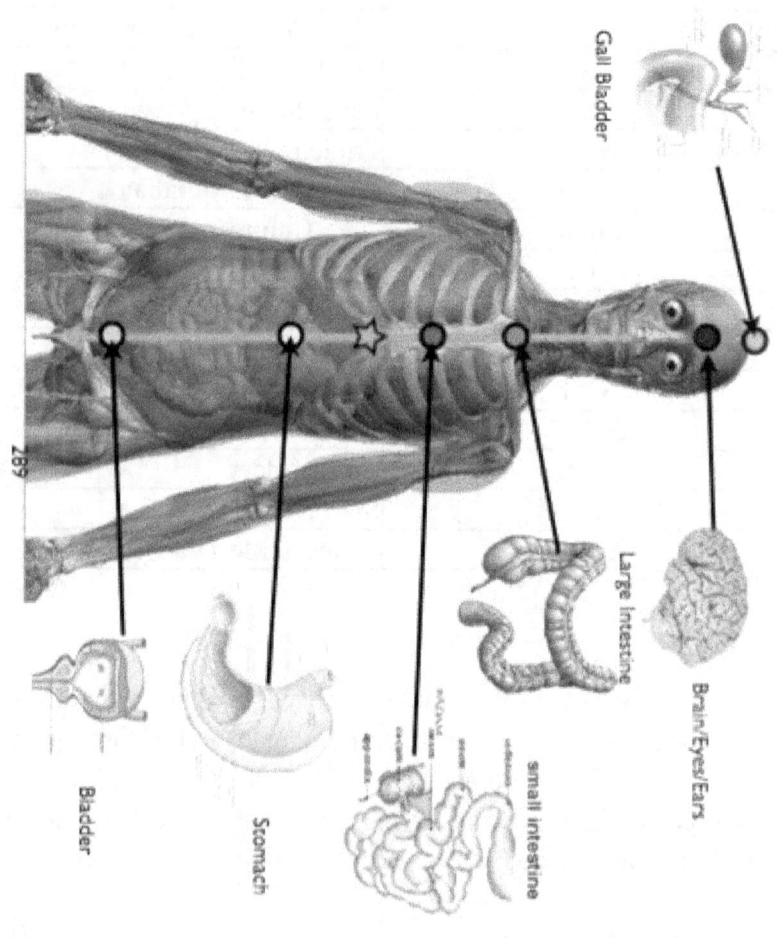

There are two unusual names in acupuncture theory that are used in the same way the names of organs are used, but they are not organs. The names are "triple burner" or "triple heater" or "sanjiao." These names are synonyms. The other unusual circuit is called the "pericardium," although it has very little to do with the covering of the heart. The triple burner is part of the yang or hollow circuitry, and the pericardium is part of the yin or capacitor circuitry. In modern anatomy, the triple burner is the sympathetic nervous system and the pericardium is the parasympathetic nervous system.

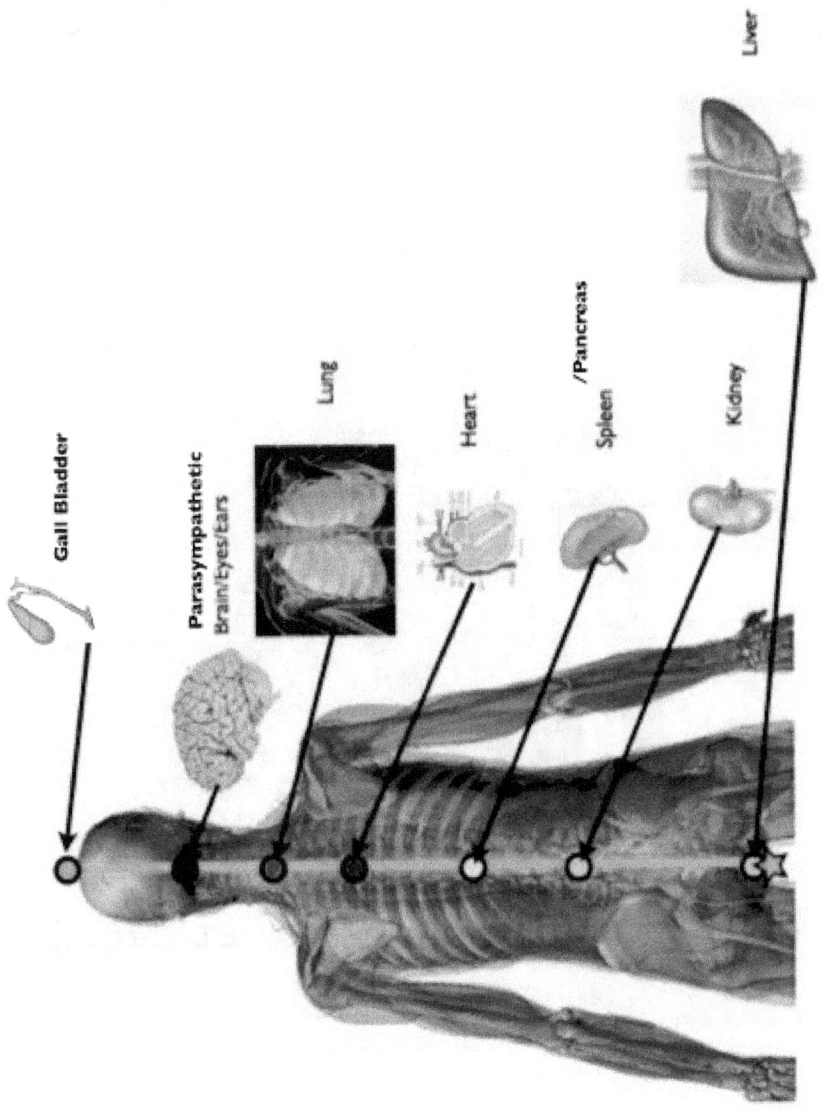

The triple burner is wired to the front BioTerminal of the skull, and the pericardium is wired to the back BioTerminal of the skull. Thus the autonomic nervous system composed of the sympathetic (triple burner) and parasympathetic (pericardium) monitor the head BioTerminals.

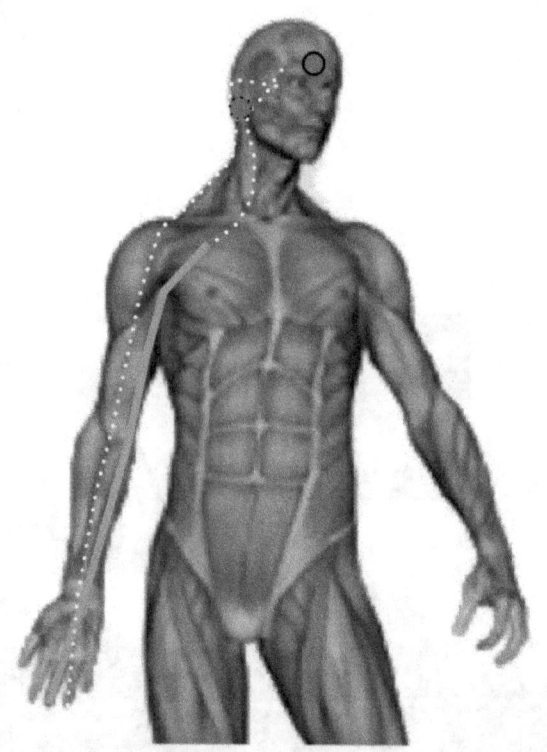

Sympathetic/Parasympathetic Tesla

The large intestine circuit is wired to the front neck BioTerminal,

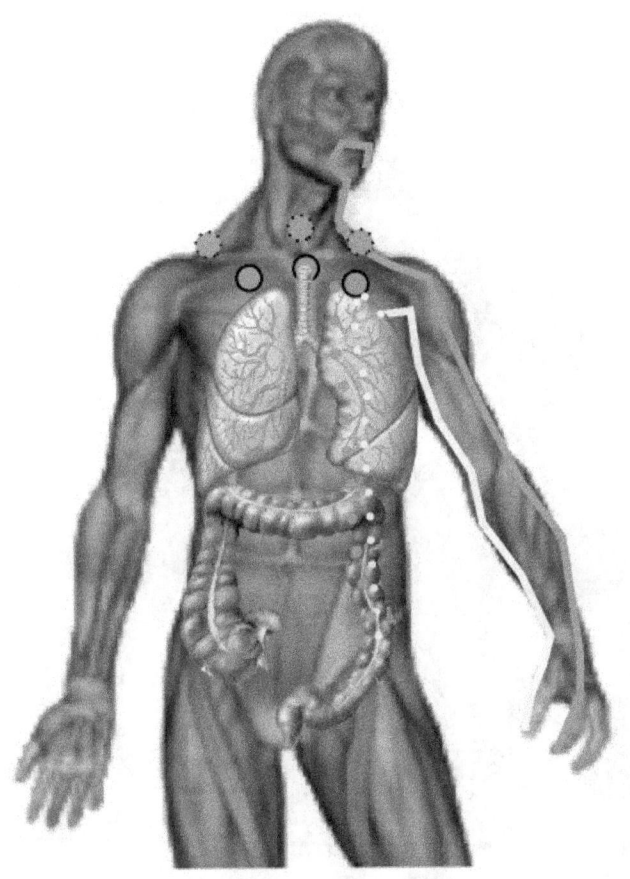

Lung/Large Intestine Tesla

and the lung circuit is wired to the back neck BioTerminal.

The small intestine circuit is wired to the front chest BioTerminal,

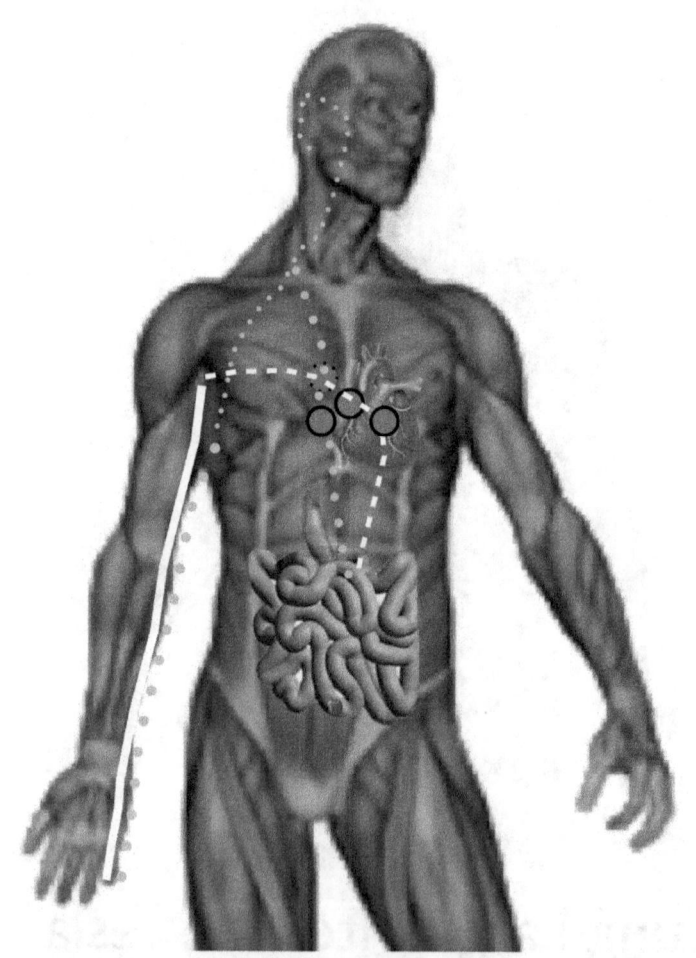

Heart/Small Intestine Tesla

and the heart circuit is wired to the back chest BioTerminal.

The stomach circuit is wired to the front abdominal BioTerminal,

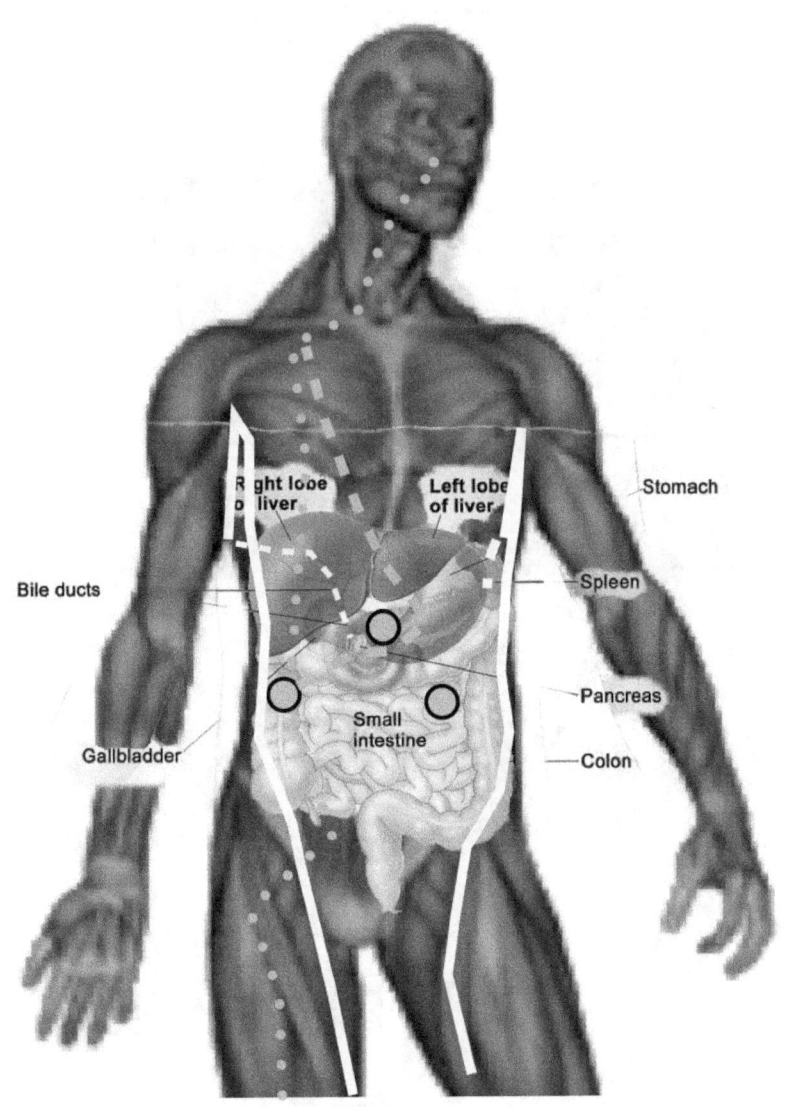

Spleen/Stomach Tesla

and the spleen circuit is wired to the back abdominal BioTerminal.

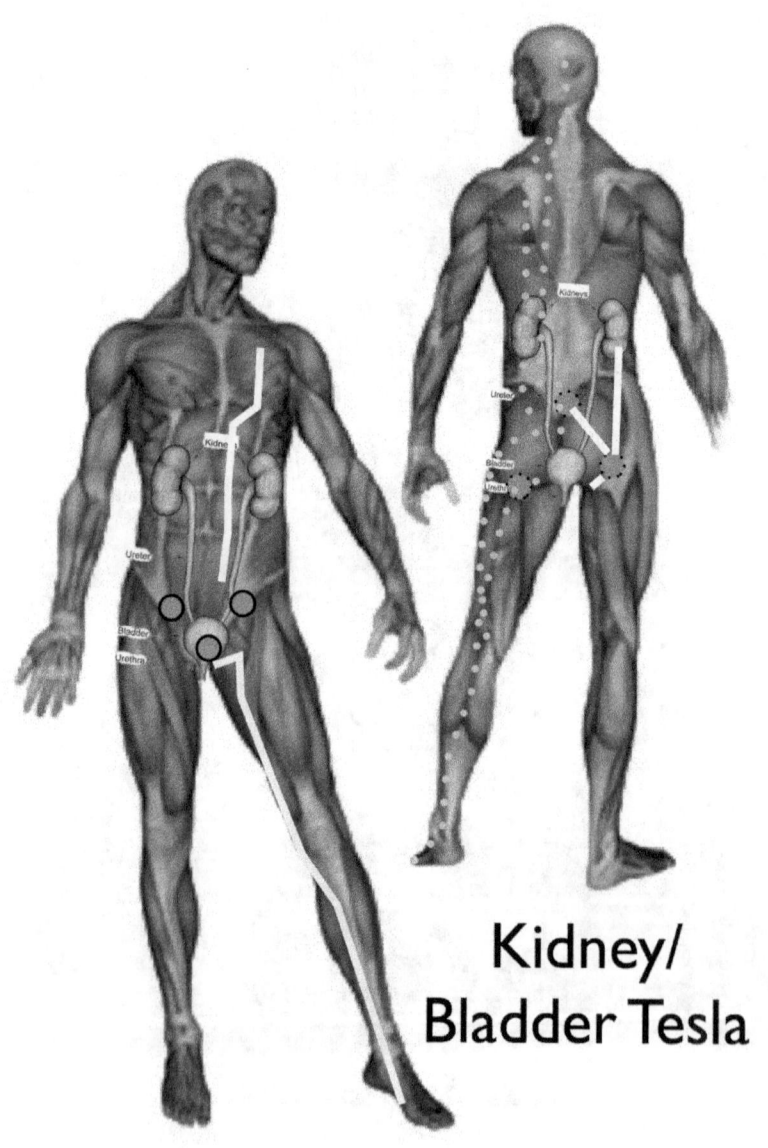

Kidney/
Bladder Tesla

The bladder circuit is wired to the front pelvis BioTerminal, and the kidney circuit is wired to the back pelvis BioTerminal.

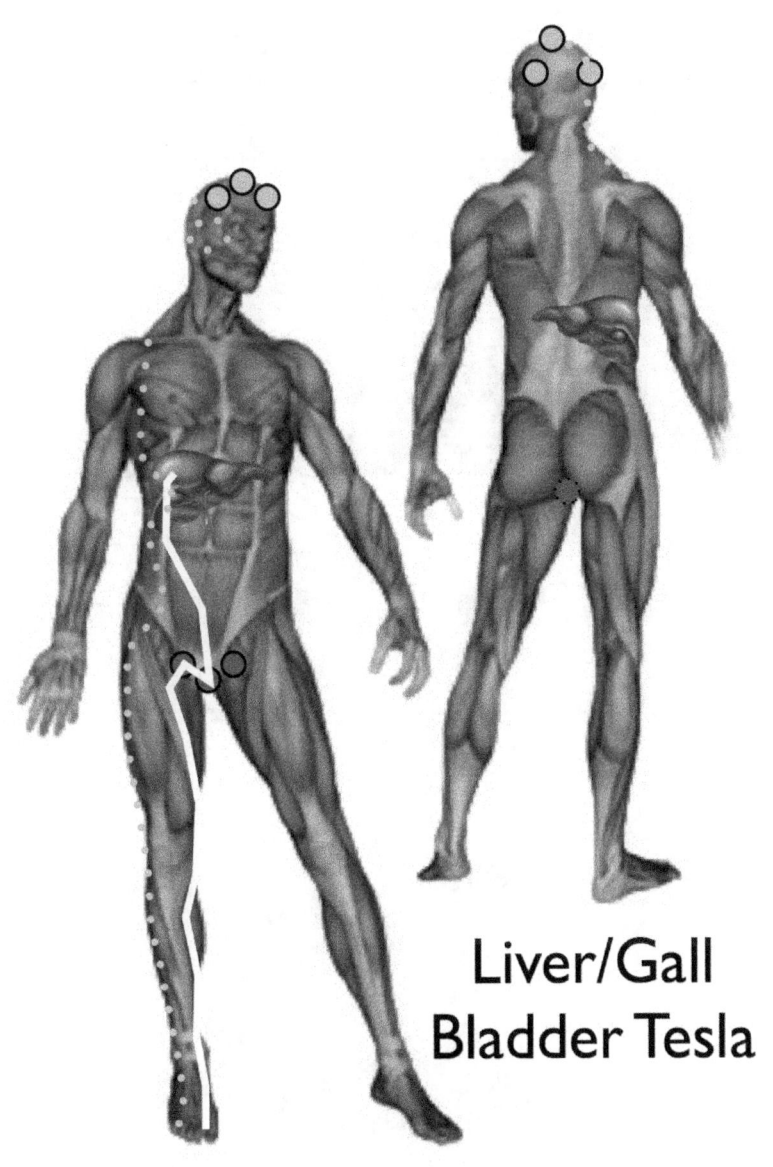

Liver/Gall Bladder Tesla

The liver circuit is wired to the crown BioTerminal, and the gall bladder circuit is wired to the base or root BioTerminal.

Remember that the liver circuit connects to the base BioTerminal, and the gall bladder circuit connects to the crown BioTerminal. I prefer to use the liver and gall bladder points on the knees instead of the classical "Luo" points for these circuits since they do not require dealing with modesty issues. Also, one can use the Mu

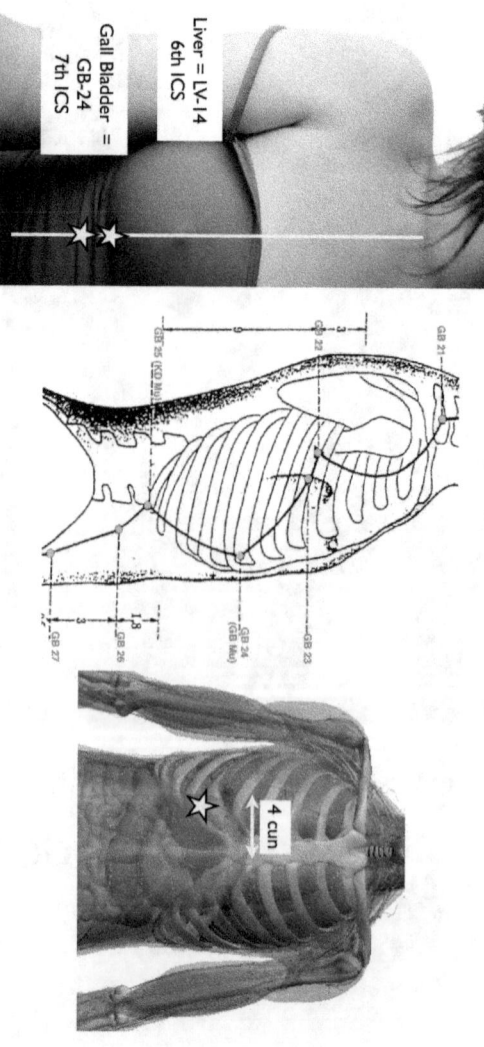

Points for liver and gall bladder.

Remember that Tesla circuits are designed to measure and adjust

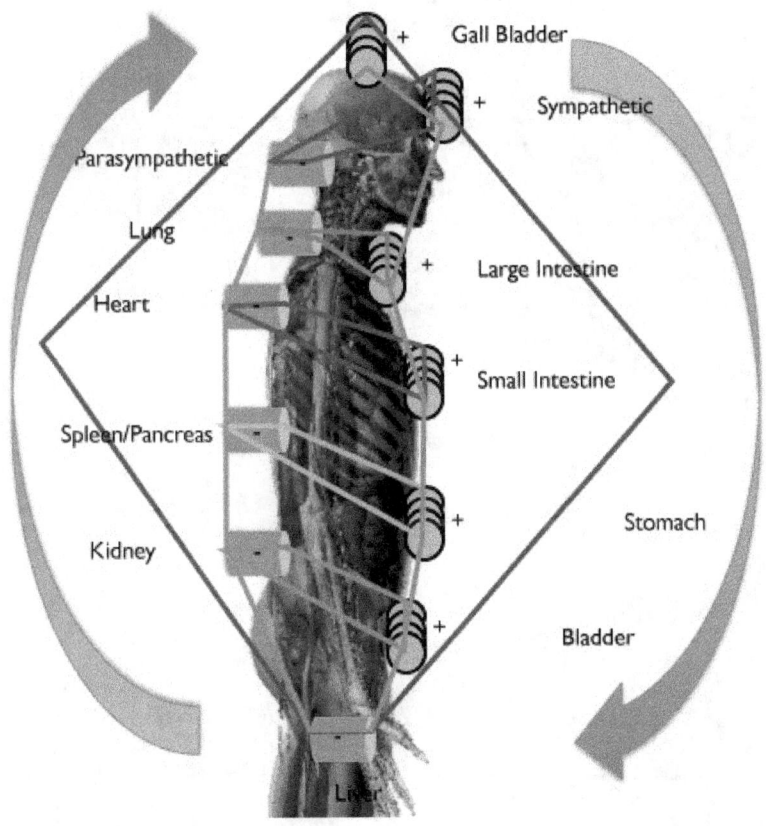

47

other circuits.

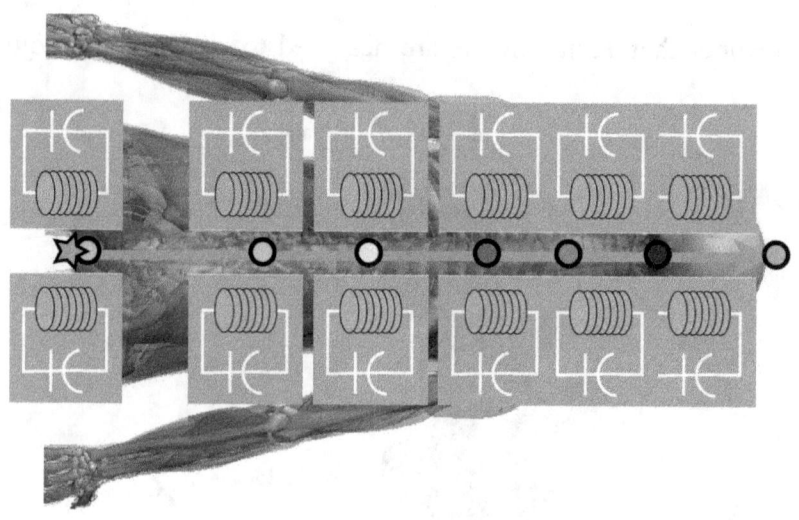

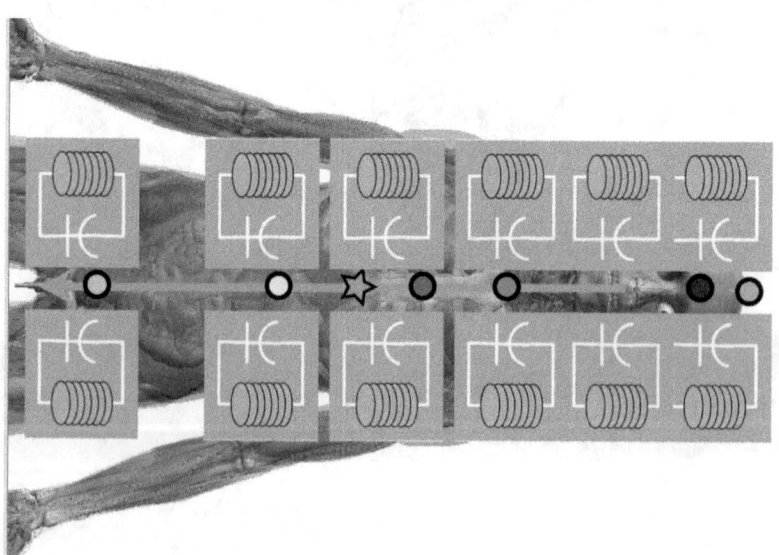

There is a Tesla circuit for each pair of organs on each side of the body. The capacitors are wired to the back and the coils are wired to the front of the body.

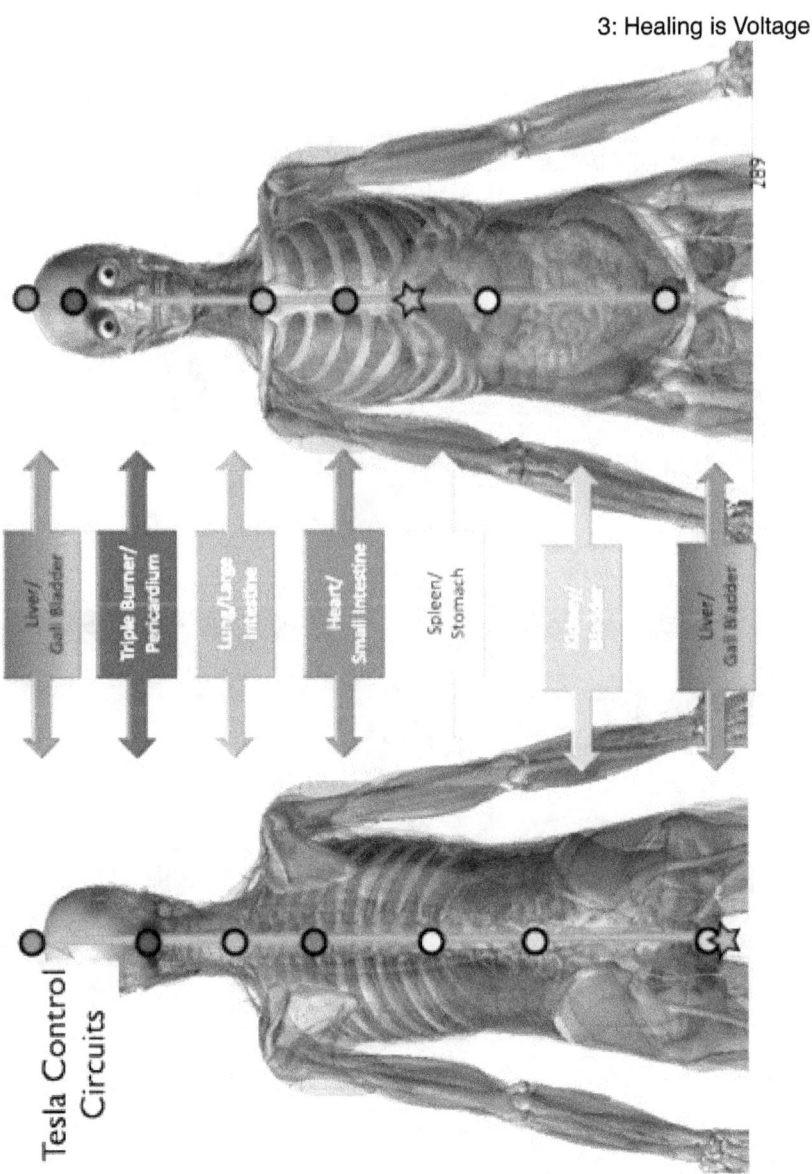

Tesla Control Circuits

Liver/
Gall Bladder

Triple Burner/
Pericardium

Lung/Large
Intestine

Heart/
Small Intestine

Spleen/
Stomach

Kidney/
Bladder

Liver/
Gall Bladder

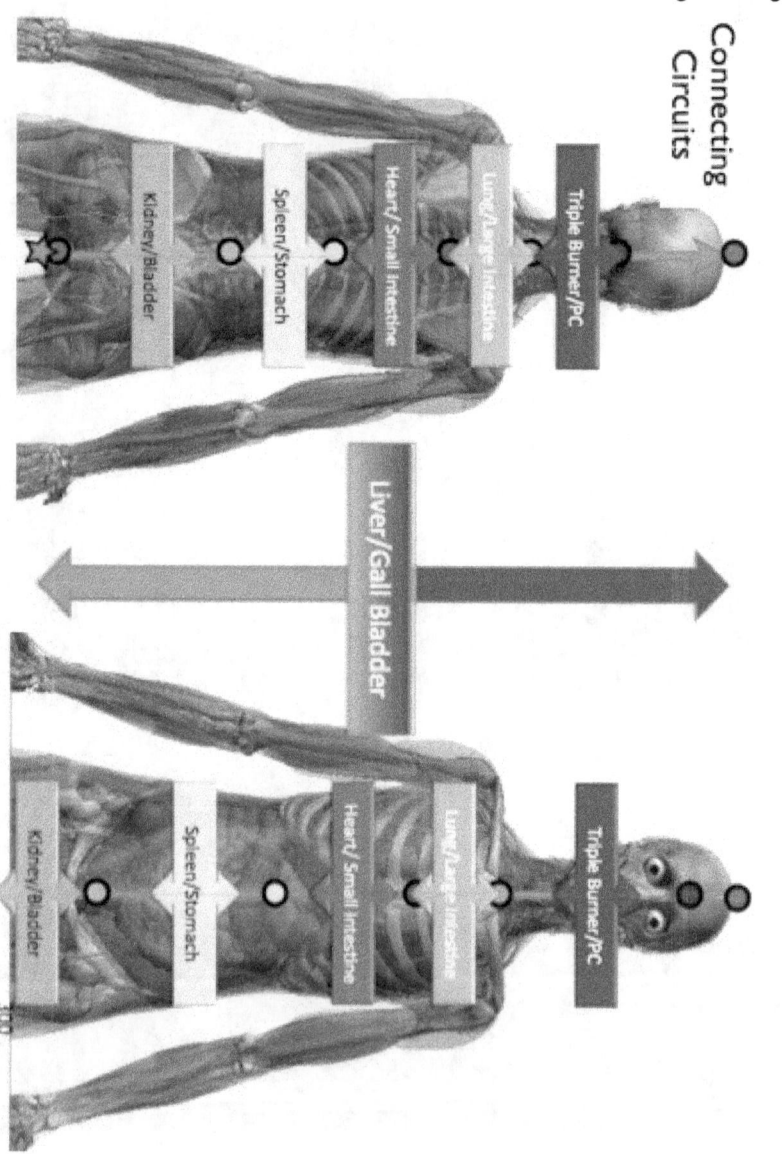

When a BioTerminal's voltage begins to drop, that is recognized

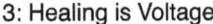

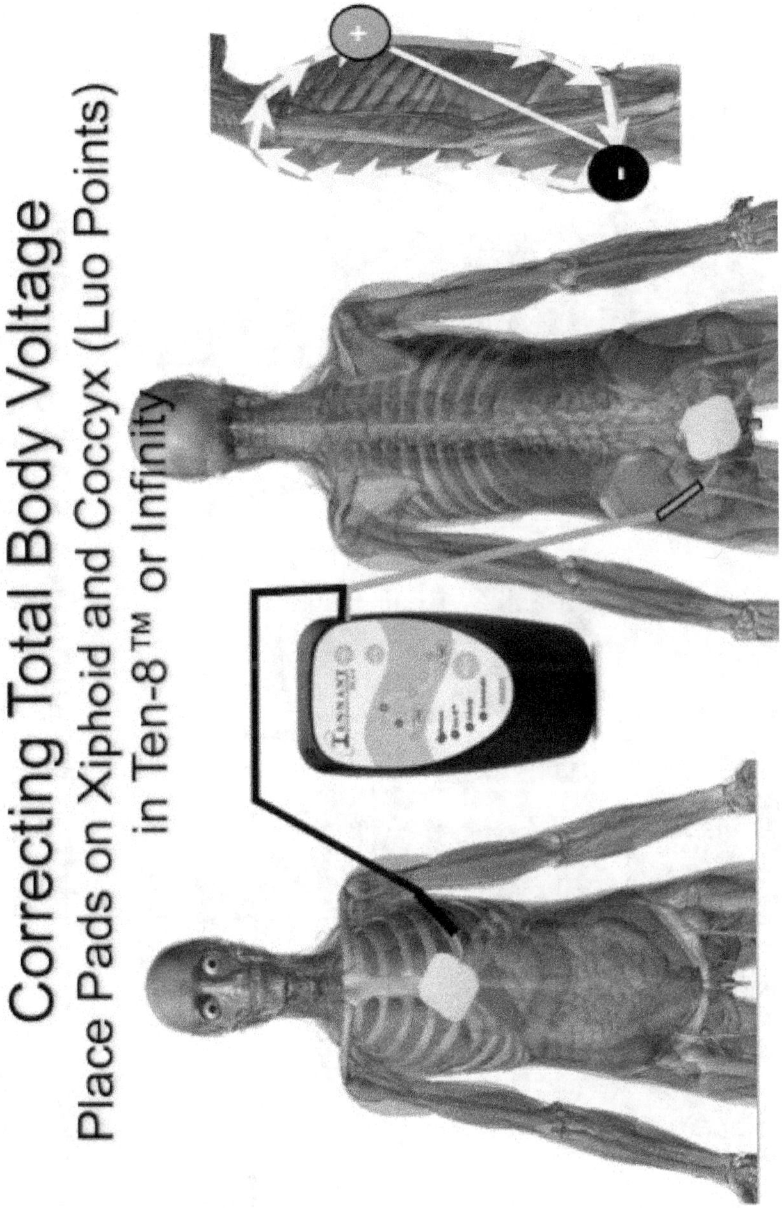

Correcting Total Body Voltage
Place Pads on Xiphoid and Coccyx (Luo Points) in Ten-8™ or Infinity

by the associated Tesla circuit. It moves electrons from the arm or leg muscles to the BioTerminal in an effort to modulate it back to normal. Thus it is important to exercise to keep the arm and leg muscle batteries charged.

When the total body voltage is low, you can use the Tennant

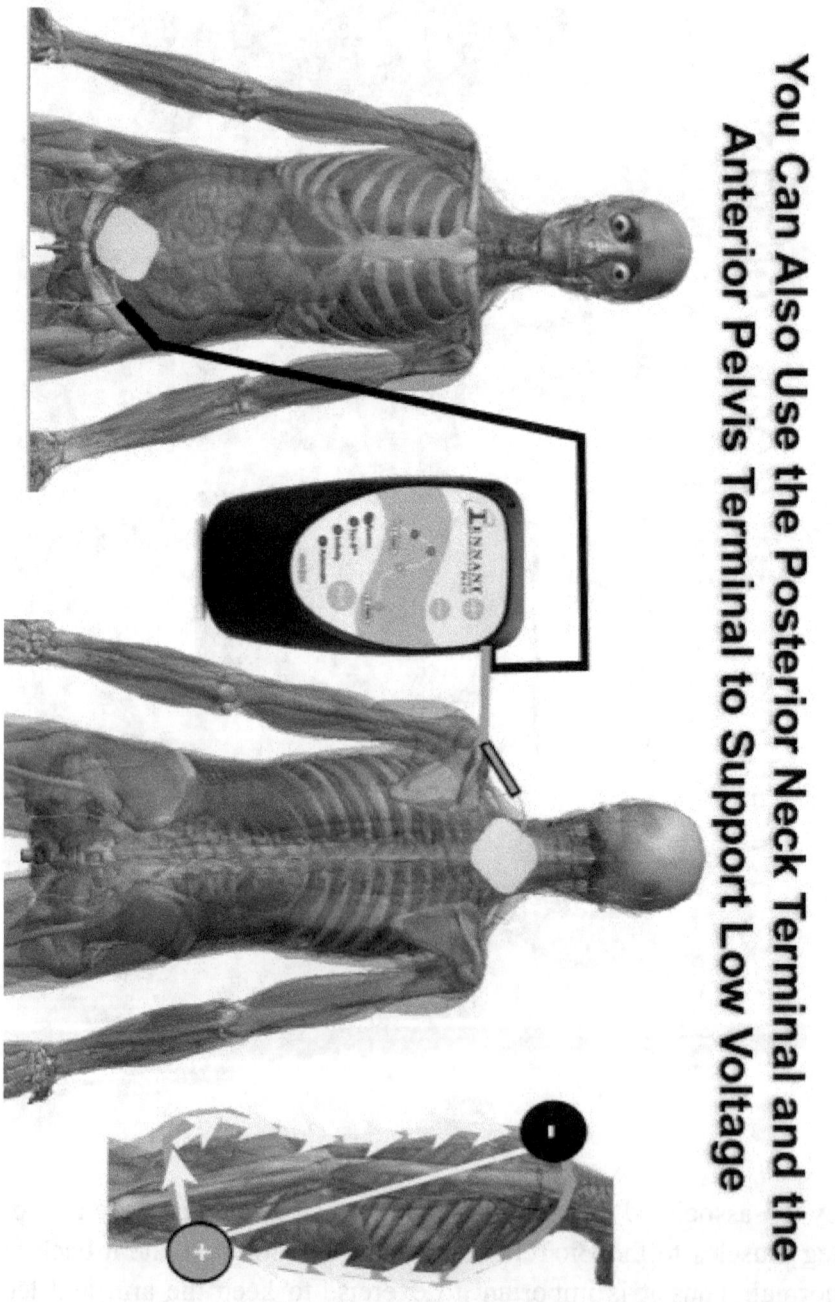

You Can Also Use the Posterior Neck Terminal and the Anterior Pelvis Terminal to Support Low Voltage

BioModulator as a portable battery charger while correcting the reasons for the low voltage. Place a patch over the supra-pubic BioTerminal and one over C-7. Attach the wire to the Tennant BioModulator and run it twenty-four hours per day until your voltages are normal.

The supra-pubic BioTerminal controls all of the yin organs (capacitors, solid organs). The BioTerminal at C-7 controls all the yang organs (hollow, coil organs).

Five Element vs. Six Element Theories

In classical acupuncture theory, there is a system called the "Five

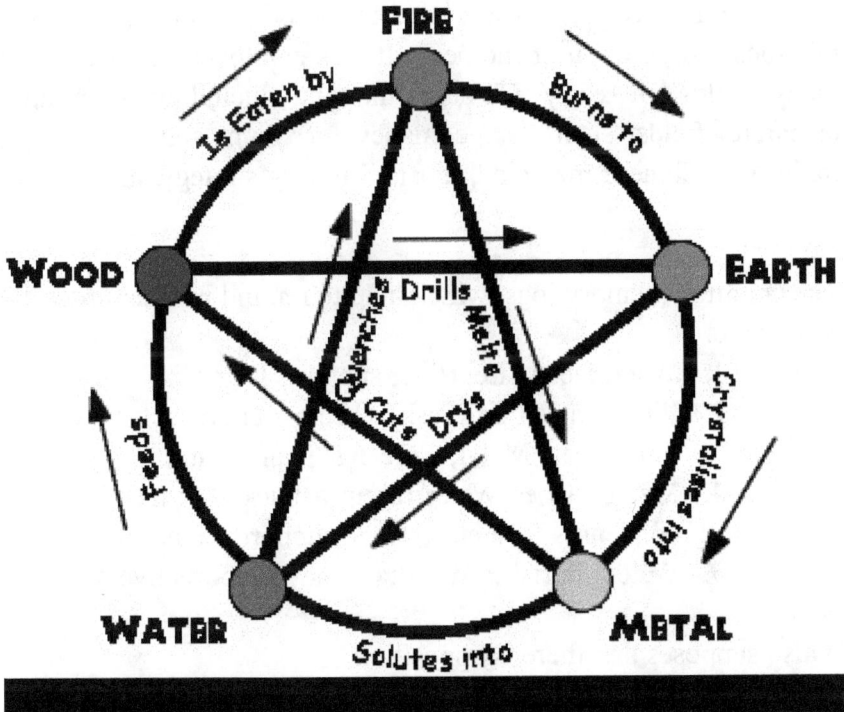

Element Theory."

"The Wu Xing," or the "Five Movements, Five Phases or Five Steps/Stages," are chiefly an ancient mnemonic device referred to in many traditional Chinese fields. It is sometimes translated as "Five Elements," but the Wu Xing are chiefly an ancient mnemonic device, hence the preferred translation of "movements," "phases," or "steps" over "elements." By the same token, Mu is thought of as "tree" rather than "wood."

The five elements are:
1. Wood = Liver and Gall Bladder
2. Fire = Heart and Small Intestine
3. Earth = Spleen and Stomach
4. Metal = Lung and Large Intestine
5. Water = Kidney and Bladder

The system of five phases was used for describing interactions and relationships between phenomena. It was employed as a device in many fields of early Chinese thought, including seemingly disparate fields such as geomancy or feng shui, astrology, traditional Chinese medicine, music, military strategy, and martial arts.

The common memory jogs, which help to remind in what order the phases are:
1. Wood feeds Fire; (liver supports heart)
2. Fire creates Earth (ash); (heart supports spleen)
3. Earth bears Metal; (spleen supports lung)
4. Metal carries Water (as in a bucket or tap, or water condenses on metal); (lung supports kidney)
5. Water nourishes Wood; (kidney supports liver)

It also supposes that there is opposition.
1. Wood absorbs Water; (liver steals from kidney)
2. Water rusts Metal; (kidney steals from lung)
3. Metal breaks up Earth; (lung steals from spleen)
4. Earth smothers Fire; (spleen steals from heart)
5. Fire burns Wood; (heart steals from liver)

Source: Wikipedia

162

This concept becomes more understandable if you look at the way

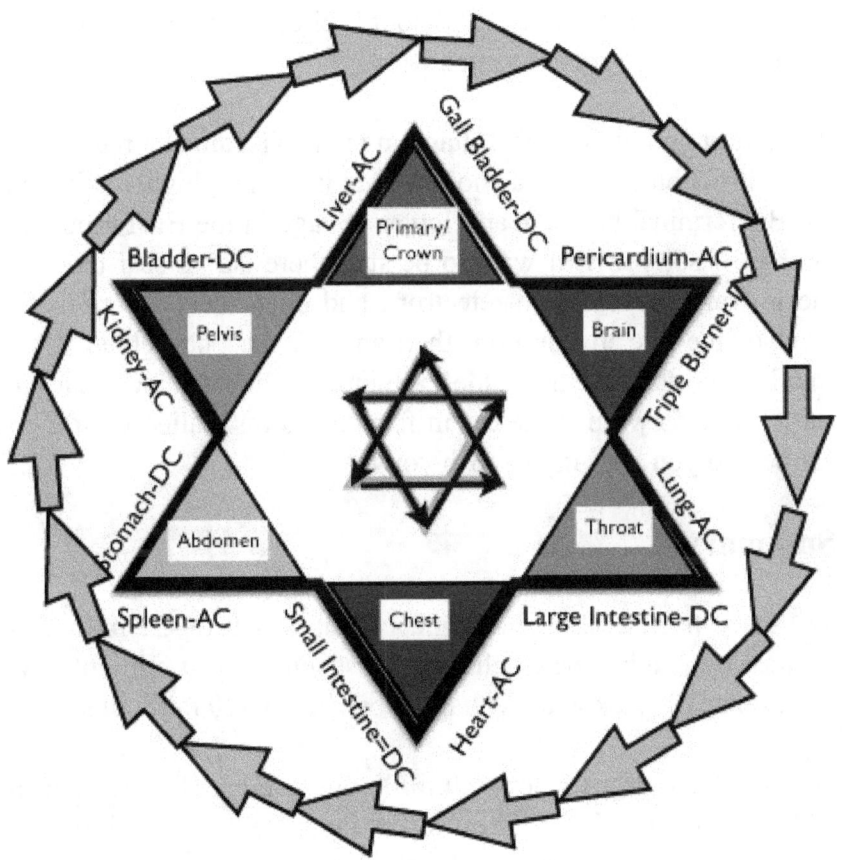

electrons flow through the acupuncture system.

I developed what I believe is a more useful system based on a six-pointed star instead of a five-star (element) theory. Start with the bladder Tesla at the posterior pelvic BioTerminal. It goes up the main cable to the primary or crown BioTerminal via the liver and gall bladder Tesla. This then connects with the head/skull BioTerminal via the pericardium and triple burner Tesla circuits. This leads us to the throat BioTerminal via the lung and large intestine Tesla. You can continue to follow the circuits in the graphic above.

If one of the BioTerminals is blocked—say by a scar—it backs up the flow of electrons to the one before it and, to some degree, to the one before that. The "detour" circuits noted above can ameliorate this to some degree.

When finding low or high voltage in the BioTerminal circuits, look to see if the blockage of a BioTerminal is causing higher voltage in the BioTerminal before it and lower voltage in the BioTerminal(s) after it. If so, you will want to be sure there isn't a scar blocking the forward movement of electrons and open the BioTerminal in front of the one in question, then amplify the one behind it and finally open the one that is the problem. It's like driving a car. You can't move forward if the car in front of you is stalled even if the car behind you is trying to push you forward.

Summary

The cells in the body are designed to run at -20 to -25 millivolts. To heal by making new cells, we must achieve -50 millivolts. We get chronically sick when voltage drops below -20 millivolts.

When voltage drops below -20 millivolts, we get chronic pain. In addition, oxygen levels drop since they are controlled by the voltage level. When oxygen levels drop, metabolism changes to where we only get two molecules of ATP instead of thirty-eight molecules per unit of fat processed. Cells struggle to function when they are getting "two miles to the gallon." In addition, the trillion or so "bugs" that are always in our bodies wake up when oxygen levels drop. They begin to "have lunch" by putting out enzymes that dissolve our cells. These enzymes enter our blood and damage cells throughout the body.

Thus chronic disease is always defined by low voltage.

To measure our voltages, we can easily use the acupuncture meridians and the BioModulator.

4 The Bowling Ball Syndrome

In traditional western medicine it is taught that the cranial bones fuse in childhood. However, it has been taught by osteopathic doctors since 1874 that the cranial bones move in a rhythmic pattern.

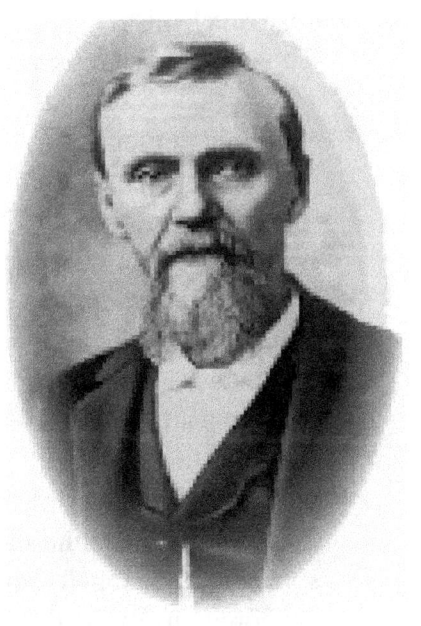

Andrew Taylor Still, MD, was a frontier doctor. He wasn't satisfied with the medicine he practiced, particularly when his own children died. He developed the concept of the importance of the movement of the spine. He established osteopathic medicine in 1874. The American School of Osteopathy in Kirksville, Missouri, awarded the first eighteen diplomas in March 1894.

According to a school statement, "Osteopathy is the knowledge of the structure, relation and function of each part of the human body applied to the adjustment or correction of whatever interferes with the harmonious operation of the same." George V. Webster, D.O. 1921.

William G. Sutherland, DO, developed cranial osteopathy. He developed the concept of the respiratory mechanism of the nervous system:

Five Phenomena of the Primary Respiratory Mechanism
1. The central nervous system (brain and spinal cord) has an inherent rhythmic motion.
2. The cerebrospinal fluid (CSF) fluctuates, or moves back and forth in a relatively closed container, the central nervous system.
3. The membranes in the head, called dura mater, surround the bones, comprise major veins in the head, and are essentially continuous with the brain. The dural membranes appear like three attached sickles, forming a "tripod" of support for the brain and the skull. They limit and control the slight motion in the bones of the head and the whole mechanism involving the cranium through the sacrum. The membranes surround the spinal cord like a large cylinder and are anchored firmly to the base of the skull and the sacrum, thus forming a core link between the two structures.
4. There are twenty-six bones in the head, and they are all in slight rhythmic motion along with the CNS, CSF, membranes, and sacrum. These bones all fit together like the gears of a watch and influence each other.
5. Since the dura mater is attached to the base of the skull and the sacrum (tailbone), as previously mentioned, the motion of the cranial mechanism is transmitted to the sacrum. The cranium and the sacrum work together as a unit.

Some credit Rollin Becker, DO, with the development of the concept of a craniosacral pump. Rollin E. Becker (1910–1996) grew up in an osteopathic household. His father, Arthur D. Becker, DO, was a prominent and respected osteopath, who served on the faculty with Dr. Andrew Taylor Still and later was dean of two osteopathic colleges. Rollin graduated from the American School of Osteopathy (later renamed the Kirksville College of Osteopathic Medicine) in 1934,

Rollin Becker, DO

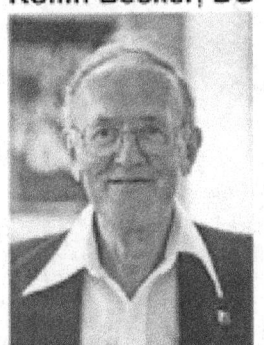

http://www.stillnesspress.com /doc/rollin_becker.htm

and following a few years in Oklahoma, he moved to Michigan, where he practiced for thirteen years.

In 1944, after about a decade in Michigan, he met William Garner Sutherland, DO, and in 1948, he first served on the teaching faculty at one of Dr. Sutherland's courses.

Dr. Becker moved to Texas in 1949, where he practiced until 1989. Throughout that time, he continued to serve Sutherland and his work. Becker was the president, from 1962 through 1979, of the Sutherland Cranial Teaching Foundation, an educational organization dedicated to perpetuating the teachings of W.G. Sutherland.

In the years following Sutherland's death in 1954, Becker played a crucial role in keeping his work alive. He went on to inspire generations of osteopathic teachers and students. http:// stillnesspress.com/doc/rollin_becker.htm

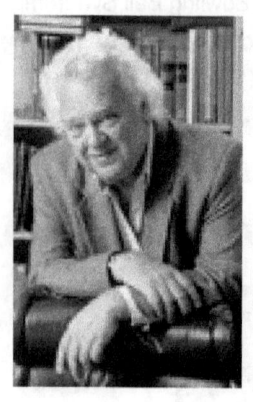

John Upledger, DO, a student of Sutherland and a contemporary of Becker, helped develop the science of craniosacral therapy in 1975. He also began studies that prove that the cranial bones move with the pulse of the nervous system. The studies listed below detail his research.

"Radiographic Evidence of Cranial Bone Mobility," Sheryl Lynn Oleski, BS, Gerald H. Smith, DDS, and William T. Crow, DO, *Cranio: The Journal of Craniomandibular Practice*; January 2002, V20N1, 34.

"Cranial Bone Movement," Heisey, R., and Adams, T., *Journal of the American Osteopathic Association.*

"Parietal Bone Mobility in the Anesthetized Cat," [see comments] Adams, T., Heisey, R.S., Smith, M.C., and Briner, B.J., *J Am Osteopath Assoc* (1992 May), 92(5): 599–600, 603–10, 615–22 ISSN: 0003-0287.

To quantify parietal bone motion in reference to the medial sagittal suture, a newly developed instrument was attached to the surgically exposed skull of anesthetized adult cats. The instrument differentiated between lateral and rotational parietal bone movements around the fulcrum of the suture. Bone movement was produced by external forces applied to the skull and by changes in intracranial pressure associated with induced hypercapnia, intravenous injections of norepinephrine, and controlled injections of artificial cerebrospinal fluid into the lateral cerebral ventricle. Responses varied considerably among test animals.

Generally, lateral head compression caused sagittal suture closure, small inward rotation of the parietal bones, increased intraventricular pressure, transient apnea, and unstable systemic arterial blood pressure. Graded increases in intracranial volume produced stepped increases in pressure, lateral expansion at the sagittal suture, and outward rotation of the parietal bones. We attribute variations in animal response largely to differences in intracranial and suture compliance among them. Cranial suture compliance may be an important factor in defining total cranial compliance.

Craniosacral Pump

**The Dura over the Sphenoid,
Down the Spine and to the Sacrum Forms the
CranioSacral Pump**

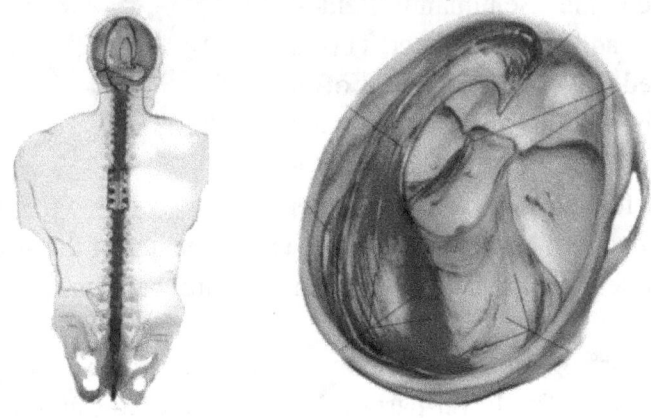

The dura attaches over the sphenoid, down the spine and to the sacrum. This forms a closed hydraulic system. There is a switch in the central joint (medial sagittal suture) that controls formation of cerebrospinal fluid. When the skull bones touch, the switch is on and fluid is deposited inside the dura. This causes the dural balloon to expand. Eventually this pulls the skull bones apart and the switch is opened. This discontinues the formation of cerebrospinal fluid.

Soon the cerebrospinal fluid leaks out of the dural balloon via the veins, and the dural balloon becomes smaller. This allows the skull bones to come back into contact. This reactivates the switch causing fluid to again be produced. This re-expands the dural balloon until again the bones separate causing the switch to open and fluid production to cease.

As this process continues, a vortex movement of fluid is formed inside the dural balloon moving cerebrospinal fluid and its nourishment around the brain and down the spinal cord.

Whenever fluid moves within a magnetic field, electrons are generated. For example, when a river runs downhill within the earth's magnetic field—called the Schumann field—electrons are added to the water. This is accompanied by the formation of a vortex in the middle of the river. Each of us has experienced walking in a stream and feeling the vortex of water 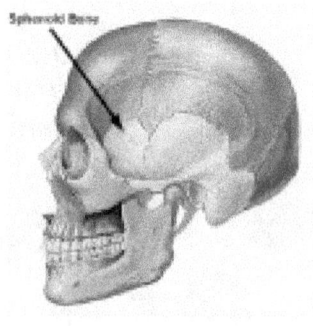 moving against our ankles as we approach the center of the stream. This same phenomenon happens within our dural balloon.

The upper part of the dural balloon is attached to the sphenoid bone of the skull. The lower part of the dural balloon is attached to the sacrum. When it pulses, it forms the craniosacral pump. As the sphenoid and sacrum move, the cerebrospinal fluid circulates through the brain and spinal cord.

When the sphenoid is de-centered and jammed, the pump stops. The nervous system must function with stagnant cerebrospinal fluid.

The

Robert Boyd, DO and Wife, Vera

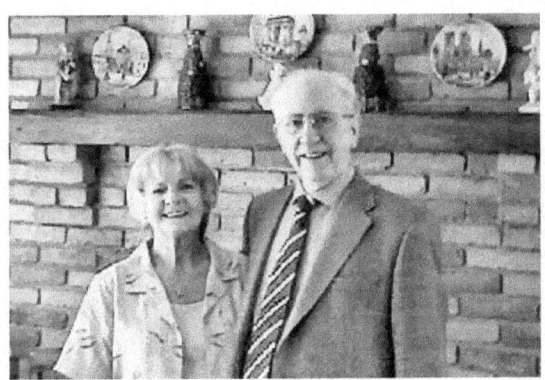

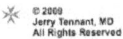
61

"Bowling Ball Syndrome" was described by Robert Boyd, DO, from Ireland. ("An Introduction to Bio-cranial Therapy," Bio-cranial Institute, Charlotte, N.C.) Boyd stated that the head weighs about the same as a bowling ball. Because it weighs so much, the body will always put the upper cervical vertebra under the center of gravity of the head to keep the head upright.

When the sphenoid bone (keystone) is moved, the other cranial bones follow. This moves the center of gravity of the skull causing the compensatory changes:
1. The two sides of the face are asymmetrical.
2. The jaw moves to one side causing TMJ
3. One eyelid is droopy (ptosis) and the opposite cheek is flattened
4. One ear canal is lower than the other
5. Obstruction of the ocular canal can increase intraocular pressure and decrease visual fields
6. Kinking of the Eustachian tubes can lead to increased ear infections
7. Sinus obstruction
8. Nasal obstruction

171

9. Snoring
10. C1-2 move to one side causing persistent headaches and neck aches
11. The entire spine is curved causing extrusion of disks
12. One shoulder is higher than the other making one arm seem short
13. One scapula is higher than the other giving pain in the interscapular area during driving and other use of the arms
14. The pelvis is rotated giving low back pain and disk extrusion
15. The rotated pelvis makes one leg relatively shorter than the other. This places more weight on one hip-knee-ankle making those joints wear out. The shift of weight to one side makes one clumsier.
16. The locking of the craniosacral pump causes the entire nervous system to use stagnant cerebrospinal fluid resulting in a general decrease in its function
17. Migraine headaches

Boyd described the "Bowling Ball Syndrome" in osteopathic terms. He developed a mechanical means of attempting to correct the Bowling Ball Syndrome that he called bio-cranial therapy. It involves placing one hand under the occiput and pinning the shoulder to the table. The head is moved in a certain arc to the maximum extension of the trapezius muscle and then a little farther. This pulls backward on the occipital bone. The occipital bone is attached to the sphenoid. This re-centers the sphenoid.

Trapezius Muscle

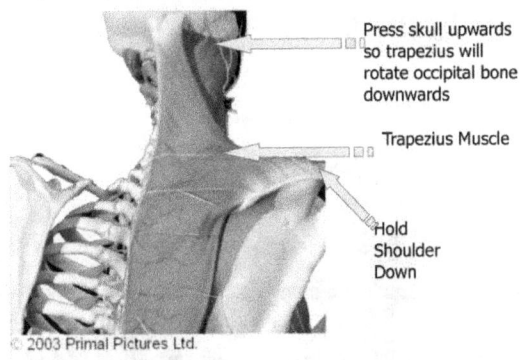

Press skull upwards so trapezius will rotate occipital bone downwards

Trapezius Muscle

Hold Shoulder Down

© 2003 Primal Pictures Ltd.

D e a n

NeuroCranial Restructuring

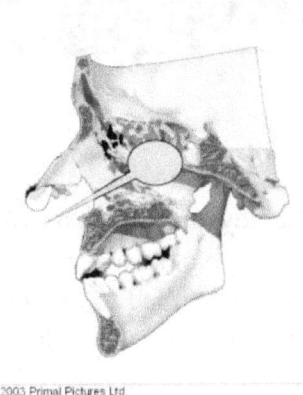

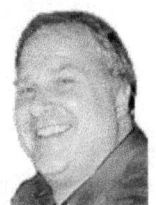

Dean Howell, ND teaches the placement of a balloon through the nostril and under the sphenoid to move it.

© 2003 Primal Pictures Ltd.

Howell of Seattle teaches placing a balloon through a nostril into the pharynx under the sphenoid. When the balloon is inflated quickly, it moves the sphenoid upward and re-centers it. He calls this neuro-cranial restructuring.

I was amazed by the results of correcting the Bowling Ball

173

Syndrome when it was demonstrated to me by Doug Hays, DC! As I began to consider how it worked, I found a different perspective than the one taught by Boyd.

Keystone

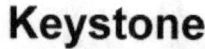

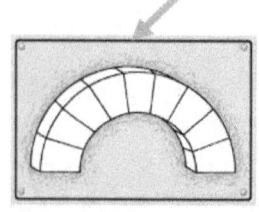

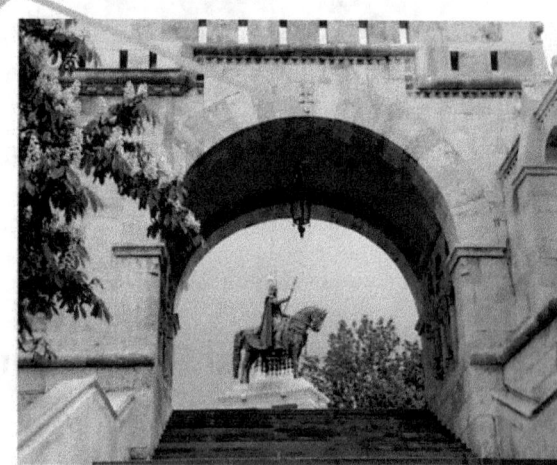

If one stacks up stones to form an arch, the piece inserted at the top of the arch is known as the keystone. The keystone, because of its shape, keeps the arch standing by causing the blocks in the arch to push against each other. When extra weight is applied to the top of the arch, the keystone helps to direct the force sideways through the other blocks.

Bowling Ball Syndrome

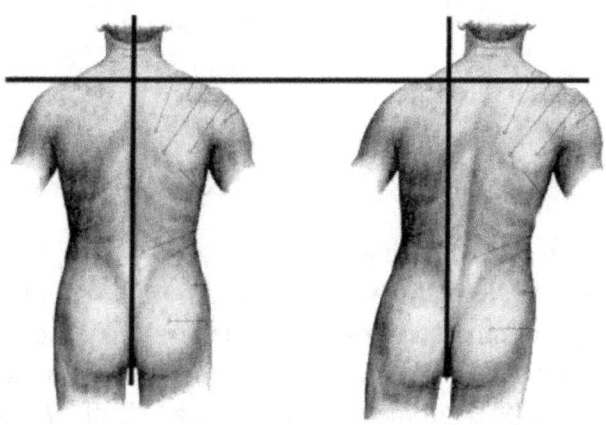

The sphenoid bone is the keystone for the skull. The other cranial bones rest on the sphenoid. The position of the sphenoid (keystone) dictates the position of all other skull bones. The sphenoid bone is often moved by trauma (birth trauma and accidents). Thus the position of the sphenoid bone dictates the center of gravity of the skull.

When it shifts, causing the other cranial bones to shift as well, it moves the center of gravity of the skull. This causes the brain to tell the neck, particularly the upper cervical vertebra, to move to get under the center of gravity of the skull so it won't fall over. This dictate from the brain changes the anatomical alignment of the whole body!

Alexander Revenko, MD, is a Russian neurologist involved with the SCENAR device. He described a technique using the SCENAR in acute settings to pulse the trapezius, calling it "Little Wings."

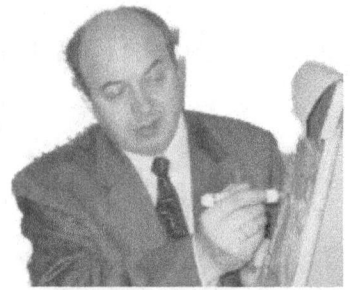

Alexander Revenko, MD

I described a technique using the SCENAR in default settings to create a strong contraction of the trapezius to simulate bio-cranial therapy. It is more complete and less painful than bio-cranial therapy. The technique involves placing the SCENAR in the same location as "Little Wings" on the side of the neck. The power is then increased until one gets an intense spasm of the trapezius for five seconds. This pulls intently on the occipital bone. Through its attachment to the sphenoid, the sphenoid is re-centered. This is performed on both sides of the neck to be certain the sphenoid is centered.

Autonomic "Reset Button"

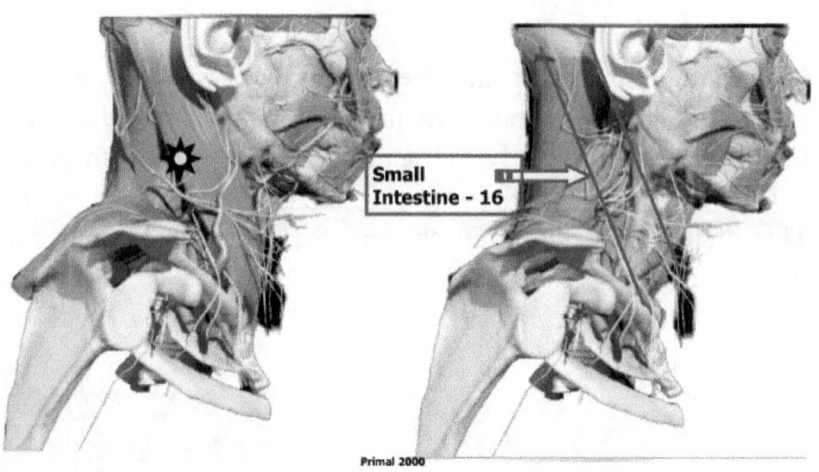

Small Intestine - 16

Primal 2000

The mechanical correction of the Bowling Ball Syndrome with the SCENAR is very annoying to the patient. I found that the same correction could be achieved energetically with the Tennant BioModulator®. This is done at a power setting that is not annoying to the patient using the mode called Infinity. It is the preferred method.

Immediately after correcting the Bowling Ball Syndrome with the Tennant BioModulator, the ears become level and the pelvic rotation is gone. It takes about 30 to 60 minutes for the cranial bones to completely re-center and the ptosis to disappear. It takes twenty-four hours for the shoulders to become even.

The craniosacral pump begins pumping immediately, but it often is irregular for about one hour. This can be tested by having the patient stand with eyes closed. Before correcting the Bowling Ball Syndrome, they will stand very still. After correction, they begin to sway back and forth about twelve times per minute.

In over ninety percent of the patients, the correction is complete and permanent unless another head trauma occurs. In those patients with low total body voltage, it slips back out and must be re-corrected.

Brain Waves and the Bowling Ball

The brain has four "gears" like an automobile:
1.   Delta = sleep
2.   Theta = not awake, not asleep
3.   Alpha = daydreaming
4.   Beta = thinking

Whenever the brain malfunctions (infection, trauma, metabolic), it produces excess second gear (theta waves) as an adaptive mechanism to help prevent seizures. This adaptive mechanism is both helpful (prevents seizures) and harmful (makes you function in second gear). (*National Head Injury Syllabus,* Head Injury Frontiers, Margaret Ayers, p. 380, 1987)

Most EEG devices apply Fourier mathematics to the data before it is presented. The Neuropathways EEG device developed by Margaret Ayers shows actual data 1/1,000 second after it occurs in the brain. Since you see the real data, you can see patterns of infection, closed head injury, open head injury, glucose metabolism insufficiency, and allergy. In addition, one can see the average voltage for each type of wave. Normal for theta and beta is two microvolts. (http://www.neuropathways.com/default.htm)

Nineteen patients were examined with the Neuropathways EEG device before and after correcting the Bowling Ball Syndrome electronically. The reduction of theta waves ranged from two percent to five percent with an average reduction of fifteen percent with one treatment.

Autonomic Nervous System

The autonomic nervous system consists of two parts, the sympathetic and parasympathetic systems. The sympathetic system is known as the "fight or flight" system and the parasympathetic system is known as the "eat, sleep, and heal" system.

Assume there is a deer in the forest. He thinks he hears a mountain lion. His sympathetic system turns on and his parasympathetic system turns off. As the sympathetic system activates, his pupils dilate, his ears stand erect, his bronchioles open wider, blood moves from his G.I. tract to his muscles effectively shutting down the digestive system, and his muscles are at attention while he figures out if he is going to be required to fight the lion or run away. As you can see, during sympathetic-on the things necessary to see better, hear better, move more air into and out of the lungs, and put all senses on high alert are affected. At the same time, the digestive system is shut down so its resources can be transferred to the muscles.

Now assume the lion does not show up. The sympathetic system turns down and the parasympathetic system turns back on. Pupils go back to normal size, ears lay down, the bronchioles relax, and the digestive system turns back on. The deer munches on some grass, takes a nap, and starts the healing process.

An important thing to notice is that the digestive system cannot work effectively while you are in sympathetic-on.

A significant difference between the deer and humans is that humans often get stuck in sympathetic-on. While in this mode, the digestive system doesn't function well, sleep is difficult, and healing cannot occur.

When you have the Bowling Ball Syndrome, you are stuck in sympathetic-on.

Almost everyone suffering from chronic illness has the Bowling Ball Syndrome. An amazing thing that happens when you correct it is that it balances the sympathetic and parasympathetic systems. Thus not only does the correction cause your posture and anatomical alignment to be corrected, it takes you out of sympathetic-on and balances your autonomic nervous system. This allows you to enter parasympathetic-on with the ability to have normal digestion, to sleep better, and to heal.

I know of no other therapy that will do this. The five-minute correction of the Bowling Ball Syndrome benefits patients more than any other therapy I know of. It is important that each patient with chronic disease be checked to see that their "bowling ball" has been corrected every day. It is easy for people to learn how to correct the Bowling Ball Syndrome for themselves using the Tennant BioModulator®.

179

5 Nutrition

The key to making chronic disease better is making a single cell work. If you give the body the things a single cell needs to work, the body often has the power to heal all of the cells of the body. That means you get well!

A cell is made up of a cell membrane and the inside, called the cytoplasm. The cell membrane is made of fats. It controls the cell and is consider the "brain" of the cell. That means you must have the proper fats to make those membranes. About twenty percent of your body is this fat, so if you weigh two hundred pounds, you need forty pounds of perfect fat to be healthy. Since cells replace themselves on an average of about eight weeks, you would need to absorb about five pounds of fat per week to stay healthy!

The cytoplasm of the cell is made up of proteins assembled from amino acids. There are eight amino acids that the body can't make (ten in children). Thus they are called essential amino acids. You must eat enough protein and have stomach acid to break the proteins into amino acids to fill this need.

To be used, proteins and fats need vitamins and minerals. To date, I have never seen a patient with a chronic disease that is not mineral deficient, and most are vitamin deficient as well.

Cells need the following to be healthy:

1. Water with voltage (alkaline water)
2. Fats to make cell membranes
3. Amino acids to make the cytoplasm (the "machinery") inside cells
4. Vitamins to allow the body to make the fats and proteins work

5.   Minerals to make the fats and proteins work, as on-off switches, and to keep your pH in the operating range
6.   Oxygen
7.   Sunshine
8.   Voltage is the same as pH. The body must have voltage to function (the same as saying you must have an alkaline pH). The body normally runs at pH of 7.35–7.45, which is the same as -20 to -25 mV.

The next important thing to recognize is the importance of your liver/gallbladder. The gallbladder is a storage tank for the bile made by the liver. It often becomes filled with sludge and doesn't function normally. This sludge becomes a breeding ground for all sorts of infections. They produce poisons called "neurotoxins" that make you sick. However, you need your gallbladder because the liver can't make bile fast enough to allow you to absorb the fat you need to keep healthy. The key is to clean it, not to remove it. (If you have already had it removed, you will need to take bile supplements the rest of your life.)

The liver is in charge of:
1.   Processing your digested food so that it can be used by the body to make new cells and to keep things working.

2.   Getting the toxic things out of your body.

3.   Controlling the immune system so you can keep infections under control.

If your liver is sick, you lose these processes resulting in chronic disease.

The liver contains 35,000 square meters (about the surface of seven football fields) of membrane surface used to accomplish these things. These membranes are made of fat. If you don't eat enough fat of the proper kind or if you eat fats that have been processed so they are similar to plastic, these membranes don't work correctly. (These "plastic fats" are called "partially hydrogenated" fats and canola oil.)

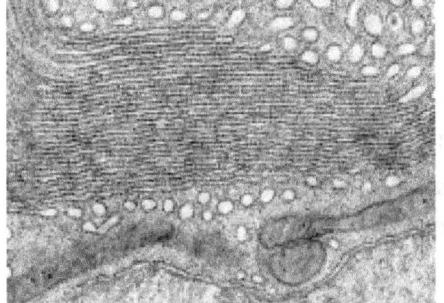

When the liver gets clogged up with debris because the membranes are made of plastic, it tries to "wash" itself with cholesterol. A high cholesterol level means your liver is trying to clean itself—much like you would try to clean the filter from your air conditioner—or that you have inadequate hormones (made from cholesterol) and the liver is trying to give you the raw materials to make them. If you interfere with that process with drugs and continue to give your body only plastic fats to repair itself, you are doomed to chronic diseases of all types.

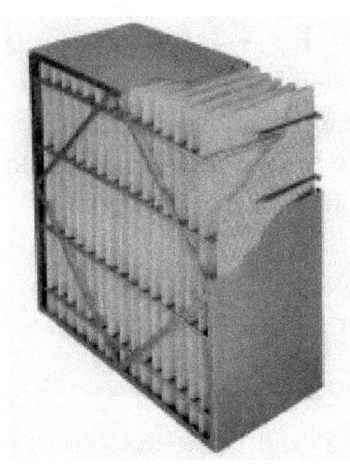

Once the liver cleans and repairs itself, the rest of the body can begin to heal. The liver will begin to supply the nutrients needed, begin to remove toxic chemicals (pesticides, pharmaceuticals, etc.), and turn on the immune system to get rid of infections. Thus your initial efforts should be to clean up and repair your liver/gall bladder. It normally takes eight to sixteen weeks for the liver to replace itself with all new cells.

Remember that the leading cause of death in the United States is reactions to pharmaceuticals. Just listen to the drug advertisements on TV and you will realize that all drugs have side effects. You should have the goal of getting off your drugs. However, do not do that without guidance. Stopping drugs suddenly often causes the body to have a bad reaction. The primary exception is anti-cholesterol drugs. You should stop them immediately. They are all liver toxic and prevent the liver from cleaning itself. Your cholesterol level will go to normal as you clean the liver, give it the fat it needs to repair itself, and correct your thyroid function.

To be healthy, you must stop eating anything that says "partially hydrogenated" or canola oil. You will have to stop eating fried foods and cheese in restaurants because these almost always are made of partially hydrogenated oils. In addition, you must stop using all forms of artificial sweeteners such as aspartame, Splenda, saccharine, xylitol, and others ending in "–ol." All of these are severe neurotoxins that the body doesn't know how to get rid of. Stop MSG as it is also a neurotoxin. Stop smoking. Stop eating soy. Stop drinking coffee, tea (green tea is okay), and alcohol.

Eat lots of raw milk, butter, and eggs. If they make you nauseated, that means your liver isn't making enough bile to absorb them. You will need to take ox bile and digestive enzymes with each meal until your liver can make bile on its own. You will be able to eat fats without trouble when you get your liver working again.

Eat things that don't have the toxins listed above. Try to vary your diet, with one-third protein, one-third fat, and one-third carbohydrates with the carbs from fruits and vegetables.

Let's assume that you have bought an old house that hasn't been lived in for several years. However, you love that old house and want to return it to its former glory. You dream of living in that wonderful house and of all the fun you will have in it.

Well—your body is that house.

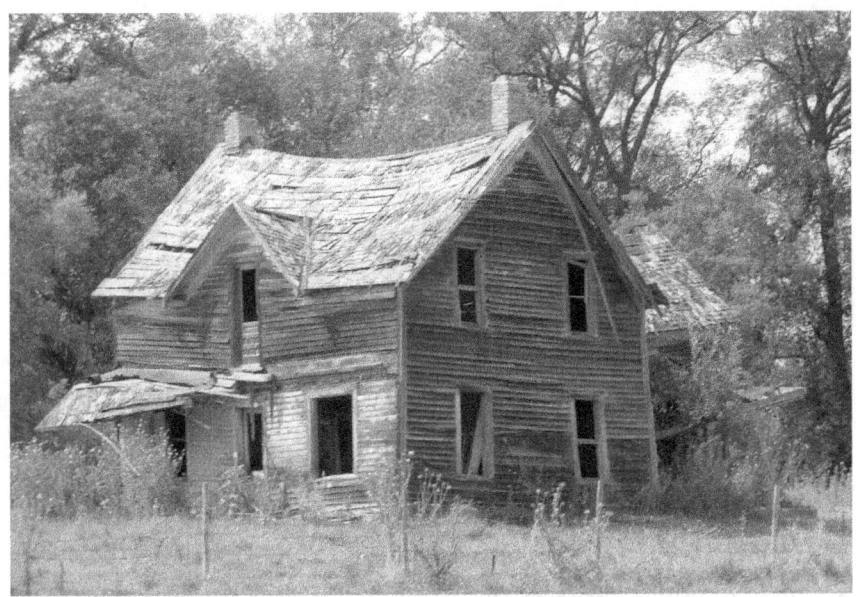

Now you have to start the process of returning it to normal. It won't happen overnight, and there are no miracle pills to make it normal. In fact, medications are simply paint. If you paint over a board eaten by termites, you may not see the holes in the board for a while, but they are still there and the rotting goes on. Medications cover up the symptoms, but the degeneration in your body continues. If you have arthritis and you take medication, the degeneration in your joints continues. You just don't feel the pain while the joints continue to rot.

So now you own the old house. What must be done before you can move in? First you will want to restore the utilities. You will need water, sewage, and electricity.

So let's get started!

Water

The body is about seventy percent to eighty percent water. Thus it is the basis of who you are and how healthy you are. Unfortunately, you have probably been led to believe that drinking things containing water is the same as drinking water—not so! When things are put into water to make the water some other drink, it changes how the water reacts in the body. If you take good water from a well or an uncontaminated stream, it will be alkaline (finding good water anywhere in the world is getting harder because of chemical contaminations). That means it contains electrons available for your body to use in its metabolism. However, if you put chlorine and/or fluoride in it, it becomes acidic. Anything that is acidic is an electron stealer. Anything that is alkaline is an electron donor.

Drinking acidic water steals electrons from your cells and damages them. Drinking water that has been made into carbonated beverages is drinking acid that is so concentrated you can use it to clean the grease off your engine or clean out your toilet! Can that possibly be good for you?

Your cells are composed of water, but it is also what your body uses to wash itself internally to clean away the garbage that gets in. Would you wash your car with coffee? Then consider washing the inside of your body with coffee or tea or sodas.

In addition, zinc is one of the most important elements in the body. Without zinc, you can't make stomach acid. Without stomach acid, you can't digest your food. Without nutrition, the body can't repair itself. In addition, without zinc, you can't make neurochemicals like serotonin, dopamine, norepinephrine, and epinephrine.

Zinc is blocked by alcohol, coffee, and tea. (Alcohol also blocks selenium.) Trying to get your fluids by drinking these substances will almost guarantee that you will become depressed. Is it any wonder so much of our population is depressed?

Many think it is healthy to drink distilled water; it is not. Distilled water pulls minerals out of your cells and into the water. You can kill yourself drinking distilled water. For example, if you put one drop of distilled water inside an eye, the cornea immediately becomes opaque and the cells inside the eye are killed as the minerals are pulled out of them.

Another problem is bottled water. Bottled water is almost always city water that has been put through a filter. It is perhaps cleaner than city water, but it is still acidic and contains many other chemicals. Many cities have tap water that has toxic levels of copper. Copper is also a zinc antagonist.

There is a problem with water bottles. The safest as far as contamination of your water is glass. However, glass has the problem of breakage.

Most water bottles are plastic. If you look on the bottom of bottled water you buy most places, you will see a triangle that contains the number one. That number relates to the kind of plastic used to manufacture the bottle. A number one usually relates 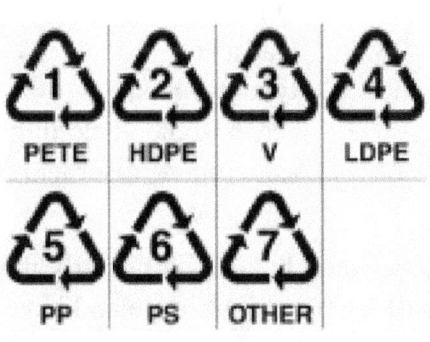 to a clear plastic that is not totally polymerized. If you leave such a bottle in the sun, the polymers from the bottle will enter the water and poison it. You probably have noticed that bottled water left in the sun tastes like plastic. What most of us didn't realize is that plastic acts like estrogen in our bodies causing hormonal imbalances and blocking zinc.

Estrogen unopposed by progesterone blocks zinc, magnesium, and vitamin B6 and leads to:

1. Increases in heart attacks and strokes
2. Aging
3. Anxiety
4. Allergies
5. Asthma
6. Breast cancer
7. Cervical cancer
8. Cold hands and feet
9. Decreased sex drive
10. Dry eyes
11. Endometriosis
12. Fat gain around hips
13. Fatigue
14. Fibrocystic breasts
15. Foggy thinking
16. Gall bladder disease
17. Hair loss
18. Headaches
19. Hypoglycemia
20. Increased blood clotting
21. Autoimmune disorders

Some water bottles, particularly those known as sports bottles, are made from polycarbonate and have a number seven on the bottom of the bottle. They contain bisphenol A. Suspected of being hazardous to humans since the 1930s, concerns about the use of bisphenol A in consumer products were regularly reported in the news media in 2008 after several governments issued reports questioning its safety, and some

retailers have removed products containing it from their shelves.

A 2010 report from the FDA raised further concerns regarding exposure of fetuses, infants, and young children. A 2008 report by the U.S. National Toxicology Program expressed "some concern for effects on the brain, behavior, and prostate gland in fetuses, infants, and children at current human exposures to bisphenol A," and "minimal concern for effects on the mammary gland and an earlier age for puberty for females in fetuses, infants, and children at current human exposures to bisphenol A.

A 2008 review has concluded that obesity may be increased as a function of BPA exposure, which "merits concern among scientists and public health officials." [30] A 2009 review of available studies has concluded that "perinatal BPA exposure acts to exert persistent effects on body weight and adiposity." Another 2009 review has concluded that "Eliminating exposures to (BPA) and improving nutrition during development offer the potential for reducing obesity and associated diseases." Other reviews have cited similar conclusions.

A 2007 review concluded that BPA, like other xenoestrogens, should be considered as a player within the nervous system that can regulate or alter its functions through multiple pathways.

A 2007 review concluded that bisphenol-A has been shown to bind to the thyroid hormone receptor and perhaps have selective effects on its functions.

A 2009 review about environmental chemicals and thyroid function raised concerns about BPA effects on triiodothyronine and concluded that "available evidence suggests that governing agencies need to regulate the use of thyroid-disrupting chemicals, particularly as such uses relate exposures of pregnant women, neonates and small children to the agents."

A 2009 review summarized BPA adverse effects on thyroid hormone action.

In 2007 and before, I had recommended the use of water bottles with the number seven on the bottom. I can no longer support that recommendation with the current studies that show the damage from bisphenol A.

It seems that the best choice for a bottle to carry water in is stainless steel.

My recommendation is that you avoid drinking anything but water. If you must drink something else, know that it is toxic to your system and be prepared for the consequences.

When people are sick, they often have decreased minerals in their bodies. Drinking water dilutes the minerals even more, leading to reduction in the voltage and making them feel worse. The answer is to restore the minerals and voltage, which allows you to drink the necessary amount of water.

Sometimes I see doctors tell their patients to drink less water because some lab test shows they have too little of something in their blood such as sodium. If you dehydrate the patient, the lab test will come back to normal but the patient feels worse. Let's assume you have two glasses of tea each containing eight ounces. One is very dark and the other is very light. If I put the light-colored one out in the sun and let some of the water evaporate, soon both glasses of tea will be the same color. If I ran a lab test on both glasses, the test might show a "normal" amount of tea in each; however, there might not be enough volume left in the dehydrated glass to do much with.

If we do that to patients, we cause their blood pressure to be too low or the inside of the cells to become too thick to function. We must correct lab results by looking at total body water, intracellular water, and extra-cellular water. Then we know if the patient has too much or too little water or too much or too little "stuff" in the water. One can tell that using a device called the Bioelectrical Impedance Analysis device.

Knowing how much water to drink is always challenging. The only sure way to know is to measure with the BIA device shown here. However, a good rule of thumb is to drink water every time you feel hungry. If you still feel hungry a few minutes after drinking, then eat. The sense of hunger is often the signal the body really wants more water.

Biological Impedance Analysis (BIA)

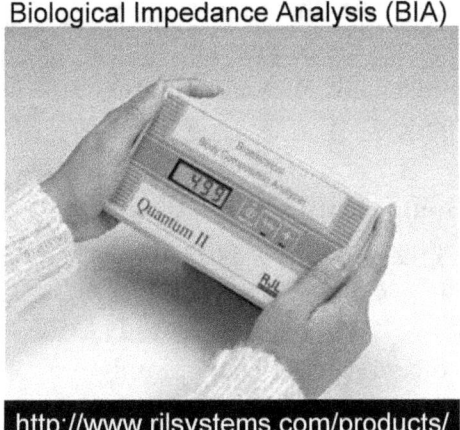

http://www.rjlsystems.com/products/

It is increasingly difficult to get good water. Our city water is an electron stealer because it contains chlorine and because it contains the treacherous fluoride, one of the worst toxins on the planet! It also contains all sorts of pharmaceuticals. Every time someone takes a medication and urinates into the toilet, some of that medication ends up in your city drinking water. It is not clear whether filters will remove these medications. It is clear that unfiltered city water contains medications that you didn't know you were drinking.

The best water system I have found is manufactured by pH-Prescription. The water tests superior to the popular ionic water devices and even removes fluoride. In addition, it is much less expensive than most other units. One can get tabletop, under sink, or whole-house models.

Some critics say that eating/drinking food/water that contains electrons has no effect on total body voltage (pH). They simply don't understand gastrointestinal physiology.

When food or water is placed into the stomach, the stomach must go to a pH of 2.0 (+280 millivolts). It does this by inserting HCl. It accomplishes this with the chemical reaction $NaCl + H2O + CO2 = HCl + NaHCO3$. This reaction requires iodine and zinc as well as vitamin B1. Note that when the stomach makes stomach acid, it inserts sodium bicarbonate (NaHCO3) into the bloodstream.

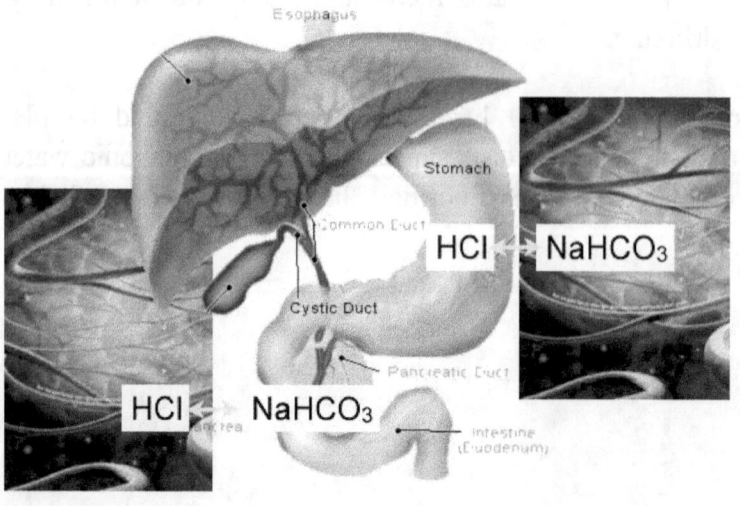

The amount of bicarbonate injected into the blood is dictated by the amount of HCl needed to achieve a pH of 2.0 (+280 millivolts). The bicarbonate is a buffer—it doesn't change the voltage of the blood but does change its ability to absorb electron stealers.

If the food/water that is consumed is alkaline, it will require more HCl to bring the pH of the stomach down to 2.0, and thus there will be more bicarbonate injected into the blood.

If the food/water that is consumed is acidic, less HCl will be required to bring the stomach to pH 2.0, and thus less bicarbonate will be injected into the blood.

This explains why eating/drinking food/water that contains electrons affects the blood. The fact that the stomach acid neutralized alkaline water does not invalidate alkaline water's benefits—it just means that more HCl will be required to bring the stomach acid to pH 2.0, and thus the blood contains more buffer.

Not having or making stomach acid has consequences. Let's say you drink a carbonated beverage. A Coca Cola has a pH of 2.5. Thus very little HCl is manufactured to bring the stomach to 2.0. Now it arrives at the small intestine. It must be alkalized since the small intestine is not able to cope with this acid. The pancreas makes sodium bicarbonate to neutralize the stomach acid. It does it by the same formula as the stomach uses, only in reverse. As it puts bicarbonate into the small intestine, it puts HCl into the blood.

If the stomach was stimulated to put bicarbonate into the blood when it made HCl, it can now be used to neutralize this HCl inserted by the pancreas. But in the cola example, no bicarbonate was injected into the blood by the stomach so there is less buffer available to deal with the HCl injected into the blood by the pancreas' need to neutralize the stomach acid it receives. Thus the total body voltage is decreased by drinking the cola.

Remember that the ability to make HCl and bicarbonate requires iodine, zinc, and vitamin B1.

So in our old house analogy, you will begin by washing out the debris inside and outside your house.

Minerals

Minerals play an important role in the body. If you think about the battery in your car, you know that if you put distilled water in it, it won't hold a charge. So it is with your body. In addition, minerals act as on-off switches in the body. This is particularly true of calcium and magnesium.

For example, to contract a muscle, calcium is necessary. To relax the muscle, magnesium is necessary. Calcium turns things on and magnesium turns things off. If you run out of one of them, you get stuck in either on or off.

Minerals and vitamins are also important in manufacturing things you need. An example is neurochemicals. To make serotonin from the protein L-tryptophan, you must have:

1. Folate
2. Calcium
3. Iron
4. Vitamin B3
5. Zinc
6. Vitamin B6
7. Magnesium
8. Vitamin C

To make dopamine and norepinephrine from the amino acid L-phenylalanine, one needs the following:

1. Folate
2. Iron
3. Zinc
4. Magnesium
5. Copper
6. Vitamin B3
7. Vitamin B6
8. Vitamin C

If you don't have calcium, magnesium, zinc, iron, copper, and the necessary vitamins, you can't make serotonin. If you don't have serotonin, you will become depressed.

The other problem is that the minerals need to be balanced. If you simply take a lot of the above minerals, you may be so out of balance that things don't work correctly.

The easiest way to tell if you need a particular mineral is to taste that mineral in solution. You will need to purchase this mineral testing/treatment kit. A mineral is dropped onto your tongue. If it tastes like water or sweet, you are deficient in it. If it tastes metallic or bitter, you don't need it. Place the ones that don't taste really bad in your morning juice. Recheck every week until each mineral deficiency is corrected. When one of the minerals starts 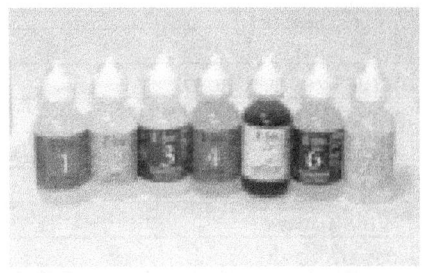 tasting really bad, you don't need any more.

Recheck your mineral level at least once every three to four months. Because our soils are so depleted of minerals, you will need to replace them periodically.

Some of the most commonly consumed water substitutes are coffee, black tea, and alcohol. All three block zinc, and alcohol

Alcohol intolerance	Zinc (30)
Asthma	Zinc (30)
Belching	Zinc (30)
Bloating	Zinc (30)
Boils	Zinc (30)
Brittle nails	Zinc (30)
Bronchitis	Zinc (30)
Colds	Zinc (30)
Conjunctivitis	Zinc (30)
Delayed healing	Zinc (30)
Depression	Zinc (30)
Dermatitis	Zinc (30)
Disrupted sleep	Zinc (30)
Dry skin	Zinc (30)
Ear infections	Zinc (30)
Early graying hair	Zinc (30)
Eczema	Zinc (30)
Fidgeting	Zinc (30)
Frequent sore throats	Zinc (30)
Gastric-esophageal reflux disease (GERD)	Zinc (30)
Gastroenteritis	Zinc (30)
Hair loss	Zinc (30)
Hay fever	Zinc (30)
Hyperactivity	Zinc (30)
Increased cholesterol	Zinc (30)
Infertility	Zinc (30)
Itchy skin	Zinc (30)
Joint pain	Zinc (30)
Joint stiffness	Zinc (30)
Loss of libido	Zinc (30)
Low blood sugar (hypoglycemic)	Zinc (30)
Low white blood cell count	Zinc (30)
Lung infections	Zinc (30)
Missed periods	Zinc (30)
Moodiness	Zinc (30)
Pimples	Zinc (30)
Pneumonia	Zinc (30)
Poor coping with stress	Zinc (30)

Poor memory	Zinc (30)
Pre-dinner tantrums	Zinc (30)
Prolonged infections	Zinc (30)
Psoriasis	Zinc (30)
Runny nose	Zinc (30)
Sinusitis	Zinc (30)
Stomach ulcers	Zinc (30)
Stretch marks	Zinc (30)
Temper outbursts	Zinc (30)
Thrush (mouth fungus)	Zinc (30)
Tinea (athlete's foot)	Zinc (30)
Warts	Zinc (30)
Arthritis	Selenium (34)
Asthma	Selenium (34)
Autoimmune diseases	Selenium (34)
Cancer	Selenium (34)
Cardiomyopathy	Selenium (34)
Depression	Selenium (34)
Diabetes	Selenium (34)
Heart disease	Selenium (34)
Hypothyroid	Selenium (34)
Increased cholesterol	Selenium (34)
Increased infections	Selenium (34)

blocks selenium. Look at the symptoms caused by a deficiency of these minerals:

Note: Zinc has an atomic number of 30 and selenium 34.

Because they prevent the absorption of zinc, drinking coffee, tea (except green tea), and/or alcohol make you susceptible to the misery of all of these things causing everything from athlete's foot to cancer! Now doesn't drinking water make more sense?

It is also important to remember that taking antacids or drugs that block stomach acid production causes you to be deficient in zinc. This makes you susceptible to all of the above things noted with zinc deficiency.

pH and Calcium

pH stands for "potential hydrogen." It is a way of talking about the amount of acid and base in our bodies. It is also a way of talking about the amount of voltage in our bodies.

pH is measured on a logarithmic scale where 0 is the most acidic and 14 is the most alkaline. Seven (7) is considered neutral.

Water ($H2O$) ionizes into hydrogen (H+) and hydroxyl (OH-) ions. When these ions are in equal proportions, the pH is a neutral 7. When there are more H+ ions than OH- ions then the water is said to be "acid." If OH- ions outnumber the H+ ions then the water is said to be "alkaline." The pH scale goes from 0 to 14 and is logarithmic, which means that each step is ten times the previous. In other words, a pH of 4.5 is ten times more acid than 5.5, one hundred times more acid than 6.5, and one thousand times more acid than 7.5.

pH is also a measure of voltage. A pH of 0 is the same as +400 mVolts. A pH of 14 is the same as -400 mVolts. Cells normally operate at a pH of 7.35 to 7.45 or -20 to -25 mVolts.

pH	0	7	14
Voltage	+400 mV	0 mV	-400 mV

Chronic disease and pain are always associated with an acidic pH, which is the same as saying that chronic disease and pain are always associated with a loss of voltage. Health is associated with the presence of voltage, which is the same as saying that healthy people have an alkaline pH.

In the body, being able to hold a charge of voltage is associated with minerals in general and calcium in particular.

When you begin your day, you "turn on the body machinery." This creates a by-product of carbonic acid. This acid must be eliminated from the body or the body loses its charge (becomes acidic). This is accomplished partly by having the carbonic acid dissociate into carbon dioxide and water. The carbon dioxide is breathed out through the lungs. However, one cannot breathe fast enough to get rid of all the carbon dioxide that needs to be eliminated, so some of it is removed by combining with ammonia from the liver and intestine to form urea nitrogen, which is then eliminated through the kidneys.

Daytime is a time of running the "machinery" and creating acids. Nighttime is a time of replacing worn-out cells and eliminating the acids created through the day that you didn't get rid of through the day.

Measurement of the salivary pH gives you an indirect indication of cellular voltage. You can think of it as how much voltage is stored in your cellular batteries. It should never be lower than 6.5. Note that the saliva pH of 6.5 suggests a cellular pH of 7.35 so there is a conversion factor of about 0.8.

Measurement of the urinary pH gives you an indication of the voltage of the extracellular and lymphatic spaces. It should also be about 6.5 after you get rid of your first morning urine. (The first morning urine represents the acid you got rid of during the night.) However, if your daytime urine pH is less than 6.5, you are dumping more acid because your extracellular space has become too acidic.

pH Color Match Guide for 5.0 to 9.0 pH Values

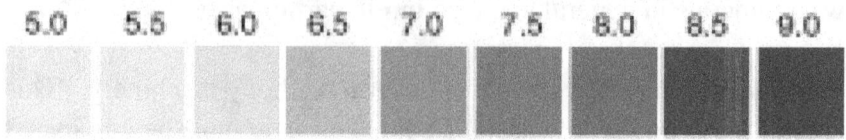

You need to be 6.5 or above once per day.

To be accurate, your salivary pH must be tested either the first thing when you wake up before you drink any water or two hours after a meal. Test it with pH strips. The graphic is printed in black and white so you don't see the colors. However, 5.0 is a tan color and 9.0 is purple. Basically the gray, blue, and purple colors are alkaline whereas the yellows and browns are acidic.

Sometimes it is difficult to decide which color is the correct one on the strip. If you want to have a more accurate way to measure pH, meters are available for about $100.

If your urine or your salivary pH falls below 6.5, you need more calcium!

Age	Male (mg.)	Female (mg.)	Pregnant (mg.)	Lactating (mg.)
Birth to 6 months	210	210		
7-12 months	270	270		
1-3 years	500	500		
4-8 years	800	800		
9-13 years	1300	1300		
14-18 years	1300	1300	1300	1300

19-50 years	1000	1000	1000	1000
>50 years	1200	1200		

This is the recommended daily intake of calcium
if you have a normal total body voltage (pH).

There are two main forms of calcium available as supplements, calcium carbonate and calcium citrate. Usually calcium carbonate is less expensive. Usually they are equally absorbed, but those with reduced stomach acid can absorb citrate better than carbonate. Carbonate is absorbed best when taken with food; citrate is absorbed equally well on an empty stomach or with food.

The amount of actual elemental calcium varies. Carbonate is forty percent calcium by weight while citrate is twenty-one percent calcium. The amount you absorb is decreased as you take more. The best absorption is when you take about 500 mg at a time, so it is better to split your doses if you take more than 500 mg/day.

Other forms that can be found are gluconate, lactate, and phosphate. Coral calcium is about one-fifth calcium carbonate. For example, 565 mg of coral calcium would contain about 110 mg of calcium carbonate.

Note that this recommendation has you taking some calcium even if your pH is above 6.5. This is advantageous if you are dealing with serious illness because microorganisms can't grow in an alkaline pH. Cancer cells have trouble growing with alkaline pH as well.

The normal human cell has a lot of molecular oxygen and a slightly alkaline pH. The cancer cell has an acid pH and lack of oxygen. Cancer cells cannot survive in an oxygen-rich environment. At a pH slightly above 7.4 (salivary pH 6.7) cancer cells become dormant, and at pH 8.5 (salivary pH 7.8) cancer cells will die while healthy cells will live. Again, the higher the pH reading, the more alkaline and oxygen rich the fluid is. Cancer and all diseases hate oxygen / pH balance. http://home.bluegrass.net/~jclark/coral_calcium.htm

Neurochemicals and Plankton

There are two basic theories of how to get people with chronic disease well and keep them that way. One is that we must find a drug that will substitute for a broken "gear" in the body or to repair the "gears" mechanically (surgery). The other is to give the body the things it needs to manufacture new cells and let it heal itself.

For those wishing to support the latter theory, it has been difficult to determine what is actually needed to make new cells. People are always saying things like they have a new herb from Africa or a fruit from China that will magically heal everything. Such findings are often useful for some but not predictable for most. My feeling has always been that our Heavenly Father would not design a body that requires unusual potions from far-away places to make us healthy.

My practice is one of "Integrative Medicine," where we see primarily people who have been sick for years and who "have tried it all." I personally suffered from viral encephalitis and a bleeding disorder that kept me incapacitated for seven years. What I have come to appreciate is that one must provide the raw materials for the body to make new cells. If one does that, even severely and chronically ill patients can heal. So what are those raw materials?

1. Water: The body is about 75% water. It needs to be clean water that is alkaline (contains voltage).
2. Fat: Every cell membrane in the body is made of two layers of fats called phospholipids.
3. Proteins: Every cell in the body contains "machinery" made up of proteins that do the work of the cell.

4. Carbohydrates: Needed primarily to provide vitamins and minerals.
5. Vitamins: To use the fats and proteins, cells need vitamins.
6. Minerals: To use the fats and proteins, cells need minerals. Minerals are also used by the body as "on-off" switches.
7. Voltage: Voltage is stored in the cell membrane of every cell to give cells the energy to work.
8. Oxygen
9. Sunshine
10. Gravity

There are very few products that provide all or even most of the raw materials needed to make new cells and sustain the existing ones. The problem is that we need all of them at the same time for things to work. For example, a protein called tryptophan is needed to make the brain chemical called serotonin. However, it takes eight vitamins and minerals for this to work. If you are missing one of them, e.g., zinc, you can't make serotonin. You may get a few of the things you need to be healthy from a product you are taking this month and a few from the product you take next month, but neither works because you didn't get them all at the same time!

One of those rare products that contains almost everything you need for life (and the rebuilding of a healthy life) is phytoplankton. It contains the ten amino acids that the body cannot make and must be consumed in our diet (essential amino acids). The essential fatty acids are also present (omega 3 and omega 6). Vitamins A (beta-carotene), B1 (thiamine), B2 (riboflavin), B3 (niacin), B5 (pantothenic acid), B6 (pyridoxine), B12 (cobalamin), C, and D (tocopherol), and major and trace minerals are all present in phytoplankton.

In short, it contains almost everything needed to sustain life. Therefore, it contains almost everything needed to restore health by providing the raw materials to make new cells that function normally. This is particularly true if we stop putting toxic materials such as artificial sweeteners and trans fats (partially hydrogenated fats) into our bodies. It is exciting to find something that seems to contain most of the things necessary to get well and stay well. It is likely that phytoplankton will change the way we think about health.

I have also found that one can replace neurochemicals with phytoplankton even when the liver is too sick to allow the person to take products with just the amino acids and vitamins/minerals necessary to make them.

Plankton works, in part, because of it contains humic and fulvic acids. The source of these substances for ocean creatures is plankton. The source of these substances for land-based creatures is supposed to be plants grown on soil that contains decayed animal and plant products. Unfortunately, our farming practices have depleted the soil of humic and fulvic. Please read the chapter devoted to this subject.

Blood Pressure

Blood pressure is related to water. Any fluid system needs…fluids! Having a normal pressure inside your vascular system is key to feeling well. The upper number of your blood pressure is called "systolic." It is a measure of the highest pressure in your system. It is the result of the heart contracting and pushing blood into the vessels. It should be between 120 and 140.

The second number is called "diastolic" pressure. It is a measure of the lowest pressure in the system and is the pressure present when the heart is between beats and is refilling itself with blood for the next pulse. It is the most important number because a persistently high pressure can damage the vessels. It should be between 80 and 90.

Some studies have shown that the most important number is the pulse pressure. That is the difference between the systolic and diastolic pressure. For example, if your blood pressure is 150/100, your pulse pressure is 50.

As you will see when we discuss heart disease and cholesterol, whatever over-expands the artery is what damages it and causes heart disease. Obviously excess pressure is what over-expands the arteries.

It is often said that blood pressure cannot be too low unless you have symptoms. That is not true. If the blood pressure is too low, you will not have enough pressure to get enough blood to your brain and you will have symptoms of chronic fatigue. When the diastolic pressure is below 80, you will often have symptoms.

Blood pressure is much like tire pressure for your car. "Cold" pressure is the pressure in your tires when the car has not been moving. It is the minimum operating pressure to make your tires work correctly. When the tires start rolling, the heat created increases the pressure in them. This is called the "hot" pressure. It is the maximum pressure experienced by the tires. If that is too high, it will damage the tire walls.

Think of systolic blood pressure as "hot" pressure and diastolic blood pressure as "cold" pressure. Your tires are designed to operate within these ranges. Too high or too low means the tires will not function correctly. So it is with blood pressure.

A major recommendation from the National Institutes of Health was published in May 2003. The National High Blood Pressure Education Program is coordinated by the National Heart, Lung, and Blood Institute (NHLBI) at the National Institutes of Health. Copies of the JNC 7 report are available on the NHLBI website at http://www.nhlbi.nih.gov or from the NHLBI Health Information Center, P.O. Box 30105, Bethesda, MD 20824-0105; Phone: 301-592-8573 or 240-629-3255 (TTY); Fax: 301-592-8563.

Blood Pressure Classification	Systolic BP	Diastolic BP
Normal	<120	and <80
Pre-Hypertension	120-139	or 80-89
Stage 1 Hypertension	140-159	or 90-99
Stage 2 Hypertension	>160	or >100

Published Abstract:

The purpose of the Seventh Report of the Joint Evaluation, and Treatment of High Blood Pressure (JNC 7) is to provide an evidence-based approach to the prevention and management of hypertension. The key messages of this report are these:

1. In those older than age 50, systolic blood pressure (BP) of greater than 140 mm mercury is a more important cardiovascular disease (CVD) risk factor than diastolic BP.
2. Beginning at 115/75 mm mercury, CVD risk doubles for each increment of 20/10 mm mercury.
3. Those who are normotensive at 55 years of age will have a 90% lifetime risk of developing hypertension.
4. Pre-hypertensive individuals (systolic BP 120-139 mm mercury or diastolic BP 80-89 mm mercury) require health-promoting lifestyle modifications to prevent the progressive rise in blood pressure and CVD.
5. For uncomplicated hypertension, thiazide diuretic should be used in drug treatment for most, either alone or combined with drugs from other classes.
6. This report delineates specific high-risk conditions that are compelling indications for the use of other antihypertensive drug classes (angiotensin-converting enzyme inhibitors, angiotensin-receptor blockers, beta-blockers, calcium channel blockers).

7. Two or more antihypertensive medications will be required to achieve goal BP (<140/90 mm mercury, or <130/80 mm mercury) for patients with diabetes and chronic kidney disease.

8. For patients whose BP is more than 20 mm mercury above the systolic BP goal or more than 10 mm mercury above the diastolic BP goal, initiation of therapy using two agents, one of which usually will be a thiazide diuretic, should be considered.

9. Regardless of therapy or care, hypertension will be controlled only if patients are motivated to stay on their treatment plan.

"Because of the new data on lifetime risk of hypertension and the impressive increase in the risk of cardiovascular complications associated with levels of BP previously considered to be normal, the JNC 7 report has introduced a new classification that includes the term 'pre-hypertension' for those with blood pressures ranging from 120-139 mmHg systolic and/or 80-89 mmHg diastolic. This new designation is intended to identify those individuals in whom early intervention by adoption of healthy lifestyles could reduce BP, decrease the rate of progression of BP to hypertensive levels with age, or prevent hypertension entirely.

Figure 11. Impact of high normal blood pressure on the risk of cardiovascular disease

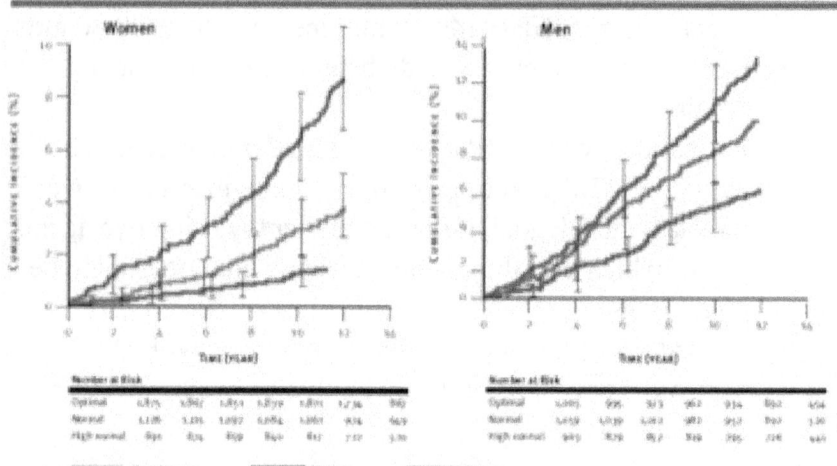

Cumulative incidence of cardiovascular events in women (panel A) and men (panel B) without hypertension, according to blood pressure category at the base-line examination.

Vertical bars indicate 95% confidence intervals. Optimal BP is defined here as a systolic pressure of <120 mmHg and a diastolic pressure of <80 mmHg. Normal BP is a systolic pressure of 120-129 mmHg or a diastolic pressure of 80-84 mmHg. High-normal BP is a systolic pressure of 130-139 mmHg or a diastolic pressure of 85-89 mmHg. If the systolic and diastolic pressure readings for a subject were in different categories, the higher of the two categories was used."

The recommendations from the Committee on Prevention and Treatment of High Blood Pressure are:

1. Treat to a BP of <140/90 unless you have diabetes or chronic kidney disease. In that case, treat to <130/80.
2. For those with BP from 120/80 to 140/90, start behavior modifications for dietary choices, exercise, stop smoking, etc.

3. For those over 140/90 (or diabetics or kidney disease with >130/80), start with a diazide diuretic as first choice medication.
4. Add additional medications as needed to reach goal BP.

Since most physicians have to see so many patients per day, it has been my experience that many skip step one of behavior modification and often start drug therapy in all patients whose blood pressure is >120/80. Also, they often choose drugs other than diuretics as the beginning medication. It has been my experience that many people with diastolic pressures <80 will have mental fog and/or dizziness because there isn't enough pressure to get adequate blood to the brain.

Several of my family members have been treated this way. When they report the symptoms to their physicians, they are told to keep taking the medications. This is the common practice of physicians treating lab results and not the patient. If a patient can't work because you have lowered their blood pressure too low, you haven't really served the patient.

I find that most patients will have a normal blood pressure in four to six months after starting the program of restoring voltage and nutrition.

One of the principle causes of too low blood pressure is dehydration. If you don't have enough fluid in the system, you can't create enough pressure. Another cause is mineral deficiency, particularly sodium and magnesium. Low blood pressure can be a symptom of a deficiency of Vitamin B5 (pantothenic acid). It can also be due to adrenal insufficiency. If your blood pressure drops instead of increasing as you stand up, that is a sign that your adrenals are not working correctly. Unstable blood pressure is often due to a lack of magnesium and/or Vitamin B1 (thiamine).

Despite the recommendations of the National Institutes of Health as discussed above, the prestigious Cochran Review has recently published (April 2010) a review of the medical literature. Their conclusion was that there is no benefit to lowering the blood pressure below 140 or 90 (systolic-diastolic) unless the patient is diabetic or has kidney disease. They found that the fewest heart attacks occur with a diastolic pressure of 86. Again we see a governmental agency with members supported by the pharmaceutical companies recommending increased use of drugs while a private organization looks at the same data and says that the drugs are not beneficial.

The substance that dilates blood vessels in the body is nitric oxide (NO). Thus the primary cause of hypertension is lack of NO. This substance has a very important role in the body as it also controls brain communication, hormones, insulin, etc. The body's ability to make it is diminished every year so that most people older thanforty0 do not have enough. It is made from the amino acid l-arginine. However, making it from l-arginine is much like the conversion of T4 to T3 that we discuss in the chapter on thyroid. If you don't have the proper vitamins and minerals, you make a fake compound that is damaging. Thus it is recommended that people over age forty do not take l-arginine. Taking it if you have had a heart attack actually increases your risk of dying of a heart attack.

The most important nutrients to take to maintain your NO levels are green leafy vegetables.

Sewage

As you clean up your old house now and in the future and wash out the debris, you will need a functional sewage system to get rid of the toxic and waste materials. One of the most important systems in the body is the large intestine. For some reason, people seem to fear the simple process of cleaning it even though very few people actually find it uncomfortable or distressing. It just means you need to be at home for a few hours.

Most traditional doctors do not believe that cleaning the intestine has any benefits. They also believe that having a bowel movement every few days is okay. This ignores the fact that healthy children and adults have multiple bowel movements per day.

Physicians will admit that many elderly have so few bowel movements that they eventually get impacted. They will acknowledge that these patients are sick but rarely think about the effects of holding toxic feces in the body for days.

For whatever reason, people routinely feel better after a colon cleanse.

Large Intestine Cleanse with Magnesium Citrate

WARNING: Drink two glasses of water before you begin. During the bowel cleaning process you will lose significant amounts of fluid. THIS IS NORMAL. It is very important that you replace this fluid to prevent dehydration. Drink large amounts of clear liquids. Drinking large amounts of clear liquids also helps ensure that your bowel will be clean and that you will not place undue stress on your kidneys. The reported complications from taking magnesium citrate are in people that failed to drink adequate fluids while taking it.

If you are diabetic, take one-half dose of insulin in the morning or as instructed by your physician.

Do not use if you have:

1. Megacolon
2. Gastrointestinal Obstruction
3. Ascites
4. Congestive Heart Failure
5. Kidney Disease
6. Children Under 5 Years of Age
7. Use with caution with Impaired Renal Function

8. Heart Disease
9. Acute Myocardial Infarction
10. Unstable Angina
11. Pre-Existing Electrolyte Disturbances
12. Increased Risk For Electrolyte Disturbances (E.G., Dehydration, Gastric Retention, Bowel Perforation, Colitis, Ileus, Inability to take Adequate Oral Fluid, Concomitant use of Diuretics or Other Medications that Affect Electrolytes)
13. Debilitated or Elderly Patients
14. Patients Taking Medications Known to Prolong the Q-T Interval (a defined part of the ECG pattern)

If you have any of these, discuss this with Dr. Tennant before taking the magnesium citrate. One can clean the colon with colonics if it is contraindicated to use magnesium citrate.

You are encouraged to drink large amounts of clear liquids to prevent dehydration. Drinking large amounts of clear liquids also helps ensure that the bowel will be clean.

DO NOT EXCEED RECOMMENDED DOSAGE, AS SERIOUS SIDE EFFECTS MAY OCCUR.

After two glasses of water, drink one-half bottle of magnesium citrate. If you do not get flushing diarrhea within thirty minutes, drink the other half with another glass of water. Drink a bottle of Gatorade after you are finished.

Probiotics

The word "probiotic" refers to bacteria that normally live in our intestines and help with digestion. They are an important part of the digestive process and need to be replaced if they are diminished in numbers by the use of antibiotics.

In addition to digestion, they are believed to assist with:

1. Competition against harmful micro-organisms including Candida, preventing colonization of pathogens through the production of inhibitory substances including acids and hydrogen peroxide and natural antibiotics
2. Enhancement of digestion of lactose (milk sugar)
3. Immune enhancement, including enhanced macrophage activity
4. Reduction in the levels of and deactivation of potential cancer-causing chemicals, particularly in the colon and direct anti-tumor activity of certain strains
5. Reduction in liver toxicity
6. Enhancement of peristalsis, digestion, regularity, and re-absorption of nutrients; in infants, promotion of healthy digestive tract colonization
7. Enhancement and balance of estrogen levels, prevention of osteoporosis through increased calcium uptake
8. Protection against food poisoning, travelers' diarrhea, allergies, skin problems
9. Enhancement of vitamin status (B, K), digestion of proteins, fats, carbohydrates

Electricity

Now that you have the water and sewage working in your old house, you need electricity. So it is with your body. When two hydrogen atoms join with an oxygen atom to form water, the first thing they do is exchange electrons. When electrons move from one place to another, this is called an electric current. All of the chemical reactions in the body depend upon voltage (movement of electrons). Every cell has its own battery pack—the cell membrane —that stores voltage and provides it to the cell as needed to keep it working.

We have discussed voltage in the body in a different chapter.

Cooking Oils

This is one of the most important parts of getting well. If you don't stop putting trans fats ("plastic fats") into your body, you will never get well! Please pay particular attention to this section.

The summary of this section is as follows: Food suppliers recognized that the major loss of profits was from spoilage. In order to stop spoilage and increase their profits, they did two things.

1. They added chemicals to the food to keep it from spoiling. These chemicals not only preserve food, they preserve the person who eats them.
2. They began to cook the fats in the food. Cooking fats at 350-380 degrees for five to six hours changes the fats into something that is one carbon atom away from plastic. You can tell this is what you are eating if the label says, "Partially Hydrogenated __." These partially hydrogenated fats are called trans fats.

When a cell in your body is worn out, it makes a new one. It looks around to see what building materials you have provided to make a new cell. If all you have given your body is plastic fat, it makes a new cell out of plastic. Remember that the cell membrane that surrounds every cell is made of fat. If you make that out of plastic, the cell doesn't work very well. It is like wrapping all your cells in cellophane.

The cell sends a message to your brain that it's hungry. Your body sends the cell some glucose and insulin. However, the glucose can't get through the "cellophane," and the cell keeps complaining that it's hungry. The body keeps sending more insulin and glucose. Much of it gets put into fat cells. Your cells keep complaining that they are hungry. Your brain keeps you eating to try to solve the hunger, but not much gets through the cellophane to the cells.

Soon you are obese and your pancreas is worn out from making so much insulin. With all that glucose in your blood stream, you are diagnosed with type II diabetes. Drugs lower the levels of sugar in your blood, but your cells are still coping with being made of plastic. Soon they begin to wear out, and you get symptoms of worn-out cells such as heart attacks, strokes, liver failure, kidney failure, blindness, chronic fatigue, etc.

Most restaurants use plastic fats for frying food. If you eat out, you must stop eating fried food or choose a restaurant that doesn't use plastic fats. Most cheese is made from plastic fats. Thus cheeseburgers and French fries are major sources of plastic fats. Fast food isn't dangerous because it's fast—it's dangerous because it's plastic.

The point you must understand is that if you insist on feeding your body plastic fats, you will never get well! However, if you give your body good fat and the other things it needs, your body will build a new you that is vibrant and healthy!

There is a lot of confusion about the type of fat to eat. Many people are becoming toxic from too much omega-3 fats (from fish oil, etc.). Your cell membranes are like your home. They need to be strong enough to be substantial but have doorways and windows to let things in and out. If you build your house out of concrete blocks with no windows or doors, it will be strong but won't work because you can't get in or out. If you build it with mostly doors and windows, the next storm will take it down.

In cells, saturated fats are strong, and unsaturated fats are porous. You need saturated fat (animal fat, for example) to make strong cells, and unsaturated fats (fish oils for example) for doors and windows. The ratio needs to be 4:1, meaning that you need to eat four times as much saturated fat as unsaturated fats or four times as many bricks as doors and windows.

215

Saturated fats have gotten a bad reputation because plastic fats are saturated. There is a difference between plastic fats and normal saturated fats.

The following discussion is for those who don't understand this problem and insist that eating fat is harmful. Remember that your body should contain about twenty percent fat since all of your cell membranes and most of your nervous system is fat. That means you need to give your body twenty-four pounds of good fat to replace the fat in your system if you weigh 120 pounds. If you weigh two hundred pounds, you will need to give your body forty pounds of good fat to get healthy!

Remember the following:

1.   There is no proven connection between cholesterol and heart disease. In fact, those dying from heart attacks generally have the lowest cholesterol levels and often have low "bad cholesterol" (LDL) levels.

2.   Eating good fat doesn't affect your cholesterol or make you obese. The liver makes as much or as little cholesterol as it wants.

3.   Eating plastic fat (trans fats) makes you obese and produces a liver and other cells that cannot function.

4.   The liver uses cholesterol to clean itself. High cholesterol means your liver filtration system is dirty and filled with toxic materials and/or that you have low levels of hormones (hormones are made from cholesterol). When the liver senses that your hormone levels are low, it makes more cholesterol to attempt to solve the problem. Why would you want to interfere with the liver's ability to clean itself by taking cholesterol-lowering drugs?

Common Name	Foods	Nomenclature	Type	Effect on membrane
Caprylic		8:00	Saturated (SFA)	Rigidity
Capric	Coconut	10:00	Saturated (SFA)	Rigidity
Lauric	Coconut, palm	10:00	Saturated (SFA)	Rigidity
Myristic	Coconut, palm	12:00	Saturated (SFA)	Rigidity
Palmitic	Palm, beef, mutton, butter, cocoa, lard, eggs	16:00	Saturated (SFA)	Rigidity
Stearic	Cocoa, beef, mutton, eggs, palm, lard	18:00	Saturated (SFA)	Rigidity
Oleic (Omega-9)	Safflower (high oleic), olive, canola, sesame, rice, butter, corn	18:1, ω-9	PUFA	Fluid
Linoleic (LA) (Omega-6)	Safflower, Sunflower, soy, oat, peanut, lard, corn	18:2, ω-6	PUFA	Fluid
Gamma-linolenic (GLA) (Omega-6)	Borage, primrose, black currant, hemp	18:3, ω-6	PUFA	Fluid
Alpha-linolenic (ALA) (Omega-3)	Flax, canola, soy, hemp	18:3, ω-3	PUFA	Fluid
Arachiodonic (AA) (Omega-6)	Eggs, butter, beef, mutton, shellfish	20:4, ω-6	HUFA	Fluid
Eicosapentaenoic (EPA) (Omega-3)	Fish oil, cold water fish	20:5, ω-3	HUFA	Fluid
Docosahexaenoic (DHA) (Omega-3)	Fish oil, cold water fish	22:6, ω-3	HUFA	Fluid
	PUFA = 2-3 double bonds			
	HUFA = >3 double bonds			
HUFA -->eicosonoids --> prostaglandins	thromboxaines			
	leukotrienes			

Fatty Acid		Omega	Source
Alpha-linolenic (ALA)		3	Flax
Eicosapentaenoic (EPA)		3	Fish
Docosahexaenoic (DHA)		3	Fish
Linoleic (LA)		6	Safflower
Gamma-linolenic (GLA)		6	Primrose
Arachiodonic (AA)		6	Egg yolk

5.   Very low cholesterol means the liver is too sick to clean itself and you will suffer major illness or death soon.

6.   To get well, you will need to eat at least twenty percent of your body weight in good fat. If you

217

weigh two hundred pounds, you will need to eat at least forty pounds of good fat to get well! Seventy-five percent of that needs to be saturated fat like animal fat and twenty-five percent needs to be polyunsaturated fat like fish oil.

7. Eating lots of butter and eggs (a stick of butter and six to twelve eggs per day) will help you get well much faster.

8. If eating fat makes you nauseated, it means your liver is too sick to use it. We will have to treat your liver so it can restore itself before you can get well.

The following is reproduced with permission from Sally Fallon with Pat Connolly and Mary G. Enig, PhD.

Nourishing Traditions: The Cookbook that Challenges Politically Correct Nutrition and the Diet Dictocrats, ProMotion Publishing, 800-231-1776, and Fallon, Sally, et al.,"Why Butter is Good for You (health aspects of dietary fat)," (Cover Story), Consumers' Research magazine, 03-01, Vol.79 (1996), 10(6). ©1996 Consumers' Research Inc.

Politically correct nutrition is based on the assumption that we should reduce our intake of fats, particularly saturated fats from animal sources. Fats from animal sources contain cholesterol, presented as the villain of the civilized diet.

Yet the textbooks tell us that fats from animal and vegetable sources provide a concentrated source of energy in the diet; they also provide the building blocks for cell membranes, for hormones, and for prostaglandins (substances that mediate important chemical processes in the body). In addition, they act as carriers for the important fat-soluble vitamins A, D, E, and K. Dietary fats are needed for conversion of carotene to vitamin A and for a host of other processes.

The theory—and it is only a theory—that there is a direct relationship between the amount of saturated fat in the diet and the incidence of coronary heart disease, as well as certain types of cancer, was proposed by a researcher named Ancel Keys in the late 1950s. Numerous subsequent studies have questioned his data and conclusions. Nevertheless, Keys' articles received far more publicity than those contradicting him. The vegetable oil industry and food processing industries, the main beneficiaries of the saturated fat/heart disease connection, began promoting and funding further research designed to support Keys' theories.

The most well-known advocate of the low-fat diet was Dr. Nathan Pritikin. Actually, Pritikin advocated eliminating sugar, white flour, and all processed foods from the diet and recommended the use of fresh raw foods, whole grains, and a strenuous exercise program; but it was the low-fat aspects of his regimen that received the most attention in the media. Adherents found that they lost weight and that their blood cholesterol levels and blood pressures declined.

The success of the Pritikin diet was probably due to a number of factors having nothing to do with a reduction in dietary fat—weight loss alone, for example, will precipitate a reduction in blood cholesterol levels—but Pritikin soon found that the fat-free diet presented many problems, not the least of which was the fact that people just could not stay on it. Those who possessed enough willpower to stay fat-free for any length of time developed a variety of health problems including low energy, difficulty in concentration, depression, weight gain, and signs of mineral deficiencies.

After problems with the no-fat regimen became apparent, Pritikin introduced a small amount of fat from vegetable sources into his diet—something like 10 percent of the total caloric intake. Today the "diet dictocrats"—essentially the public health establishment, including primarily the large health charities and the federal government—advise us to limit fats to 25-30 percent of the caloric intake (12-15 percent of the diet by weight). A careful reckoning of daily fat intake, and avoidance of animal fats, is presented as the key to perfect health.

The experts assure us the theory that animal fat consumption causes coronary heart disease is backed by abundant evidence. Most people would be surprised to learn that there is, in fact, very little evidence to support the contention that a diet low in cholesterol and saturated fat actually reduces death from heart disease or in any way increases one's life span.

Consider the following:
Before 1920, coronary heart disease was rare in America, so rare that when a young internist named Paul Dudley White introduced the German electrocardiograph to his colleagues at Harvard University, they advised him to concentrate on a more profitable branch of medicine. The new machine revealed the presence of arterial blockages, thus permitting early diagnosis of coronary heart disease, but in those days clogged arteries were a medical rarity, and White had to search for patients who could benefit from his new technology.

During the next forty years, however, the incidence of coronary heart disease rose dramatically, so much so that by the mid-'50s, heart disease was the leading cause of death among Americans. Today, heart disease causes 40 percent of all U.S. deaths.

If, as we have been told, heart disease results from consumption of saturated fats, one would expect to find a corresponding increase in animal fat in the American diet. Actually the reverse is true. During the sixty-year period from 1910 to 1970, the proportion of traditional animal fat in the American diet declined from 83 to 62 percent, and butter consumption plummeted from eighteen pounds per person per year to four pounds. During the past eighty years, dietary cholesterol intake has increased only one percent. During the same period the percentage of dietary vegetable fat in the form of margarine, shortening, and refined oils increased about 400 percent, and the consumption of sugar and processed foods increased about 60 percent.

The Framingham Heart Study is often cited as proof of the cholesterol/animal fat theory. This study began in 1948 and involved about 6,000 people from the town of Framingham, Massachusetts. Two groups were compared at five-year intervals—those who consumed little cholesterol and saturated fat and those who consumed large amounts.

Today, after forty years, the current director of this study admits: "In Framingham, Mass., the more saturated fat one ate, the more cholesterol one ate, the more calories one ate, the lower the person's serum cholesterol. ... [W]e found that the people who ate the most cholesterol, ate the most saturated fat, and ate the most calories weighed the least and were the most physically active."

The study did show that those who weighed more and had higher blood cholesterol levels were more at risk for future coronary heart disease; but weight gain and cholesterol levels had an inverse correlation with fat and cholesterol intake in the diet.

221

The Lipid Research Clinics Coronary Primary Prevention Trial (LRC-CPPT), which cost 150 million dollars, is the study most often cited by the experts to justify the low fat diet. Actually, <u>dietary cholesterol and saturated fat were not tested in this study as all subjects were already on a low-cholesterol, low-saturated fat diet. Instead, the study tested the effects of a cholesterol-lowering drug.</u>

Statistical analysis of the results indicated a 24 percent reduction in the rate of coronary heart disease in the group taking drugs compared with the placebo group; however, <u>non-heart disease deaths in the drug group increased— deaths from cancer, stroke, violence, and suicide.</u> Even the claim that a diet low in saturated fat and cholesterol reduced heart disease is suspect. <u>Independent researchers who tabulated the results of this study found no significant statistical difference in the coronary heart disease death rate between the two groups.</u> However, both the popular press and medical journals touted the LRC-CPPT survey as the long-sought proof that animal fats are the cause of heart disease, America's number one killer.

Mother's milk contains a higher proportion of cholesterol than almost any other food. It also contains over 50 percent of its calories as fat, much of it saturated fat. Both cholesterol and saturated fat are essential for growth in babies and children, especially in development of the brain. (Yet the American Heart Association is now recommending a low-cholesterol, low-fat diet for children.) Most commercial formulas are low in saturated fats and some are almost completely devoid of cholesterol. A recent study linked a low-fat diet with failure to thrive in children.

As a final example, consider the French. The French diet is loaded with saturated fats in the form of butter, eggs, cheese, cream, liver, meats, and rich pates. Yet the French have a lower rate of coronary heart disease than many other western countries. In the United States, 315 of every 100,000 middle-aged men die of heart attacks each year; in France the rate is 145 per 100,000. In the Gascony region, where goose and duck liver form a staple of the diet, this rate is a remarkably low: 80 per 100,000. This phenomenon has recently gained international attention and has been dubbed the paradox francais.

Clearly, something is wrong with the theories we read in the popular press (and used to bolster sales of low-fat concoctions and cholesterol-free foods). The notion that saturated fats per se cause heart disease as well as cancer is not only not facile, it is just plain wrong. But it is true that some fats are bad for us. In order to understand which ones, we must know something about the chemistry of fats.

Fat Chemistry. Most fat in our bodies and in the food we eat is in the form of triglycerides, that is, three fatty acid chains attached to a glycerol molecule. Elevated triglycerides in the blood have been positively linked to proneness to heart disease, but these triglycerides do not come directly from dietary fats; they are made in the liver from any excess sugars that have not been completely burned. The source of these excess sugars is any food containing carbohydrates, but particularly refined sugar and processed carbohydrates.

In simple terms, fatty acids are chains of carbon atoms with hydrogen linkages. A fatty acid is called saturated when all available carbon bonds are occupied by a hydrogen atom. Monounsaturated fatty acids have one pair of carbon atoms double bonded to each other and therefore lack two hydrogen atoms. The monounsaturated fatty acid most commonly found in our food is oleic acid, the main

223

component of olive oil. Polyunsaturated fatty acids have two or more pairs of carbon double bonds and therefore lack four or more hydrogen atoms. The two polyunsaturated fatty acids found most frequently in our foods are double unsaturated linoleic acid with two double carbon bonds (also called omega-6) and triple unsaturated linolenic acid with three double bonds (also called omega-3).

All fats and oils, whether of vegetable or animal origin, are some combination of saturated fatty acids, monounsaturated fatty acids (oleic acid), and the polyunsaturates linoleic and linolenic acid. In general, animal fats such as butter, lard, and tallow contain about 50 percent saturated fat and are solid at room temperature. Vegetable fats from northern climates contain a preponderance of polyunsaturated fatty acids and are liquid at room temperature. But vegetable oils from the tropics are highly saturated. Coconut oil, for example, is 92 percent saturated. These fats are liquid in the tropics, but hard as butter in northern climes. <u>Highly saturated tropical oils such as coconut and palm oil are not harmful, as the popular press would lead us to believe. These fats and oils have nourished healthy populations, free of heart disease, for millennia.</u> Vegetable oils are more saturated in hot climates because the increased saturation helps maintain stiffness in plant leaves. Olive oil with its preponderance of oleic acid is the product of a temperate climate. It is liquid at warm temperatures but hardens when refrigerated.

Researchers classify fatty acids not only according to their degree of saturation but also by their length.

1. Short-chain fatty acids have four to six carbon atoms (butter and coconut)

2. Medium-length fatty acids have eight to twelve (butter

and coconut)

3. Long-chain fatty acids have 14 to 18 carbon atoms (beef fat)

4. Very-long-chain fatty acids have 20 to 24 carbon atoms (fish oils, organs)

Saturated fats vary in length from short to long. Butter and coconut oil contain a large portion of short- and medium-chain fatty acids, while stearic acid, the main component of beef fat, is a long-chain fatty acid with 18 carbons. Oleic acid, linoleic acid, and linolenic acid also have 18 carbons. Very-long-chain fatty acids, such as those found in fish oils and organ tissues, tend to be highly unsaturated, with four, five, and even six double bonds.

Short- and medium-chain fatty acids have several interesting properties.
1. Longer-chain fatty acids are absorbed by the lymph system and must be acted on by bile salts.
2. Short-chain fatty acids (butter and coconut) are absorbed directly through the portal vein to the liver. As they do not need to be acted upon by the bile salts, these short-chain fatty acids supply quick energy.

In general, the body uses the longer-chain fatty acids, including the longer-chain saturated fatty acids, to construct membranes and vital hormone-like substances, to create electric potentials, and to move electric currents.

It is the longer-chain fatty acids that are stored in the adipose tissue, particularly oleic and linoleic acid. Thus butter and coconut oil, which contain a significant portion of short- and medium-chain fatty acids, do not contribute to weight gain as much as olive and vegetable oil. The short- and medium-chain fatty acids also have antimicrobial and anti-fungal properties in the intestinal tract; they have anti-tumor properties and help strengthen the immune system, while an excess of polyunsaturated fatty acids stimulate tumor growth.

Summary: (JLT)

1. Short-chain fatty acids have four to six carbon atoms (butter and coconut)
   a. Do not contribute to weight gain as much as olive and vegetable oil
   b. Have antimicrobial and anti-fungal properties in the intestinal tract
   c. Have anti-tumor properties and help strengthen the immune system,
2. Medium-length fatty acids have eight to twelve (butter and coconut)
   a. Do not contribute to weight gain as much as olive and vegetable oil
   b. Have antimicrobial and anti-fungal properties in the intestinal tract
   c. Have anti-tumor properties and help strengthen the immune system,
3. Long-chain fatty acids have 14 to 18 carbon atoms (beef fat)
   a. Absorbed by the lymph system and must be acted on by bile salts
   b. Used to construct membranes and vital hormone-like substances, to create electric potentials, and to move electric currents
   c. Stored in the adipose tissue, particularly oleic and linoleic acid
4. Very-long-chain fatty acids have 20 to 24 carbon atoms (fish oils, organs)
   a. Absorbed by the lymph system and must be acted on by bile salts

b. Used to construct membranes and vital hormone-like substances, to create electric potentials, and to move electric currents

c. Stored in the adipose tissue, particularly oleic and linoleic acid; an excess of polyunsaturated fatty acids stimulate tumor growth.

Too Many Polyunsaturates.

Unsaturated omega-3 and omega-6 fatty acids are called essential fatty acids, or EFAs, because the body cannot manufacture them, at least not in the form in which they occur. Researchers vary in their estimates of the amount of polyunsaturated fatty acids needed in the diet, giving figures as low as 0.5 percent and as high as 15 percent, but recent scientific evidence supports the lower range and has led knowledgeable researchers to recommend limiting our intake of polyunsaturates to 4 percent of the caloric total, in approximate proportions of 1.5 percent omega-3 fatty acid and 2.5 percent omega-6. (More recently, Yehuda et al. have proven that the proper ratio is 4:1 of omega-6 to omega-3 of the lower order linoleic and linolenic acids. JLT)

What we find in the American diet is a high intake of polyunsaturates—something like 10 to 30 percent of the total caloric intake. Worse, most of these polyunsaturates are in the form of omega-6 linoleic acid, with very little of vital omega-3 linolenic acid. Recent research has revealed that too much omega-6 in the diet can interfere with the enzymes that produce longer chain, highly saturated fatty acids, which are the precursors of important prostaglandins. These are localized tissue hormones that direct many processes in the cells.

When the production of prostaglandins is compromised by

excess omega-6 in the diet, coupled with too little omega-3, serious problems result including inflammation, hypertension, irritation of the digestive tract, depressed immune function, sterility, cell proliferation, cancer, and weight gain. Other studies indicate that excessive unsaturated fatty acids in the diet of infants can interfere with brain development and with learning and behavior.

In contrast, dietary saturated fats (e.g., coconut, palm, beef, butter, eggs) contribute to optimal utilization of essential fatty acids. Thus, although not called essential, saturated fats are absolutely necessary in the diet, not only for the role they play in enhancing EFA utilization, in supplying quick energy, and in their immune system enhancing characteristics, but also because of the important vitamins they carry.

A Serious Problem.

A serious problem with the polyunsaturate family, and particularly omega-3 (fish, flax, hemp), is its instability. With their double carbon bonds, these fatty acids tend to polymerize, that is, bond with each other and bond with other molecules. They are also more easily rendered rancid when subjected to heat, oxygen, and moisture as in cooking and processing. Rancid oils are characterized by free radicals in the double bond, that is, single atoms or clusters with an unpaired electron in an outer orbit.

These compounds are extremely reactive chemically. They have been characterized as "marauders" in the body, for they attack cell walls and red blood cells and cause damage in DNA/RNA strands, thus triggering mutations in tissue, blood vessels, and skin. Free radical damage to the skin causes wrinkles and premature aging; free radical damage to the tissues and organs sets the stage for tumors. Is it any wonder that tests and studies have repeatedly shown a high correlation between cancer and the consumption of polyunsaturates? New evidence links exposure to free radicals with premature aging, with autoimmune diseases such as arthritis, and to Parkinson's disease, Lou Gehrig's disease, Alzheimer's, and cataracts.

(Note that recent work shows that many sources of omega-3 like cod liver oil are severely contaminated with chemical toxins in the ocean. It is critical to only buy and use molecularly distilled omega-3 oils that have removed these carcinogens. Most health food stores do not sell these as it takes one hundred pounds of cod livers to produce ten pounds of toxin-free oil, which makes it more expensive. Use only molecularly distilled omega-3 supplements. JLT)

It is important to understand that of all substances ingested by the body, it is polyunsaturated oils that are most easily rendered dangerous by food processing, especially unstable omega-3 linolenic acid. Consider the following processes inflicted upon naturally occurring fats before they appear on our tables:

Extraction. Oils naturally occurring in fruits, nuts, and seeds must first be extracted. In the old days this extraction was achieved by a slow-moving stone press. But oils processed in large factories are obtained by crushing the oil-bearing seeds and heating them to 230 degrees Fahrenheit. The oil is then squeezed out at pressures from 10 to 20 tons per inch, thereby generating more heat. During this process the oils are exposed to damaging light and oxygen.

High-temperature processing causes the weak carbon bonds of the unsaturated fatty acids, especially triple unsaturated linolenic acid, to break apart, thereby creating dangerous free radicals. In addition, antioxidants including fat-soluble vitamin E, which protect the body from the ravages of free radicals, are neutralized or destroyed by high temperatures and pressures.

(There is a safe modern technique for extraction that drills into the seeds and extracts the oil and its precious cargo of antioxidants under low temperatures, with minimal exposure to light and oxygen. These unrefined oils will remain fresh for a long time if stored in the refrigerator in dark bottles. Extra virgin olive oil is produced by crushing olives between stone or steel rollers. This process is a gentle one that preserves the integrity of the fatty acids and the numerous natural preservatives in olive oil. If the olive oil is packaged in an opaque container, it will retain its freshness and precious store of antioxidants many months.)

Hydrogenation. This is the process that turns polyunsaturates (margarine and shortening), normally liquid at room temperature, into a fat that is solid at room temperature. To produce them, manufacturers begin with the cheapest oil (soy, corn, or cottonseed) already rancid from the extraction process. These oils are then mixed with tiny metal particles—usually nickel oxide. Nickel oxide is very toxic when absorbed and is impossible to eliminate totally from margarine. (Nickel is a severe neurotoxin. JLT)

The oil with its nickel catalyst is then subjected to hydrogen gas in a high-pressure, high-temperature reactor. Next, soap-like emulsifiers and starch are squeezed into the mixture to give it a better consistency. The oil is yet again subjected to high temperature when it is steam cleaned. This removes its horrible odor. Margarine's natural color, an unappetizing grey, is removed by bleach. Coal tar dyes and strong flavors must then be added to make it resemble butter. Finally the mixture is compressed and packaged in blocks or tubs, ready to be spread on your toast (and make "plastic cell membranes" JLT).

Forget Margarine. Margarine and other partially hydrogenated oils are even worse for you than the highly refined vegetable oils from which they are made because of chemical changes that occur during the hydrogenation process. Under high temperatures, the nickel catalyst causes the hydrogen atoms to change position on the fatty acid chain. Before hydrogenation, two hydrogen atoms occur together on the chain, causing the chain to bend slightly and creating an electron cloud at the site of the double bond. This is called the "cis" formation, the configuration most commonly found in nature. With hydrogenation, one hydrogen atom is moved to the other side so that the molecule straightens. This is called the "trans" formation, rarely found in nature.

These man-made trans fats are toxins to the body, but unfortunately your digestive system does not recognize them as such. Instead of being eliminated, the trans fats are incorporated into the body's cell membranes as if they were cis-fats; your cells actually become hydrogenated. Once in place, trans-fatty acids with their misplaced hydrogen atom wreak havoc in cell metabolism. These altered fats actually block the utilization of essential fatty acids, causing many deleterious effects ranging from sexual dysfunction, increased blood cholesterol, and paralysis of the immune system.

In the 1940s, researchers found a strong correlation between cancer and the consumption of fat, but the fats used were hydrogenated fats, not naturally saturated fats. (Until recently, the confusion between hydrogenated fats and naturally saturated fats has persisted not only in the popular press, but in scientific data bases, resulting in much error in study results.)

Consumption of hydrogenated fats is associated with a host of other serious diseases, not only cancer but also atherosclerosis, diabetes, obesity, immune system dysfunction, low birth weight babies and birth defects, sterility, difficulty in lactation, and problems with bones and tendons. Yet hydrogenated fats continue to be promoted as health foods. Margarine's popularity represents a triumph of advertising over common sense. Your best defense is to avoid it like the plague.

Go Butter. The media's constant attack on saturated fats is extremely suspect. Claims that butter causes chronic high cholesterol values have not been substantiated by research, although some studies show that butter consumption causes a small temporary rise. (Other studies have shown that stearic acid, the main component of beef fat, actually lowers cholesterol.) Margarine, on the other hand, provokes chronic high levels of protective cholesterol and has been linked to both heart disease and cancer. Butter has received so much adverse propaganda that we have lost sight of the fact that it has long been a valuable component of many traditional diets containing the following vital nutrients:

- Fat-Soluble Vitamins

  These include vitamins A (retinol), D, and E, as well as all their naturally occurring constituents needed to obtain maximum effect. Butter is America's best source of these essential vitamins. In fact, vitamin A from butter is more easily absorbed and utilized than from other sources. (These fat-soluble vitamins are relatively stable and survive the pasteurization process.) These vitamins act as catalysts to mineral absorption. Without them, we are not able to utilize properly the minerals we ingest, no matter how abundant they may be in our diets.

The only good source of fat-soluble vitamins in the American diet, one sure to be eaten, is butterfat. Butter added to vegetables and spread on bread and cream added to soups and sauces ensures proper assimilation of the minerals and water-soluble vitamins in vegetables, grains, and meat.

- Arachidonic Acid

    This is a polyunsaturate containing four double carbon bonds and is found in small amounts in animal fats but not in vegetable fats. Arachidonic acid is a precursor to important prostaglandins and other vital substances. (Arachidonic acid makes up seventeen percent of cell membranes and there is no vegetable source for it, meaning that total vegans cannot have normal cells. JLT)

- Short- and Medium-Chain Fatty Acids

    Butter contains about 15 percent short- and medium-chain fatty acids. This type of saturated fat, as mentioned, is absorbed directly from the small intestine to the liver, where it is converted to energy. These fatty acids also have antimicrobial, anti-tumor, and immune system supportive properties, especially 12-carbon lauric acid, a medium-chain fatty acid not found in other animal fats. Highly protective lauric (coconut and palm oil) should be called a conditionally essential fatty acid because it is one saturated fat that the body does not make itself. We must obtain it from one of two dietary sources: butter or tropical oils. Propionic acid and butyric acid, very-short-chain fatty acids, are all but unique to butter. These have anti-fungal properties as well as anti-tumor effects.

- Omega-6 and Omega-3 Polyunsaturates

    These occur in butter in small but equal amounts. This balance between linoleic and linolenic acid prevents the kind of problems associated with over-consumption associated with omega-6 (or omega-3 JLT) fatty acids.

- Conjugated Linoleic Acid

    Butterfat also contains a form of rearranged linoleic acid called CLA that has strong anticancer properties.

- Lecithin

    Lecithin is a natural component of butter. It is known to assist in the proper assimilation and metabolization of cholesterol and other fat constituents.

- Cholesterol

    Mother's milk is high in cholesterol because it is essential for growth and development. Cholesterol is also needed to produce a variety of steroids that protect against cancer, heart disease, and mental illness.

- Glycosphingolipids

    This special category of fat protects against gastrointestinal infections, especially in the very young and the elderly. For this reason, children who drink skim milk have diarrhea at rates three to five times greater than children who drink whole milk.

- Trace Minerals

    Many trace minerals are incorporated into the fat globule membrane of butterfat, including manganese, zinc, chromium, and iodine. In mountainous areas far from the

234

sea, iodine in butter protects against goiter and other thyroid problems. Butter is extremely rich in selenium, a vital antioxidant, containing more per gram than herring or wheat germ.

In summary, our choice of fats and oils is one of extreme importance. Most people, especially infants and growing children, benefit from more fat in the diet rather than less. But the fats we eat must be chosen with care. Avoid all processed foods containing partially hydrogenated fats and polyunsaturated oils. Instead use extra virgin olive oil and unrefined flaxseed oil in salad dressings. Acquaint yourself with the merits of coconut oil for baking. And finally, use good old-fashioned butter, not margarine, with the happy assurance that it is a wholesome—indeed, an essential— food for you and your whole family.

© 1996 Consumers' Research Inc. "Why Butter Is Good For You (Health Aspects of Dietary Fat)." (Reproduced here with permission of Ms. Fallon; JLT)

Polyunsaturated fats (PUFA) are extremely vulnerable to damage from heat, so they are not suitable for high-temperature cooking. These oils are best used in salad dressings, sauces, and dips. To add flavor to grains and stir-fry dishes, sprinkle the cooked food with flaxseed oil just before serving.

For high temperature cooking, use extra virgin olive oil or organic coconut butter.

In July 2002, the National Academy of Sciences' Institute of Medicine, which advises the government on health policy, made official what many researchers have argued for years: Trans fat worsens blood-cholesterol levels and almost surely increases the risk of heart disease. The institute concluded that people should consume as little trans fat as possible.

That report has helped push the government and the food industry to start taking aggressive steps to address this long-neglected threat to public health. The Food and Drug Administration (FDA) could be close to finalizing a rule that would require trans-fat labeling on packaged foods. Canada instituted such a requirement early this year as part of its mandatory nutrition-labeling system. Labeling not only will help consumers cut back on trans, it will also be "a profound disincentive for manufacturers" to use partially hydrogenated oils," says Marion Nestle, PhD, professor and chair of New York University's department of nutrition and food studies, and author of "Food Politics: How the Food Industry Influences Nutrition and Health."

To figure the amount of trans-fatty acid in packaged food by using the new U.S. labels

1. Find the amount of "Total Fat" on the label.
2. Find the amounts of "Saturated Fat," "Polyunsaturated Fat," and "Monosaturated Fat." (These are found on the label, listed directly under "Total Fat" and slightly indented. If one or the other is not listed, that particular food does not contain it.)
3. Add these three together. If there are only two listed, add them together or use one amount if only one is listed.
4. Subtract the total amount of #3 from the amount of #1.
5. The answer is the amount of trans-fatty acid in that product.

Trans fats are one carbon atom away from being plastic. This "near-plastic" fat ends up in your cell membranes. Thus when you eat trans fats, you become mostly plastic! Is it any wonder why your cells don't work well and you don't feel good when your cells are made of "near-plastic"?

http://www.consumerreports.org/main/detailv2.jsp?CONTENT

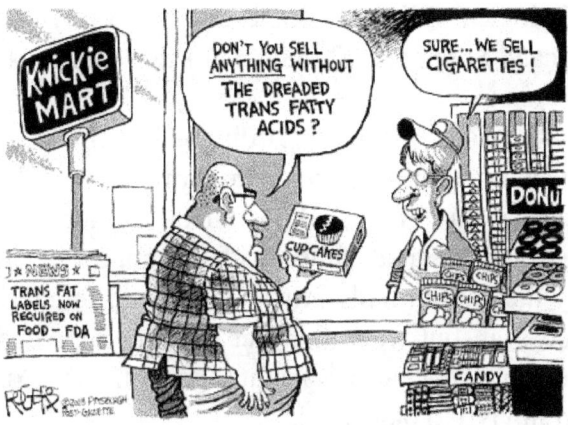

%3C%3Ecnt_id=300681&FOLDER%3C%3Efolder_id=162689

Here is a summary of a few facts regarding canola oil:

1. It is genetically engineered rapeseed.
2. Canada paid the FDA the sum of $50 million to have rapeseed registered and recognized as "safe." (Source: Young Again and others)
3. Rapeseed is lubricating oil used by small industry. It has never been meant for human consumption.
4. It is derived from the mustard family and is considered a toxic and poisonous weed, which when processed, becomes rancid very quickly.
5. It has been shown to cause lung cancer
6. It is very inexpensive to grow and harvest. Insects won't eat it.
7. Some typical and possible side effects include loss of vision, disruption of the central nervous system, respiratory illness, anemia, constipation, increased incidence of heart disease and cancer, low birth weights in infants and irritability.

Here is a review article about canola oil (rapeseed oil) and its toxic effects from a Swedish medical journal:

"Physiopathological Effects of Rapeseed Oil: a Review," Borg, K. Acta Med Scand Suppl (1975), 585: 5–13 ISSN: 0365-463X

"Rapeseed oil has a growth retarding effect in animals. Some investigators claim that the high content of erucic acid in rapeseed oil alone causes this effect, while others consider the low ratio saturated/monounsaturated fatty acids in rapeseed oil to be a contributory factor. Normally erucic acid is not found or occurs in traces in body fat, but when the diet contains rapeseed oil erucic acid is found in depot fat, organ fat, and milk fat. Erucic acid is metabolized in vivo to oleic acid.

The effects of rapeseed oil on reproduction and adrenals, testes, ovaries, liver, spleen, kidneys, blood, heart, and skeletal muscles have been investigated. Fatty infiltration in the heart muscle cells has been observed in the species investigated. In long-term experiments in rats erucic acid produces fibrosis of the myocardium. Erucic acid lowers the respiratory capacity of the heart mitochondria. The reduction of respiratory capacity is roughly proportional to the content of erucic acid in the diet, and diminishes on continued administration of erucic acid.

The lifespan of rats is the same on corn oil, soybean oil, coconut oil, whale oil, and rapeseed oil diet. Rats fed a diet with erucic acid or other docosenoic acids showed a lowered tolerance to cold stress (+4 degrees C). In Sweden, erucic acid constituted 3-4% of the average intake of calories up to 1970 compared with about 0.4% at present."

1.   Generally rapeseed has a cumulative effect, taking almost ten years before symptoms begin to manifest. It has a tendency to inhibit proper metabolism of foods and prohibits normal enzyme function. Canola is a trans-fatty acid, which has shown to have a direct link to cancer. These trans-fatty acids are labeled as hydrogenated or partially

hydrogenated oils. Avoid all of them!

2.   According to John Thomas' book Young Again, twelve years ago in England and Europe, rapeseed was fed to cows, pigs, and sheep that later went blind and began attacking people. There were no further attacks after the rapeseed was eliminated from their diet.

Source: David Dancu, ND, http://www.karinya.com/canola.htm

Milk

One of the three total foods capable of supporting life is raw milk; however, when milk is heated to pasteurize it, the proteins are destroyed. When it is homogenized, it is blown through nozzles to break the long fat chains into short, broken pieces of fat. Thus pasteurized, homogenized milk is no longer milk but instead contains toxic proteins and fat particles.

Most people who think they are "lactose intolerant" are really just sensitive to the toxic brew we call milk that is available in grocery stores.

The state of Maryland was considering prohibiting people who own cows from drinking their own milk or from forming cooperatives so people who buy a portion of a cow could consume raw milk. This rebuttal letter written by Sally Fallon puts it all into perspective. I reproduce it here with her permission.

RESPONSE TO LETTER FROM TED ELKINS, DEPUTY DIRECTOR,

OFFICE OF FOOD PROTECTION AND CONSUMER HEALTH SERVICES,

MARYLAND DEPARTMENT OF HEALTH AND MENTAL

HYGIENE

The following are comments and clarifications to a letter from Ted Elkins, Deputy Director, Office of Food Protection and Consumer Health Services, sent to citizens who submitted comments to oppose the Notice of Proposed Action to amend Regulation .06 under COMAR 10.15.06.Production, Processing, Transportation, Storage and Distribution of Milk.

To summarize, Mr. Elkin has made a series of statements unsupported by references and scientific studies. He has ignored many relevant findings concerning the safety and health benefits of raw milk and the increasing evidence of disease caused by pasteurized milk. He has not reported on evidence of bias in reports on alleged problems with raw milk and has withheld discussion of the numerous incidents of food-borne illness in many commonly consumed foods, thus perpetuating the double standard that uninformed health officials have applied to raw milk. The citizens of Maryland deserve accurate information, not unsubstantiated boilerplate allegations.

"The State of Maryland and other federal and state health agencies have documented a long history of the risks to human health associated with the consumption of raw milk. Clinical and epidemiological studies from the Food and Drug Administration (FDA), state health agencies, and others have established a direct causal link between gastrointestinal disease and the consumption of raw milk."

While several incidents of food-borne illness in recent years have been attributed to the consumption of raw milk, no positive correlation in these cases was established, and government reports on these cases show strong evidence of bias. For example, in 1983, a reported outbreak of Campylobacter in raw milk led to the passage of anti-raw milk legislation in the state of Georgia. However, extensive testing failed to find Campylobacter or any other pathogens in any milk products from the dairy. All safety measures had been followed faithfully.

In spite of this lack of evidence, the author of the official report concluded: "The only means available to ensure the public's health would be proper pasteurization before consumption." (American Journal of Epidemiology, 1983 Vol. 114, No 4) Ironically, just 4 years later, a massive outbreak of over 16,000 culture-confirmed cases of antimicrobial-resistant Salmonella typhimurium was traced to pasteurized milk from one dairy in Georgia (JAMA 1987 Dec. 11; 258(22): 3269-74). Yet health officials still allow the sale of pasteurized milk in Georgia.

Another example concerns a November 2001 outbreak of Campylobacter in Wisconsin, which local health officials and the Centers for Disease Control blamed on raw milk from a cow-share program in Sawyer County. According to an official report, posted on the CDC website, 70-75 persons became ill from Campylobacter infection during the 12 weeks following November 10, 2001. However, independent investigators determined that the number of afflicted was over 800. Only 24 of 385 cow-share owners became ill. Most had consumed hamburger at a local restaurant. There was no illness in the remaining 361 cow-share owners and most of those who became ill did not consume raw milk.

Health workers at local hospitals showed a clear evidence of bias by testing only those who said they had consumed raw milk; others who reported in sick but had not drunk raw milk were sent home without investigation. Most importantly, independent lab tests found no Campylobacter in the raw milk (www.realmilk.com). This outbreak is one that health officials almost always emphasize when arguing against the consumption of raw milk; yet the evidence of the case points to the fact that raw milk was not the cause of the outbreak.

"The microbial flora of raw milk may include human pathogens present on the cow's udder and teats."

Standard sanitary procedures can completely eliminate the presence of human pathogens in human milk. Organic Pastures Dairy in California produces raw milk for retail sales. The dairy and the state have conducted routinely tests for several years and have never found a human pathogen in the raw milk they produce (www.organicpastures.com).

The intrinsic safety of raw milk stands in sharp contrast to the dangers inherent in other foods. For example, a 1978 survey found Salmonella in many "health food" products, including soy flour, soy protein powder, and soy milk powder. The authors of the report concluded that "The occurrence of this pathogen in three types of soybean products should warrant further investigation of soybean derivatives as potentially significant sources of Salmonella (Applied and Environmental Microbiology, Mar 1979, pp. 559-566).

While raw milk often gets the blame for food-borne illnesses, Campylobacter is best known for contaminating meats. For example, a study carried out during 1999–2000 found that 70.7 percent of chicken and 14.5 percent of turkey samples from Washington, D.C., grocery stores was infected with Campylobacter. (Zhao C., et al., Applied and Environmental Microbiology, 2001:67(12): 5431-5436). Maryland law does not require pasteurization of chicken and turkey, which is highly likely to contain human pathogens, yet has taken steps to deny access to raw milk, which seldom if ever contains human pathogens.

If the goal of the state of Maryland is to eliminate our exposure to human pathogens, perhaps health department officials should take steps to ban the use of coins and cookware. E. coli has been shown to survive on coins for 7–11 days at room temperature; Salmonella enteritidis can survive 1–9 days on pennies, nickels, dimes and quarters; and Salmonella enteritidis can also survive on glass and Teflon for up to 17 days (Jiang and Doyle, Journal of Food Protection 1999; 62(7): 805-7).

The truth is that humans are exposed to pathogens on a daily basis —on surfaces, in our water, and in the food we eat. To single out raw milk as a source of pathogens shows extreme bias against the only food that is intrinsically safe and that furthermore contains many components that support our immunity to pathogens.

"Further, the intrinsic properties of milk, including its pH and nutrient content, make it an excellent medium for the survival and growth of pathogenic bacteria."

This statement reveals the complete ignorance of over 40 years of science indicating that raw milk does not support the survival and growth of pathogenic bacteria. Milk contains numerous components that fight against pathogens and strengthen the immune system. These include:

1. Lactoperoxidase, an enzyme that uses small amounts of H_2O_2 and free radicals to seek out and destroy bad bacteria. It is found in all mammalian secretions, such breast milk, tears, and saliva. Lactoperoxidase levels are much higher in the milk of animals than humans. For example, lactoperoxidase levels are 10 times higher in goat milk than in human breast milk. So effective is lactoperoxidase in fighting pathogens that other countries are looking into using lactoperoxidase instead of pasteurization to ensure safety of commercial milk (British Journal of Nutrition (2000), 84, Suppl. 1. S19-S25; Indian Journal Exp Biology Vol. 36, August 1998: 808-810; 1991 J Dairy Sci 74: 783-787; Life Sciences, Vol. 66, No 23: 2433-2439, 2000).

2. Lactoferrin, an enzyme that steals iron away from pathogens and carries it through the gut wall into the blood stream and also stimulates the immune system. Lactoferrin also ensures complete assimilation of iron by the infant.

3. Polysaccharides, special sugars that encourage the growth of good bacteria in the gut; protect the gut wall

4. Medium-chain fatty acids, special types of fats that disrupt cell walls of bad bacteria; levels are so high in goat milk that the test for the presence of antibiotics had to be changed.

5. Enzymes that disrupt bacterial cell walls

6. Antibodies that bind to foreign microbes and prevent them from migrating outside the gut; initiate immune response (British Journal of Nutrition (2000) 84. Suppl. 1, S3-S10, S11-S17).

7. White blood cells that produce antibodies against specific bacteria, producing immunity for life in the infant

8. B-lymphocytes, compounds that kill foreign bacteria and call in other parts of the immune system

9. Macrophages, components that engulf foreign proteins and bacteria

10. Neutrophils, which kill infected cells; mobilize other parts of the immune system

11. T-lymphocytes, components that multiply if bad bacteria are present while producing immune-strengthening compounds

12. Lysosyme, which kills bad bacteria by digesting their cell walls

13. Hormones and growth factors, which stimulate the maturation of gut cells thereby preventing "leaky" gut

14. Mucins, which adhere to bad bacteria and viruses, preventing those organisms from attaching to the mucosa

and causing disease

15. Oligosaccharides, special types of sugars that protect other protective components from being destroyed by stomach acids and enzymes; they bind to bacteria and prevent them from attaching to the gut lining and have other functions just being discovered.

16. B12 binding protein, a component that reduces the levels of vitamin B12 in the colon, which harmful bacteria need for growth; this compound also ensures complete assimilation of B12 by the infant.

17. Bifidus factor is a complex of good bacteria that promotes growth of Lactobacillum bifidis, a helpful bacteria in a baby's gut, which helps crowd out dangerous germs.

18. Fibronectin, which increases antimicrobial activity of macrophages and helps to repair damaged tissues (J Pediatr 1994 Feb.; 124(2): 193-8; Curr Med Chem 1999 Feb.; 6(2): 117-27)

Most of these components are completely inactivated by pasteurization (Scientific American, December 1995; The Lancet, Nov. 17, 1984), making pasteurized milk highly susceptible to contamination. Mr. Elkin's statement, that "the intrinsic properties of milk, including its pH and nutrient content, make it an excellent medium for the survival and growth of pathogenic bacteria," applies only to pasteurized milk, not to raw milk.

It is of interest to note that, until recently, the medical profession claimed that breast milk was sterile. Research conducted over the last 20 years indicates that breast milk contains pathogens, often at very high levels. It is actually beneficial for breast milk to contain pathogens because the bioactive components in milk program the baby to have immunity for life to any pathogens with which he comes in contact (J Appl Microbiol. 2003; 95(3): 471-8; Neonatal

Netw. 2000 Oct.; 19(7) 21-5; J Hosp Infec. 2004 Oct; 58(2): 146-50; J Nutr. 2005 May; 135(5): 1286-8; Curr Med Chem. 1999 Feb; 6(2): 117-27; Adv Exp Med Biol. 2004; 554: 145-54; Scientific American. Dec. 1995; Lancet. 1984 Nov. 1 7; 2(841 2): 111-3; Lancet. 1984 Nov. 17; 2(8412): 111-3; Cent Afr J Med. 2000 Sep; 46(9): 247-51; Eur J Pediatr. 2000 Nov.; 159(11): 793-7; J Dairy Sci 1991 ;74:783-787).

Maryland health officials do not require breast-feeding mothers to pasteurize their milk before giving it to their babies; yet these same officials discourage mothers who are unable to breast feed from giving their infants the most appropriate and immune-building substitute—raw milk from another mammal such as a cow or goat.

A 1994 study found that premature infants fed raw human milk had lower rates of infection compared to those fed pasteurized human milk (Lancet, November 17, 1984). In fact, pasteurization of human milk for babies carries considerable risk. A recent outbreak of Pseudomonas aeruginosa in a neonatal intensive care unit caused by a contaminated milk bank pasteurizer resulted in 31 cases of infection and 4 deaths (Arch Dis Child Fetal Neonatal Ed. 2003 Sep; 88(5): F434-5).

The intrinsic safety of raw milk has been proven in several published reports showing that raw milk passes the "challenge test." That is, when pathogenic bacteria are introduced to raw milk, their numbers rapidly decline; subsequent testing reveals no pathogens even though they were introduced in large numbers. For example, Lactoperoxidase in raw milk has been shown to kill added fungal and bacterial agents (Life Science 2000 66(25): 2433-9; Indian Journal of Experimental Biology 1998; 36: 808-11).

In a challenge test, raw goat milk killed Campylobacter jejuni (Hygiene (London) 1985 Feb.; 94(1): 31-44).

When Campylobacter was added to raw milk at 4 degrees C at levels of 13,000,000 per ml, levels were less than 10 per ml nine days later (Doyle, et al. Applied and Environmental Microbiology, 1982; 44(5): 1154-58). The anti-microbial properties of raw milk are even more active when milk is not refrigerated. Researchers found that bovine strains of Campylobacter were decreased by 100 cells per ml and poultry strains decreased by 10,000 cells per ml in 48 hours in raw milk at room temperature (37 degrees C) (Dicer KS. Mikrobiyol Bul 1987 Jul; 21(3): 200-5).

Most recently, the University of California conducted challenge tests on Organic Pastures raw milk in California, finding that pathogens added to raw milk disappeared completely within 36 hours (www.organicpastures.com).

"On August 10, 1987, FDA published 21 CFR Part 1240.61, a final regulation mandating the pasteurization of all milk and milk products in final package form for direct human consumption. This regulation addresses milk shipped in interstate commerce and became effective September 9, 1987. In the Federal Register notification for the final rule to 21 CFR Part 1240.61, FDA made a number of findings including the following: 'Raw milk, no matter how carefully produced, may be unsafe.'"

This statement may be part of the official record, but it contradicts other statements published by the U.S. government. A study carried out over 19 years and posted on the Centers for Disease Control website gives the incidence of food-borne illness from raw milk at 1.9 cases per 100,000 people, 1973–1992 (American Journal Public Health, Aug. 1998, Vol. 88., No 8). This report cites many incidents reputed to be caused by raw milk but not necessarily proven; the actual rate of illness caused by raw milk, on a per-consumer basis, may in fact be much lower.

Based on the same CDC website, the incidence of food-borne illness from all foods including pasteurized milk during the period 1993–1997 is 4.7 cases per 100,000 people (U.S. Census Bureau 1997 population estimate 267,783,607). Based on the CDC website, the incidence of reported food-borne illness from other foods (not including milk) are 6.4 cases per 100,000 people per year from 1993 to 1997. Therefore, the incidence of food-borne illness from consuming raw milk is at least 2.5 times lower than the incidence of food-borne illness from consuming pasteurized milk and at least 3.5 times lower than the incidence of food-borne illness from consuming other foods.

Thus the statement published in the Federal Register is false; raw milk is safer than any other food in the food supply. If a food is to be taken out of the food supply because it "may be unsafe," then we would have nothing left to eat. Raw salads, fruits, vegetables, shellfish, eggs and meat, plus pasteurized milk, soy products, baby formula, and mayonnaise have all caused proven outbreaks of illness. Yet these foods remain in the food supply, putting the citizens of Maryland at continued risk.

According to our government, food-borne diseases cause approximately 76 million illnesses, 325,000 hospitalizations and 5,000 deaths per year; the most common source of these infections is fruits, vegetables, and salads. For example, in 1997, there were 1,104 reported cases of food-borne illness from salads and 719 from fruits and vegetables while only 23 from milk, mostly pasteurized milk (MMWR Vol. 45, No SS-5).

"It has not been shown to be feasible to perform routine bacteriological tests on the raw milk itself to determine the presence or absence of all pathogens and thereby ensure that it is free of infectious organisms."

This statement would not hold up in a court of law. Today it is completely feasible to perform routine bacteriological tests on raw milk; these can be performed at the farm and are very inexpensive. There is even a test for E. coli O157:H7 that can be carried out on the farm and costs only $8 per test. It is shameful that health officials of the state of Maryland are unfamiliar with these tests.

"Opportunities for the introduction and persistence of Salmonella on dairy premises are numerous and varied, and technology does not exist to eliminate Salmonella infection from dairy herds or to preclude re-introduction of Salmonella organisms. Moreover recent studies show that cattle can carry and shed S. dublin organisms for many years and demonstrated that S. dublin organisms cannot be routinely detected in cows that are 'mammary gland' shedders."

This statement applies only to large confinement herds. It has proven completely possible to eliminate pathogens from dairy premises when cows are raised on pasture and reasonable sanitary protocols are followed. Over several years of testing, not a single human pathogen has been found on the premises of Organic Pastures dairy in California, not in the manure and not in the milk (www.organicpastures.com).

"During this rule making process, the American Academy of Pediatrics and numerous other organizations submitted comments in support of the proposed regulation. In deciding upon mandatory pasteurization, FDA determined that pasteurization was the only means to assure the destruction of pathogenic microorganisms that might be present."

This statement is completely false. Pasteurization does not ensure the destruction of pathogenic microorganisms in milk. A study published in 2002 found evidence of Mycobacterium paratuberculosis in many samples of pasteurized cow's milk (Appl Environ Microbiol 2002 May; 68(5): 2428-35). M. paratuberculosis has been associated with Crohn's disease.

Other studies indicate that B. cereus spores, botulism spores, and protozoan parasites survive pasteurization (Elliott Ryser, Public Health Concerns. In: Marth, E., Stelle, J., eds. Applied Dairy Microbiology, New York, Marcel Dekker, 2001).

Furthermore, the U.S. government has documented numerous outbreaks of food-borne illness from pasteurized milk. These include:

1. 1945–1,492 cases for the year in the U.S.
2. 1945–1 outbreak, 300 cases in Phoenix, AZ
3. 1945–Several outbreaks, 468 cases of gastroenteritis, 9 deaths in Great Bend, KS
4. 1976–Outbreak of Yersinia enterocolitica in 36 children, 16 of whom had appendectomies, due to pasteurized chocolate milk
5. 1978–1 outbreak, 68 cases in AZ
6. 1982–over 17,000 cases of Yersinia enterocolitica in Memphis, TN
7. 1982–172 cases, with over 100 hospitalized from a three-southern-state area.
8. 1983–1 outbreak, 49 cases of Listeriosis in Massachusetts
9. 1984–August, outbreak of S. typhimurium, approximately 200 cases, at one plant in Melrose Park, IL
10. 1984–November outbreak S. typhimurium at same plant in Melrose Park, IL
11. 1985–March, outbreak, 16,284 confirmed cases at same plant in Melrose Park, IL
12. 1985–197,000 cases of antimicrobial-resistant Salmonella infections from one dairy in California
13. 1985–1,500+ cases, Salmonella culture confirmed, in Northern Illinois
14. 1987–Massive outbreak of over 16,000 culture-confirmed cases of antimicrobial-resistant Salmonella typhimurium traced to pasteurized milk in Georgia
15. 1993–2 outbreaks statewide, 28 cases Salmonella infection
16. 1994–3 outbreaks, 105 cases, E. coli and Listeria in California
17. 1993-1994–outbreak of Salmonella enteritidis in over 200 due to pasteurized ice cream in Minnesota, South Dakota, and Wisconsin
18. 1995–1 outbreak, 3 cases in California
19. 1995–outbreak of Yersinia enterocolitica in 10 children, 3

hospitalized due to post-pasteurization contamination
20. 1996–2 outbreaks Campylobacter and Salmonella, 48 cases in California
21. 1997–2 outbreaks, 28 cases Salmonella in California

The fact that Mr. Elkins does not present the full story by enumerating the many outbreaks of food-borne illness in pasteurized milk provides clear evidence of bias on the part of a Maryland health official.

"This decision was science-based, involving epidemiological evidence. FDA and the Centers for Disease Control and Prevention in Atlanta have documented illnesses associated with the consumption of raw milk, including 'certified raw milk' and have stated that the risks of consuming raw milk far outweigh any benefits."

It is obvious that this decision was not science-based and that it contradicts the epidemiological evidence provided by our government agencies.

"Based on research, which has failed to demonstrate a significant difference between the nutritional value of pasteurized and unpasteurized milk, the FDA and CDC reiterate that the health risks associated with raw milk consumption far outweigh the benefits."

Mr. Elkins seems to be unaware of numerous studies showing the benefits of raw milk over pasteurized. For example, studies carried out during 1935 and 1940 at Randleigh Farm, a research facility in upstate New York, found that rats fed raw milk had better growth and denser bones than those fed pasteurized milk. The rats on pasteurized milk developed hairless patches due to vitamin B6 deficiency and on autopsy showed poor integrity of internal organs (Annals of Randleigh Farm).

These studies confirm the findings of Francis Pottenger who noted that the organs of cats fed raw milk were in excellent condition, with creamy yellow subcutaneous tissue of high vascularity. The heart size of raw milk-fed cats was moderate, the liver in good condition, the intestines firm, and the uterus well supported. By contrast the internal organs of pasteurized milk-fed cats were inferior, with slight fatty atrophy of the liver, inferior condition of the heart, lack of intestinal tone, and moderate distention of the uterus. The skin of the pasteurized milk-fed cats had a purplish discoloration due to congestion and the fur was of poor quality (Pottenger's Cats, Price-Pottenger Nutrition Foundation).

During 1930–31, Dr. Ernest Scott and Prof. Lowell Erf of Ohio State University carried out rat studies that compared the effects of a diet of whole raw milk with one of whole pasteurized milk. Rats fed whole raw milk had good growth, sleek coats, and clear eyes. The rats had excellent dispositions and enjoyed being petted. By contrast, rats fed whole pasteurized milk had rough coats, slow growth, anemic, and loss of vitality and weight. They were very irritable, often showing a tendency to bite when handled (Jersey Bulletin 1931 50: 210-21 1; 224-226, 237).

Studies of guinea pigs carried out by Dr. Rosalind Wulzen and Paul N. Harris, Department of Zoology, Oregon State College, are particularly revealing. Animals fed whole raw milk had excellent growth and no abnormalities. By contrast, those fed pasteurized milk had poor growth, muscle stiffness, emaciation, and weakness and death within one year. Autopsy revealed atrophied muscles streaked with calcification and calcium deposits under the skin, in the joints, the heart, and other organs (American Journal of Pathology Vol. XX VI, Jul-Nov 1950 pp. 595-615).

As for pasteurized milk, many recent studies document the association of pasteurized milk with diabetes (Br J Nutr 2006 Mar; 95(3): 603-8; Diabetes 2000 Jun; 49(6): 91 2-7), frequent ear infections (J Pediatr Rio J 2006 Mar-Apr; 82(2): 87-96; Rev Alerg Mex 2001 Sep-Oct; 48(5): 141-4; Acta Paediatr 2000 Oct; 89(10):

1174-80; Acta Otolaryngol 1999; 1 19(8): 867-73) and asthma (Ann Allergy Asthma Immunol 2002 Dec; 89(6 Suppl 1): 33-7; J Allergy Clin Immunol 2001 Nov.; 108(5): 720-5; West J Nurs Res 1996 Dec; 18(6): 643-54; Pediatr Pulmonol Suppl 1995; 1 1: 59-60). Of interest is a 2002 study showing that "farm milk," that is raw milk, had a protective effect against this debilitating and even lift-threatening condition (Lancet 2002 Feb. 1 6; 359(9306): 623-4).

The scientific literature contains many case histories of recovery from these conditions by eliminating pasteurized milk from the diet. Meanwhile reports of recovery from these and other conditions by consuming raw milk are accumulating. The growing numbers of Maryland consumers—especially growing children— who cannot tolerate pasteurized milk deserve to have a choice for raw milk.

"Numerous documented outbreaks of milk-borne disease involving Salmonella and Campylobacter infections have been directly linked to the consumption of raw milk in the past 20 years. Since the early 1980s, cases of raw milk-associated campylobacteriosis have been reported in the states of Arizona, California, Colorado, Georgia, Kansas, Maine, Montana, New Mexico, Oregon, and Pennsylvania. An outbreak of salmonellosis, involving 50 cases, was confirmed in Ohio in 2002. Recent cases of E. coli O1 57:H7, Listeria monocytogenes, and Yersinia enterocolitica infections have also been attributed to raw milk consumption."

It would be helpful if Mr. Elkins would provide references so that they could be evaluated for legitimacy and bias. Given the double standard applied to raw milk, it is likely that many of these cases were merely reported, not proven. The 2002 Ohio outbreak that he cites was a case in which health officials demonstrated clear evidence of bias. According to the CDC report, "The source for contamination was not determined; however, the findings suggest that contamination of milk might have occurred during the milking, bottling, or capping process."

There were many possible vectors of illness on the dairy besides raw milk—besides providing raw milk, the dairy also operated a petting zoo. There have been several incidents of illness contracted by children visiting a petting zoo, cases that have nothing to do with raw milk. Based on this one incident, in which raw milk was not proven the culprit, the dairy, which had been in business for decades without incident, caved in to health department pressure and stopped the sale of raw milk.

"State health and agricultural agencies utilize the U.S. Public Health Service/FDA Pasteurized Milk Ordinance (PMO) as the basis for the regulation of Grade 'A' milk production and processing. The PMO has been sanctioned by the National Conference on Interstate Milk Shipments (NCIMS) and provides a national standard of uniform measures that is applied to Grade 'A' dairy farms and milk processing facilities to ensure safe milk and milk products. Section 9 of the PMO specifies that only Grade 'A' pasteurized milk be sold to the consumer."

This issue is a red herring. The individual states do not need to follow the PMO. The PMO is a choice, not an obligation. California, the top milk-producing state, does not follow the PMO but created its own regulations. Furthermore, the state can accept the PMO but have exceptions in certain areas, as does Colorado. In any event, PMO regulations do not prohibit consumers from drinking raw milk. It must be stressed that neither the federal government nor the individual states prohibit the consumption of raw milk. Such laws would be inherently unconstitutional, depriving citizens the right to liberty and property without due process of law.

"In summary, since raw milk may contain infective doses of human pathogens, its consumption increases the risk of a variety of illnesses. Even when milk is produced and handled under sanitary conditions, the only proven, reliable method of reducing the level of human pathogens in milk and milk products to safe levels is pasteurization. The FDA has strongly advised against the consumption of raw milk. As the state agency responsible for health of the citizens of Maryland, the Department of Health and Mental Hygiene cannot, in good conscience, condone or encourage the sale of raw milk."

As we have demonstrated in this letter, raw milk does not contain "infective doses of human pathogens" and its consumption does not "increase the risk of a variety of illnesses." Pasteurization does not guarantee a safe product and the risk of contracting food-borne illness from raw milk is lower than the risk of contracting food-borne illness from pasteurized milk. The statements made in writing by Mr. Elkins would not hold up in a court of law and are an insult to Maryland consumers.

But in any event, Maryland consumers are not asking for legalization of the sale of raw milk, but only confirmation of the right to drink the raw milk from their own cows, which is a public policy of the state of Maryland. Maryland consumers are not asking the Department of Health and Mental Hygiene to condone or encourage the sale of raw milk, but merely insisting that the state of Maryland support the rights of its citizens to enter into contractual agreements guaranteed by Maryland law (title 16, Section 401), which recognizes the right of an owner of dairy livestock to contract with another for the boarding and care of that livestock. MDHMH is interfering in areas where it has no jurisdiction whatsoever and is overstepping the bounds of its regulatory authority.

Sally Fallon, President
The Weston A. Price Foundation
May 23, 2006

Sugar

Eating sugar, especially processed sugar, causes the release of insulin. High levels of constant insulin are toxic and cause prolonged inflammation in the body.

Two large studies have been done that looked at the effects of more or less insulin on long-term death rates. The first was called the ACCORD trial and included 10,251 patients. The second, called the NICE-SUGAR Study, included 6,104 patients. Both trials proved that higher insulin activity was associated with higher death rates.

> "Intensive Glycemic Control in the ACCORD and ADVANCE Trials," Dluhy, R.G., and McMahon, G.T., N Eng J Med. (2008), 358: 2560–2572.

> As compared with standard therapy, the use of intensive therapy to target normal glycated hemoglobin levels for 3.5 years increased mortality and did not significantly reduce major cardiovascular events. These findings identify a previously unrecognized harm of intensive glucose lowering in high-risk patients with type II diabetes.

> "Normoglycemia in Intensive Care Evaluation: NICE SUGAR STUDY, N Eng J Med. 2009; 360: 1283–1297 March 26, 2009)

> In this large, international, randomized trial, we found that intensive glucose control increased mortality among adults in the ICU: a blood glucose target of 180 mg or less per deciliter resulted in lower mortality than did a target of 81 to 108 mg per deciliter.

Every cell in the body is designed to run primarily on fat except the nerves. They are designed to run primarily on glucose. This includes the brain.

When you eat carbohydrates, they are digested to glucose, and this causes the pancreas to put out insulin. The glucose is used to fill up the liver. The liver can hold about one and a half hours worth of glucose for the brain. The remainder is placed into fat cells.

One of the problems is that insulin turns glucose into fat, but it cannot turn fat back into glucose. Thus once glucose becomes fat, insulin cannot access that energy storage for placing glucose in the liver.

Let's say your liver is full of glucose. Then an hour goes by. Your brain "looks" down at the liver and says, "Oh my! There are only thirty minutes worth of fuel left for me—hurry and eat a Snickers bar and drink a Coke so I don't run out of fuel!" Your brain encourages you to eat rapidly digested carbohydrates.

When you eat proteins, a part of them is converted to glucose. However, eating protein causes the pancreas to make glucagon instead of insulin. The glucagon fills the liver with glucose and then deposits the rest in fat cells. However, there is a big difference between glucagon and insulin. Glucagon can turn the fat back into glucose. So when the hour goes by and the brain notices that the liver is getting low on fuel, it doesn't really care because it realizes that you have a two-year supply of glucose in that belly that hangs over your belt. With glucagon present, it isn't worried that it will run out of fuel, so it doesn't insist on you eating some carbs.

This is the basis of the Atkins diet. It isn't necessarily the healthiest way to eat because an all-protein diet isn't giving you the vitamins, minerals, and other nutrients you get from eating fruits and vegetables. However, it does explain why it works. It also explains why Americans have become so obese since doctors have begun recommending a low-fat, low-protein, high-carbohydrate diet filled with pasta, bread, fruits and vegetables.

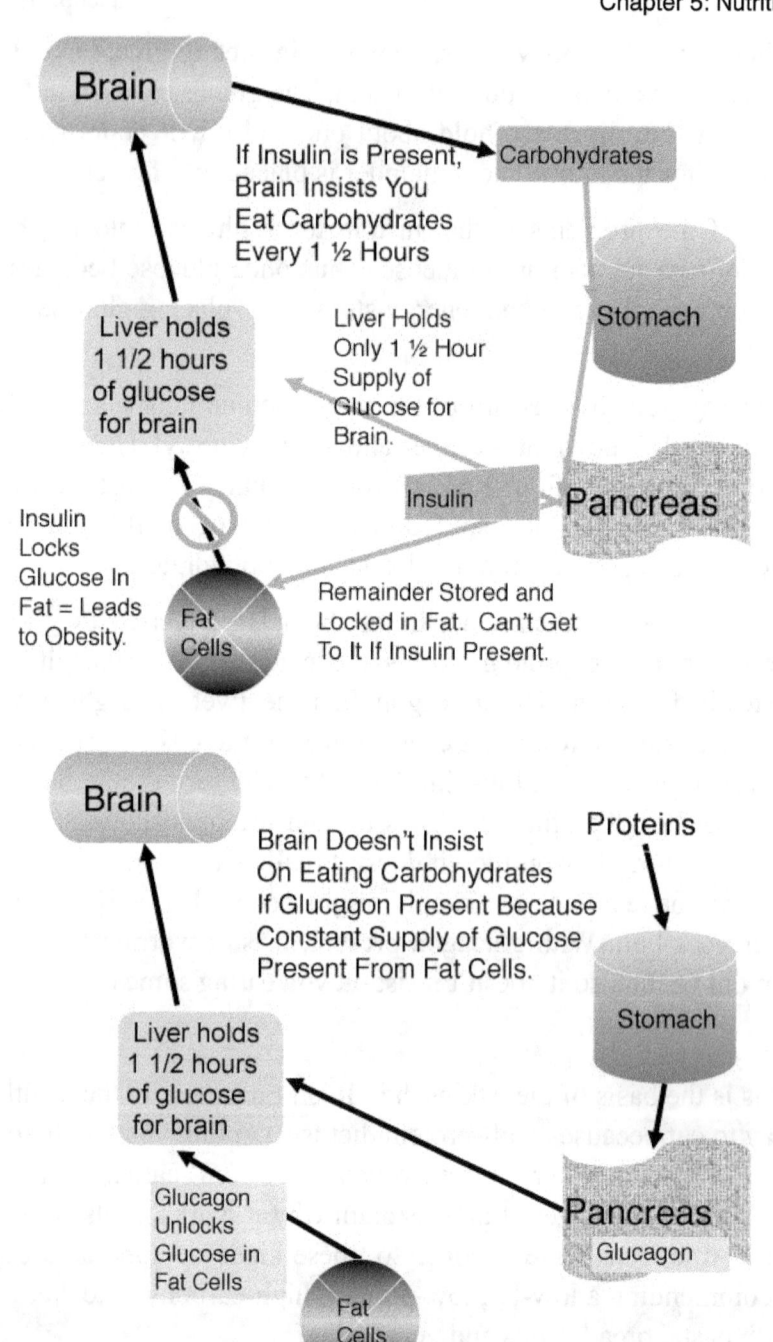

Tennant

258

Symptoms of Insulin Resistance (Type II Diabetes)

Here is a list of some of the most common symptoms of people with insulin resistance. Many symptoms manifest themselves immediately following a meal of carbohydrates, and others are more or less always present. Keep in mind that these symptoms may also be related to other problems.

1. Fatigue. The most common feature of insulin resistance is that it wears people out. Some are tired just in the morning or afternoon, others are exhausted all day.
2. Brain fogginess. Sometimes the fatigue of insulin resistance is physical, but often it's mental. The inability to focus is the most evident symptom. Poor memory, loss of creativity, and poor grades in school often accompany insulin resistance, as do various forms of "learning disabilities."
3. Low blood sugar. Mild, brief periods of low blood sugar are normal during the day, especially if meals are not eaten on a regular schedule. But prolonged periods of this "hypoglycemia," accompanied by many of the symptoms listed here, especially physical and mental fatigue, are not normal.
4. Feeling agitated, jittery, and moody is common in insulin resistance, with almost immediate relief once food is eaten.
5. Intestinal bloating. Most intestinal gas is produced from carbohydrates in the diet. Insulin resistance sufferers who eat carbohydrates suffer from gas—lots of it.
6. Sleepiness. Many people with insulin resistance get sleepy immediately after eating a meal containing more than twenty percent to thirty percent carbohydrates. This means typically a pasta meal, or even a meat meal that includes potatoes or bread and a sweet dessert.
7. Increased weight and fat storage. For most people, too much weight is too much fat. In males, a large abdomen is the more obvious and earliest sign of insulin resistance. In females, it's prominent buttocks.

8. Increased triglycerides. High triglycerides in the blood are often found in overweight persons. But even those who are not overweight may have stores of fat in their arteries as a result of insulin resistance. These triglycerides are the direct result of carbohydrates in the diet being converted by insulin.

9. Increased blood pressure. It is a fact that most people with hypertension have too much insulin and are insulin resistant. It is often possible to show a direct relationship between the level of insulin and blood pressure: as insulin levels elevate, so does blood pressure.

10. Depression. Because carbohydrates are a natural "downer," depressing the brain, it is not uncommon to see many depressed persons who also have insulin resistance.

http://www.healingdaily.com/detoxification-diet/insulin.htm

A huge problem is the widespread use of high fructose corn syrup, particularly in our epidemic of obesity.

"Intake of Sugar-sweetened Beverages and Weight Gain: a Systematic Review," Malik, V.S., Schulze, M.B., and Hu, F.B., Am J Clin Nutr. (2006 Aug), 84(2): 274–88, Department of Nutrition, Harvard School of Public Health, Boston, Massachusetts

Abstract:

Consumption of sugar-sweetened beverages (SSBs), particularly carbonated soft drinks, may be a key contributor to the epidemic of overweight and obesity, by virtue of these beverages' high added sugar content, low satiety, and incomplete compensation for total energy. Whether an association exists between SSB intake and weight gain is unclear. We searched English-language MEDLINE publications from 1966 through May 2005 for cross-sectional, prospective cohort, and experimental studies of the relation between SSBs and the risk of weight gain (i.e., overweight, obesity, or both). Thirty publications (15 cross-sectional, 10 prospective, and 5 experimental) were selected on the basis of relevance and quality of design and methods.

Findings from large cross-sectional studies, in conjunction with those from well-powered prospective cohort studies with long periods of follow-up, show a positive association between greater intakes of SSBs and weight gain and obesity in both children and adults. Findings from short-term feeding trials in adults also support an induction of positive energy balance and weight gain by intake of sugar-sweetened sodas, but these trials are few. A school-based intervention found significantly less soft-drink consumption and prevalence of obese and overweight children in the intervention group than in control subjects after 12 months, and a recent 25-week randomized controlled trial in adolescents found further evidence linking SSB intake to body weight.

The weight of epidemiologic and experimental evidence indicates that a greater consumption of SSBs is associated with weight gain and obesity. Although more research is needed, sufficient evidence exists for public health strategies to discourage consumption of sugary drinks as part of a healthy lifestyle.

In our house analogy, it is likely that rats have built a nest in your old home. There will be spider webs, ants, mice, crickets, termites, etc. These pests will damage your home and steal your food if you don't get rid of them. So it is with our bodies. Heavy metals in our tissues and biotoxins (chemicals that damage our cells) will have concentrated in our livers and gall bladders because those organs try to remove these pests from our bodies—often unsuccessfully.

Most of these toxic things are fat-soluble (dissolved in the fat of our bodies). This is particularly true of our cell membranes and our brains, endocrine glands, and livers. Since they are fat-soluble, they tend to get stored and concentrated in our livers and gall bladders. Bacteria, viruses, and fungi then tend to grow in our gall bladders and produce more toxins. In this manner, our livers and gall bladders become a "rat's nest" that must be cleaned out for us to start feeling better.

Gall Bladder

There are many misconceptions about the gall bladder. Note the following facts:

1. The gall bladder is a very important organ, not something to be disposed of if it annoys you. The same symptoms of pain, bloating, and heartburn occur in 50 to 100 percent even after you have had your gall bladder removed. More than 500,000 North Americans have their gall bladders removed every year.

2. The liver makes 1 1/2 quarts of bile per day to digest fats. Since the liver can't make bile fast enough to digest a fatty meal, the gall bladder is necessary to store bile. Without the gall bladder, you can't do a good job of digesting fats. Since every cell membrane in the body is made of fat, if you can't digest the fats, you can't repair your cells (heal) without help.

3. Forty percent of Americans have abdominal pain, bloating, loose stools, and symptoms often thought to be from the stomach (heartburn due to gas pushing stomach acid into the esophagus), fever and chills, nausea and vomiting, and yellowing of the skin—all due to gall bladder malfunction.

4. The most likely people to make gallstones are fair complexion, female, fat, fertile (previous pregnancies), and over forty (known as the "five Fs").

5. Gall stones are more common in people who eat a low fat

diet, obesity, take oral contraceptives, and take calcium, estrogen, antibiotics, and non-steroidal anti-inflammatory drugs.

Here are some ways to help clean the gall bladder:

1. Gall bladder flush: The first thing in the morning, drink one teacup of grapefruit juice with two tablespoons of extra virgin olive oil. Do not drink or eat anything else for thirty minutes. At bedtime, take two more tablespoons of extra virgin olive oil and a teacup of either grapefruit or prune juice. Repeat the morning and evening juice/oil for seven days. Also, each day for seven days, drink one quart of apple juice to soften any stones.

2. Taurine is an amino acid needed to make bile. You will need to take 1000 mg/day. In studies, 100 percent of those taurine-deficient developed gallstones. In those given taurine supplements, the formation of gallstones dropped to zero.

3. Vitamin C: Take 2000 mg/day.

4. You should plan on taking vitamin C long term.

If you have had your gallbladder removed, you will need to take bile salts (ox bile) 500 mg every time you eat.

Liver Cleanup

The liver, the largest solid organ, is the body's detoxification center and a vast center for metabolic activity including:

1. Lipid/carbohydrate/protein metabolism
2. Blood synthesis
3. Bilirubin metabolism
4. Urea cycle
5. Ammonia detoxification

6. Biliary processes
7. Bile and cholesterol synthesis
8. Oxidative energy metabolism
9. Hormone metabolism
10. Immune function (Kupffer cells)
11. Clearance of drugs (pharmaceuticals)
12. Processing of nutrients, toxins, and bile acids from the intestine.

The liver's detoxification processes has three distinct phases. The purpose is to change fat-soluble toxins into water-soluble products that can be excreted from the body. Conversion of cholesterol into bile is a primary process in the elimination of wastes. Thus high cholesterol often is a symptom of the liver attempting to clear toxins from the body and should not be interrupted with anti-cholesterol drug therapy:

Phase I: polarity is increased by a process called oxidation or hydroxylation using enzymes called PP450 oxidases. It requires oxygen as toxins are burned or oxidized. Elevation of very long chained fatty acids is indicative of interruption of Phase I.

Phase II: toxins are made more water soluble using oxidation, reduction, hydrolysis, dehalogenation, methylation, sulfation, glucuronidation, peptide conjugation, acetylation, and glutathione conjugation.

Phase III: toxins ported from cells for removal via gallbladder and kidneys.

When detoxification is occurring, nitrogen may be retained involving albumin, uric acid, BUN, or creatinine. Ammonia levels rise due to impaired ability to convert ammonia into urea.

I prefer to use essential oils to help support and clean the liver along with bile to allow fat to be absorbed to make new liver cells.

Remember that the liver replaces itself every eight weeks and weighs 4.6 pounds—that takes a lot of fat. If you can't make adequate bile because your liver is dirty or you don't have a gall bladder, it will be difficult for you to absorb enough fat to keep your liver working correctly.

Liver Cleanse: Make a tea and drink every bedtime for three months: Place 5–7 drops of Dr. Tennant's Liver Cleanse Essential Oils into a cup of hot water. Add one tablespoon of coconut oil and 1–3 teaspoons of local raw honey. You may drink hot or add ice.

NOTE: Therapeutic essential oils come from plants. The fragrance of each oil can be made in a laboratory, but they have no therapeutic effects. Essential oils contain mixtures of hundreds of compounds. For example, orange oil has thirty-four alcohols (a form of chemical that the body needs), thirty esters, twenty aldehydes, fourteen ketones, ten carboxylic acids, and thirty-six terpenes. This cannot be duplicated in a lab. Do not purchase your oils at a health food store since 95 percent of oils there have no therapeutic effect! You can get the oil blend for a liver cleanse by calling my office at 972-580-1156.

Oral butyrate therapy addresses both control of nitrogen in states of increased blood ammonia and interruption of abnormal lipid metabolism. It also clears what are called "renegade fats" from the liver. If essential oil therapy is not adequate to achieve normal liver function, taking butyrate capsules is often helpful. It tastes bad and often leaves an aftertaste, but it works.

Vitamin B12

According to John V. Dommisse, MD, an expert in vitamin B12 (cyanocobalamin) deficiency and therapy, the psychiatric conditions most associated with vitamin B12 deficiency include toxic brain syndrome, paranoia, violence, and depression. There is a well-documented association between B12 deficiency and dementia. In an article entitled "Subtle Vitamin B12 Deficiency in

Psychiatry: A Largely Unnoticed but Devastating Relationship?" published in Medical Hypotheses 2, Dommisse expresses the opinion that most cases of so-called "Alzheimer's dementia" ("idiopathic dementia") are actually cases of B12 deficiency. According to Dommisse, B12 deficiency can cause depression and even, in certain cases, bipolar-1 disorder (manic-depressive illness) and, more commonly, bipolar-2 disorder (cyclothymic personality).

Says Dommisse: "The third most common psychiatric manifestation of this deficiency is violent behavior, yet how often is this deficiency ever sought or treated in criminal cases of violent behavior? I have witnessed numerous cases of rage attacks, temper outbursts, domestic violence, etc., where the violence ceased after the patient's B12 deficiency was diagnosed and properly treated."

The fourth and last major psychiatric effect of this deficiency is paranoid ideation and even paranoid psychosis (but not schizophrenia).

Fatigue is another symptom of vitamin B12 deficiency but the medical community has been slow to recognize the connection. "Even after major articles, like that of Lindenbaum in the New England Journal of Medicine in 1988," says Dommisse, "fatigue is still not recognized as a prominent feature of B12 deficiency syndrome. Peripheral neuropathy is another non-psychiatric condition that can result from this and other B vitamin deficiencies. However, by the time the deficiency is recognized (serum level below 200 pg/ml), just as in the case of the dementia, the neuropathy may well have become irreversible. Then the treating physician will say, 'See, B12 treatment does not reverse dementia (or neuropathy)!'"

A major point by this author is that the range used to establish serum vitamin B12 deficiency in conventional medicine (less than 200 to 400 pg/ml) is far too low. When peripheral neuropathy occurs in this range, it is often permanent. The author suggests that 1,000 to 2,000 pg/ml may be the optimal range. The hydroxy- and methyl- forms of vitamin B12 are generally recommended.

Cyanocobalamin at high doses has never been shown to be toxic. Oral doses of 1,000 to 5,000 ug daily have been used in cases of pernicious anemia to maintain these patients' vitamin B12 levels. Oral doses of 1,000 to 2,500 ug after both breakfast and supper seem the best way to maintain very high levels of serum vitamin B12.

Symptoms of B12 deficiency include:

Anemia	Schizophrenia
Pale, smooth tongue	Dizziness
Brown spots over joints	Sore tongue
Paranoia	Irritability
Bursitis	Temper outbursts
Poor memory	Mood swings
Dementia	Tingling
Psychosis	Nausea
Depression	Violence
Restlessness	Negative thinking
Diarrhea	Weakness

Any child with violent tendencies, especially when accompanied by fatigue and neuropathy, should be tested for vitamin B12 deficiency. An acute condition can be treated with oral supplements or vitamin B12 injections. In the long term, the best protection is a diet rich in animal foods.
http://www.westonaprice.org/children/childviolence.html

One should be mindful of the relationship between B12 and folate (folic acid). Both are needed for methylation, and a deficiency of either can produce anemia. Always correct both if deficient. If the blood test for homocystein is high, always use the methyl forms of

B6, B12, and folate.

Glutathione

Glutathione is known as the master antioxidant (electron donor), the director of the immune system, and the director of detoxification.

Glutathione is critical in the management of your voltage. When an electron donor gives up its electrons, the donor can become a stealer. Glutathione readily supplies the electrons to restore your electron donor to its donor status so it can help again.

Glutathione is not significantly absorbed from the gut, so taking it doesn't help. However, it is made in every cell in the body by assembling the amino acids cysteine, glycine, and glutamine. Thus the key is for you to be sure to consume those amino acids.

Poor diet, pollution, toxins, medications, stress, trauma, aging, infections, and radiation all deplete your glutathione.

Glutathione has multiple functions:
1. It is the major antioxidant produced by the cells, participating directly in the neutralization of free radicals and reactive oxygen compounds, as well as maintaining exogenous antioxidants such as vitamins C and E in their reduced (electron donor) forms.
2. It detoxifies many foreign compounds and carcinogens, both organic and inorganic.
3. It is essential for the immune system to exert its full potential, e.g.:
   a. Modulating antigen presentation to lymphocytes, thereby influencing cytokine production and type of response (cellular or humoral) that develops
   b. Enhancing proliferation of lymphocytes thereby

increasing magnitude of response
   c. Enhancing killing activity of cytotoxic T cells and NK cells
   d. Regulating apoptosis, thereby maintaining control of the immune response
4. It plays a fundamental role in numerous metabolic and biochemical reactions such as DNA synthesis and repair, protein synthesis, prostaglandin synthesis, amino acid transport, and enzyme activation. Thus every system in the body can be affected by the state of the glutathione system, especially the immune system, the nervous system, the gastrointestinal system, and the lungs. – Wikipedia
5. It is necessary for converting T4 to T3 (thyroid hormones). It is also necessary to transfer electrons from the cell membrane to the mitochondria.

Supplementing has been difficult, as research suggests that glutathione taken orally is not well absorbed across the gastrointestinal tract. In a study of acute oral administration of a very large dose (3 grams) of oral glutathione, Witschi and coworkers found that "it is not possible to increase circulating glutathione to a clinically beneficial extent by the oral administration of a single dose of 3g of glutathione."

However, plasma and liver glutathione concentrations can be raised by oral administration of S-adenosylmethionine (SAMe), glutathione precursors rich in cysteine include N-acetylcysteine (NAC) and whey protein, and these supplements have been shown to increase glutathione content within the cell.

N-acetylcysteine is available both as a drug and as a generic supplement. Alpha lipoic acid has also been shown to restore intracellular glutathione. Melatonin has been shown to stimulate a related enzyme, glutathione peroxidase, and silymarin, an extract of the seeds of the milk thistle plant (Silybum marianum) has also demonstrated an ability to replenish glutathione levels.

Low glutathione is also strongly implicated in wasting and negative nitrogen balance, notably as seen in cancer, AIDS, sepsis, trauma, burns, and even athletic overtraining. Glutathione supplementation can oppose this process and in AIDS, for example, result in improved survival rates. – Wikipedia

The least expensive way to restore and maintain your glutathione levels is to drink raw milk or make milkshakes from non-denatured whey protein. This usually means that the whey was obtained from non-pasteurized (raw) milk.

Summary

We get well and stay well by making new cells that work. To make a new cell requires -50 millivolts of energy and the raw materials to make a cell. If you have toxic things or infections nearby, the new cell will be damaged as well.

We are going to discuss the primary things that reduce voltage:
1. Hypothyroidism
2. Lack of stomach acid
3. Dental infections
4. Scars
5. Lack of exercise

The primary rule you should remember is that anything you put into the body that cannot be used to make a new cell or provide voltage for that cell must be eliminated from the body at some cost to the system. That includes chemicals used as pharmaceuticals or preservatives in our food, toxins in our environment, materials used for dental fillings that leech chemicals like mercury, chemicals in things we put on our skin like soap and cosmetics, dirty air we breathe, etc.

The basic diet must be one that has not been raised/cultivated with chemicals and has not been processed to increase the shelf life. Do most of your shopping around the perimeter of the grocery store where you find produce. If it contains something you can't pronounce, don't consume/use it.

Stop Consuming Toxins

1. Stop smoking
2. Stop drinking coffee, black tea, alcohol
3. Stop eating artificial sweeteners
4. Stop eating MSG
5. Stop eating soy
6. Stop eating plastic fats (partially hydrogenated) and canola oil
7. Get chloride filter for water and stop using fluoridated toothpaste
8. Stop using microwave

Bibliography

For an extensive bibliography, contact the author at jtenn@tennantinstitute.com or see Healing is Voltage, the textbook written by the author.

6 Hypothyroidism

In this chapter, we are going to discuss the causes of a major epidemic in the United States. The symptoms of the epidemic— obesity, hypertension, diabetes, high cholesterol, heart attacks, depression, etc.—are well known. However, the root causes of

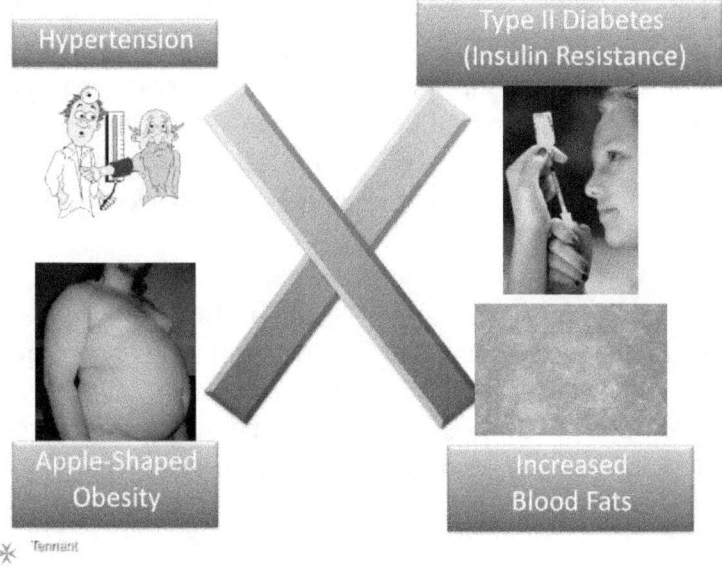

these miseries are not well known.

To discuss hypothyroidism, we must first discuss metabolic syndrome X and iodine deficiency as this understanding is necessary to understand hypothyroidism. Most doctors agree that what is called metabolic syndrome X is responsible for most of the illnesses in the United States. So what is metabolic syndrome X?

The symptoms and features of metabolic syndrome X are:
1. Fasting hyperglycemia – diabetes mellitus type II or impaired fasting glucose, impaired glucose tolerance, or insulin resistance
2. High blood pressure

273

3. Central obesity (also known as visceral, male-pattern or apple-shaped adiposity), overweight with fat deposits mainly around the waist
4. Decreased HDL cholesterol and elevated triglycerides

Obesity

Obesity requires some special attention. When you are bigger around the waist than around your hips, you are said to have "apple obesity." This type of obesity is associated with illnesses such as heart attacks, strokes, diabetes, gall bladder disease, and cancer. When you are bigger around your hips than around your waist, you are said to have "pear obesity." This is associated with hormonal imbalances but is not as likely to cause heart attacks, strokes, and cancer.

A major contributor to obesity is MSG. Leptin is a hormone released to tell your brain that you are full. MSG damages the brain so that it does not recognize leptin. Thus you always feel hungry. MSG is put in foods because it is addicting and makes you want to eat more, resulting in more profits for the food manufacturers.

MSG is hidden in foods by calling it "other spices." Additives that always contain MSG:
1. Textured protein
2. Autolyzed yeast
3. Hydrolyzed oat flour

Metabolic syndrome is an epidemic that also includes stress, anger, heart attacks, ADHD, migraine headaches, and childhood and adult obesity with depression.

Traditional medicine has not found a solution for metabolic syndrome X except for diet and exercise. Often diet and exercise alone will not reduce blood pressure, correct diabetes, correct blood lipids, or allow you to lose weight. Metabolic syndrome X often proceeds to fibromyalgia. Doctors typically prescribe pills to lower blood pressure, pills to lower blood sugar, pills to lower cholesterol, and a band around your stomach without asking why you got these illnesses in the first place.

It is my opinion that metabolic syndrome X is simply type II hypothyroidism. After six to twelve months of therapy for hypothyroidism, most cases of hypertension, diabetes, high cholesterol, and obesity return to normal without other therapies. Studies have also shown that eighty percent of arthritics will be normal.

A significant cause of obesity is lack of stomach acid. We discussed this in the chapter on nutrition.

Another significant cause of obesity is consuming high fructose corn syrup, especially in sodas. One soda a day increases your weight one pound per month. If you gain twelve pounds per year, in five years you are sixty pounds overweight just from one soda per day!

Another cause of obesity is high glycemic index foods. These are foods that are rapidly digested and results in a spike of insulin. The excess glucose is stored in fat cells and the body cannot use this glucose when insulin is present as discussed in the chapter on nutrition. The high glycemic index foods are primarily the white foods: white flour, white rice, white sugar and white potatoes. Instead you should eat whole grain flour, whole grain rice, stevia, and sweet potatoes.

As we will discuss later in this chapter, metabolic syndrome with insulin resistance is often the result of an increase in rT-3 relative to T-3. This is associated with obesity as well.

Iodine Deficiency

Most people know that the thyroid uses lots of iodine to make thyroid hormone. The thyroid gland gets to use iodine before other parts of the body. However, most people don't know that every gland in the body that secretes something needs large amounts of iodine. Iodine is the "truck" that carries the secretion from inside the cell to outside the cell. Thus most cysts in the body are due to iodine deficiency as the secretions are accumulated inside the cells to form cysts.

A partial list of cells that secrete is given below.
1. Thyroid: has highest concentration
2. Salivary glands
3. Cerebrospinal fluid and brain
4. Intestinal mucosa (esophagus, stomach, small intestine, large intestine)
5. Choroid plexus
6. Breasts
7. Ovaries
8. Vagina and uterus
9. Prostate
10. Ciliary body of the eye
11. Nose, sinuses, mouth
12. Substantia nigra of the brain
13. Conjunctiva of the eye
14. Stomach acid
15. Digestive enzymes in pancreas
16. Liver and gall bladder
17. Skin
18. Bone marrow
19. Pancreas
20. Adrenal glands
21. Kidney
22. Lung

Note that this list is the same organs that typically get cancer!

The Japanese consume a lot of seaweed and thus a lot of iodine. They have the least amount of cancer of anyone on the planet. The only kind of cancer they have in excess is stomach cancer. Iodine is inactivated by nitrates (found in processed meats like bologna and hot dogs), and when they eat processed meats, this inactivates the iodine in their stomachs, allowing them to get stomach ulcers and stomach cancer. It is apparent that iodine is protective against cancer.

Iodine kills all single-celled organisms like viruses, bacteria, fungi, and protozoa.

Jean Lugol, a Paris physician, in 1829 discovered that iodine is more soluble in water that contains potassium iodide. This is the basis for "Lugol's solution." Lugol's solution implies that it is water based. "Tincture of iodine" means it is in an alcohol base whereas Lugol's solution is water based.

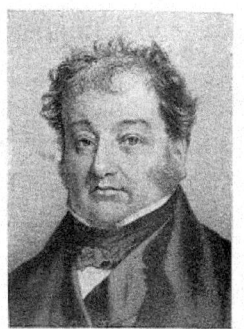

Iodine is bactericidal even at dilutions of 1:170,000! Microorganisms do not develop resistance to iodine.

Iodine is so important in brain development that iodine deficiency is the leading cause of intellectual impairment in the world! (ADD/ADHD?)

Hypothyroidism is one of the leading causes of violent behavior in the world.

It was suggested by Campbell in the "China Study" that the reduction in cancer and heart disease in Asia was due to a vegetarian diet, but the differences may well be in the amount of iodine consumed and not in the amount of meat eaten. The China

Study was an epidemiological survey and not a study in which one group gets one substance and other group gets a placebo.

The parts of the body exposed to the outside world have iodine levels thirty times the blood level. Iodine is the immune system's "bug killer." That is, it is the bug killer for bugs trying to enter the body. For example, if you breathe in a flu virus and you have enough iodine in the lining of your nose, it will kill the virus before it has a chance to enter the system.

Once a microorganism is in the body, it is attacked by white blood cells. Neutrophils, a type of white blood cells, contain hydrogen peroxide to kill the bacteria. Vitamin C creates hydrogen peroxide in the body, increasing the efficiency of the immune system.

Drinking Lugol's solution or taking dehydrated Lugol's in capsule form is the best treatment for food poisoning as it kills the bacteria.

Lugol's solution will inactivate snake venoms.

Nitrates (hot dogs, bologna, processed meats) inactivate iodine and allow Helicobacter pylori to grow in the stomach and cause stomach ulcers/cancer.

If large foreign proteins are ingested, they are inactivated by iodine preventing them from becoming allergens. Iodine is necessary to make stomach acid. Humans should never absorb proteins. We must only absorb amino acids to make our own proteins. When we don't have stomach acid because we are deficient in iodine, zinc, and vitamin B1, we absorb whole proteins. The immune system recognizes that the body didn't make these proteins and assumes they are invaders. It makes antibodies to attack them. Having enough iodine to make stomach acid thus helps prevent food allergies.

The energy in fats is contained in their double bonds. These double bonds are protected by iodine.

Fetal iodine is five times the level in the mother. Low maternal iodine can lead to miscarriage, birth defects, failure to thrive, mental retardation, etc.

There are only micrograms of iodine in table salt and some of the companies are using bromine instead of iodine because it is cheaper (and toxic). Sea salt contains almost no iodine! Adults need 12–15 milligrams of iodine per day! Because of our farming practices, there is very little iodine in our soils. About the only people in the United States with normal levels of iodine are those who eat seaweed frequently.

Every person should be taking iodine to prevent infections and cancer. One can take it orally since it doesn't go into the large intestine to kill the good bacteria. It isn't well absorbed through the skin.

The easiest way to take iodine is as Lugol's solution dehydrated into capsule form. Generally, they are in 12.5 mg capsules. It is often necessary to take 50 mg per day for three to four months to allow the body to catch up from its deficiency. Then take one capsule of 12.5 mg/day.

Remember that you need iodine to protect you against infections and cancer whether your thyroid is functioning normally or not. You also need it to make every organ that secretes something work.

Up to ninety percent of the American population has undiagnosed hypothyroidism! This epidemic is causing havoc with our mental and physical health. It is easily and inexpensively treated. The primary cause is fluoride in our water and dental products and lack of iodine. Soy also shuts down the entire endocrine system including the thyroid.

I can't urge you strongly enough to read the web site http:// poisonfluoride.com/pfpc/index.html. You will quickly discover how toxic fluoride is and that the symptoms of hypothyroidism and fluoride poisoning are the same. See the following table. What you will see is that the symptoms of hypothyroidism and fluoride poisoning are indistinguishable.

The numbers are references to medical articles from which the data was taken. The left column is hypothyroid symptoms and the right is fluoride poisoning symptoms. Note they are essentially the same!

The reference list takes up about twenty pages so they are not included in this book. If you want them, go to the website listed above.

FLUORIDE POISONING	THYROID DYSFUNCTION (Iodine Deficiency)
Abnormal Sweating (18)	Abnormal Sweating (154, 155, 156)
Acne (2,3)	Acne (52)
FLUORIDE POISONING	THYROID DYSFUNCTION (Iodine Deficiency)
ADHD/Learning Disorders (4,7)	ADHD/Learning Disorders (54)
Allergies (2)	Allergies (52)
Alopecia (Hair-loss)(18)	Alopecia (151)
Alzheimer's Disease (5,6,46)	Alzheimer's Disease (98)
Anaphylactic Shock (2))	Anaphylactic Shock (124
Anemia (15)	Anemia (67)
Apnea (Cessation of breath)	Apnea (52)
Aorta Calcification (2)	Aorta Calcification (100)
Asthenia (Weakness) (18)	Asthenia (97)
Asthma (2)	Asthma (129)
Atherosclerosis (3)	Atherosclerosis (59)

Arthralgia (2)	Arthralgia (58)
Arthritis (8, 13)	Arthritis (52, 58)
Ataxia (2)	Ataxia (66)
Autism (169)	Autism (170, 171)
Back Pain (2)	Back Pain (153)
Behavioral Problems (3)	Behavioral Problems (54)
Birth Defects (5)	Birth Defects (53)
Blind Spots (3)	Blind Spots (52)
Body temperature disturbances (13)	Body temperature disturbances (52)
Breast Cancer (5)	Breast Cancer (147)
Cachexia (wasting away)(2)	Cachexia (133)
Carpal Tunnel Syndrome (5)	Carpal Tunnel Syndrome (52)
Cataracts (2)	Cataracts (69)
FLUORIDE POISONING	THYROID DYSFUNCTION (Iodine Deficiency)
Change in blood pressure (2)	Change in blood pressure (52)
Chest pain (26)	Chest pain (52)
Cholelithiasis (Gallstones)(2)	Cholelithiasis (134)
Chronic Fatigue Syndrome (2)	Chronic Fatigue Syndrome (52)
Collagen breakdown (3)	Collagen Breakdown (99)
Cold Shivers (13)	Cold Shivers (52)
Coma (1,3)	Coma (65)
Concentration Inability (13,8)	Concentration Inability (52)
Constipation (52)	Constipation (52)
Convulsions (2)	Convulsions (81)

Crying easily for no apparent reason (18)	Crying easily for no apparent reason (52)
Death (3)	Death (123)
Decrease in Testosterone (32)	Decrease in Testosterone (96)
Dementia (2)	Dementia (54)
Demyelinizing Diseases (2, 35)	Demyelinizing Diseases (137)
Dental Abnormalities (2)	Dental Abnormalities (86)
Dental Arch smaller (27)	Dental Arch smaller (95)
Dental Crowding (23)	Dental Crowding (93)
Dental enamel more porous (29)	Dental enamel more porous (96)
Dental Fluorosis (Mottling of teeth)	Mottling of teeth (172)
Delayed Eruption of Teeth (28)	Delayed Eruption of Teeth (86)
Depression (8)	Depression (52, 97, 152)
Diabetes Insipidus (36a,b)	Diabetes Insipidus (120)
FLUORIDE POISONING	THYROID DYSFUNCTION (Iodine Deficiency)
Diabetes Mellitus (2)	Diabetes Mellitus (64)
Diarrhea (8)	Diarrhea (53)
Dizziness (8,13)	Dizziness (52)
Down's Syndrome (10)	Down's Syndrome (54)
Dry Mouth (2)	Dry Mouth (52)
Dyspepsia (8)	Dyspepsia (157)
Dystrophy (3)	Dystrophy (79)
Early/Delayed Onset of Puberty(14)	Early/delayed Onset of Puberty (53)
Eczema (2)	Eczema (115, 116)
Edema(3)	Edema (97)

Epilepsy (2)	Epilepsy (121)
Eosinophilia (15)	Eosinophilia (55)
Excessive Sleepiness (8)	Excessive Sleepiness (52)
Eye, ear and nose disorders (8)	Eye, ear and nose disorders (52)
Fatigue (2,13)	Fatigue (52)
Fearfulness (1,18)	Fearfulness (71)
Fever (13)	Fever (96)
Fibromyalgia (2)	Fibromyalgia (143)
Fibrosarcoma (3)	Fibrosarcoma (144)
Fibrosis (3)	Fibrosis (76a,b)
Fingernails:Lines/Grooves (1)	Fingernails:Lines/Grooves (97)
Fingernails:Brittle (1,3)	Fingernails:Brittle (97)
Forgetfulness (3)	Forgetfulness (97)
Gastro-disturbances (8)	Gastro-disturbances (52)
FLUORIDE POISONING	THYROID DYSFUNCTION (Iodine Deficiency)
Gastric Ulcers (2)	Gastric Ulcers (92)
Giant Cell Formation	Giant Cell Formation (135)
Gingivitis (19, 173)	Gingivitis (72)
Goiter (2)	Goiter (52)
Growth Disturbances (1)	Growth Disturbances (53)
Headache (2)	Headache (118)
Hearing Loss (5)	Hearing Loss (165)
Heart Disorders	Heart Disorders (52)
Heart Failure (3)	Heart Failure (109, 110)

Heart Palpitations (13)	Heart Palpitations (52)
Hepatitis (2)	Hepatitis (136)
Hemorrhage (1,2)	Hemorrhage (85)
Hives (3)	Hives (108)
Hoarseness (18)	Hoarseness (97)
Hyperparathyroidism (2)	Hyperparathyroidism (82)
Hypertension (8)	Hypertension (52, 60)
Hypoplasia (40)	Hypoplasia (150)
Immunosuppression (3)	Immunosuppression (52)
Impotence (3)	Impotence (97)
Incoherence (8)	Incoherence (54)
Infertility (2,3)	Infertility (87)
Inflammatory Bowel Disease	Inflammatory Bowel Disease (142)
Inner Ear Disorders (2,5)	Inner Ear Disorders (139)
Irritability (18)	Irritability (160)
FLUORIDE POISONING	THYROID DYSFUNCTION (Iodine Deficiency)
Joint Pains (8)	Joint Pains (52)
Kidney Failure (2)	Kidney Failure (125)
Lack of Energy (8)	Lack of Energy (52)
Lack of Coordination (2)	Lack of Coordination (52)
Loss of Appetite (2)	Loss of Appetite (97)
Loss of Consciousness (2)	Loss of Consciousness (138)
Loss of IQ (25)	Loss of IQ (83)
Loss of Spermatogenesis (33)	Loss of Spermatogenesis (102)

Low Birth Weight (5)	Low Birth Weight (158)
Lung Cancer (3)	Lung cancer (145)
Lupus (3)	Lupus (101)
Magnesium Deficiency (2)	Magnesium Deficiency (94)
Memory Loss (13)	Memory Loss (52)
Mental Confusion (20)	Mental Confusion (52,54)
Migraine (8)	Migraine (52)
Moniliasis (candidiasis) (162)	Moniliasis (candidiasis) (161)
More fluorosis/high altitudes (30,31)	More hypothyroidism/high altitudes (96)
Mouth Sores (2)	Mouth Sores (87)
Myalgia (Muscle Pain) (2)	Myalgia (58)
Myotrophy (Muscle wasting) (2)	Myotrophy (58)
Multiple Sclerosis (4)	Multiple Sclerosis (126)
Muscle Cramps (3)	Muscle Cramps (58)
Muscle Stiffness (3)	Muscle Stiffness (58)
FLUORIDE POISONING	THYROID DYSFUNCTION (Iodine Deficiency)
Muscle Weakness (2)	Muscle Weakness (57)
Musculoskeletal Disease (3)	Musculoskeletal Disease (80,57)
Nausea (8,13)	Nausea (52)
Osteoarthritis (2)	Osteoarthritis (62)
Osteoporosis (2)	Osteoporosis (62)
Osteosarcoma (22b)	Osteosarcoma (104)
Optic Neuritis (2)	Optic Neuritis (68)

Oral Squamous Cell Carcinoma (22)	Oral Squamous Cell Carcinoma (103)
Otosclerosis	Otosclerosis
Parkinson's Disease (5)	Parkinson's Disease (110,111)
Pins & Needles (18)	Pins & Needles (52)
Polydipsia (2)	Polydipsia (64)
Polyneuropathy (2)	Polyneuropathy (57)
Polyurea (2)	Polyurea (64)
Pyelocystitis (2)	Pyelocystitis (63)
Premature Delivery (16)	Premature Delivery (52)
Pruritis (Itchy Skin) (3)	Pruritis (113)
Pulmonary Edema (2)	Pulmonary Edema (114)
Recurring Colds (18)	Recurring Colds (52)
Respiratory Complications (13,8)	Respiratory Complications (52)
Restlessness (13)	Restlessness (52)
Retinitis (2)	Retinitis (128)
Rhinitis (38)	Rhinitis (6)
FLUORIDE POISONING	THYROID DYSFUNCTION (Iodine Deficiency)
Schizophrenia (18)	Schizophrenia (163, 164)
Scleroderma (3)	Scleroderma (74)
Skin Pigmentation (2)	Skin Pigmentation (97)
Secondary teeth erupt later (16)	Secondary teeth erupt later (86)
Sensitive to light (1,17)	Sensitive to light (52)
Seizures 913)	Seizures (88)
Shortness of Breath (13)	Shortness of Breath (52)

SIDS (16)	SIDS (54)
Sinus Infections (2,8)	Sinus Infections (52)
Swallowing Difficulties (Dysphagia) (13)	Swallowing Difficulties (52)
Swelling in Face (Angioedema) (3)	Swelling in Face (97)
Telangiectasia (166)	Telangiectasia (167, 168)
Testicular Growth/Alteration (2, 42)	Testicular Growth/Alteration (102)
Thirst (13)	Thirst (89)
Thrombosis (39)	Thrombosis (122, 141a,b)
Thyroid Cancer (22)	Thyroid Cancer (87)
FLUORIDE POISONING	THYROID DYSFUNCTION (Iodine Deficiency)
Tinnitus (8)	Tinnitus (52)
Tingling Sensations(18)	Tingling Sensations (52)
Visual disturbances (13,8)	Visual Disturbances (52)
Ulcerative Colitis (41)	Ulcerative Colitis (142)
Urticaria (2)	Urticaria (105, 106, 107)
Uterine Bleeding (2)	Uterine Bleeding (91)
Uterine Cancer (23)	Uterine Cancer (77)
Vaginal Bleeding (5)	Vaginal Bleeding (90)
Vas Deferens Alterations (5)	Vas Deferens Alterations (146)
Vertigo (8)	Vertigo (52)
Vitiligo (white spots/skin) (2)	Vitiligo (73)
Weak Pulse (13)	Weak Pulse (52)
Weight Disturbances (2)	Weight Disturbances (52)
Zinc Deficiency (2)	Zinc Deficiency (94)

How Does the Thyroid Work?

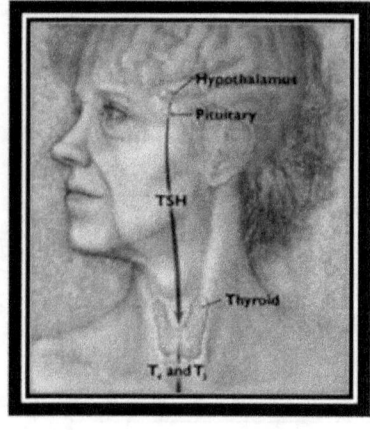

Thyroid Stimulating Hormone
TSH

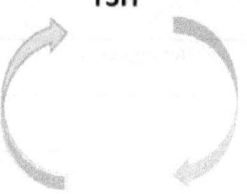

Thyroid Hormone
T4 ➤ T3

The pituitary gland produces thyroid stimulating hormone (TSH). It causes the thyroid gland to produce thyroid hormone (T-4). This thyroid hormone is converted to the active form T-3.

When more T-3 and T-4 are present, the pituitary stops making TSH. Thus they are in a "teeter-totter" or feedback relationship.

When we do blood tests, we expect the TSH, T-3, and T-4 to be in the normal range when the thyroid is functioning normally. If the TSH is high, we would assume the T-3 and T-4 are too low and the pituitary is trying to correct the situation. This would be called type I hypothyroidism.

If the TSH is low and the T-3 and T-4 are high, we would diagnose hyperthyroidism (overactive thyroid). Thus TSH tends to be the opposite of the T-3 and T-4 if you are not balanced.

We doctors tend to order these tests. If they are normal, we tell you that your thyroid is functioning just fine and don't consider that your physical findings are diagnostic of hypothyroidism. I am going to tell you why the lab tests haven't been working.

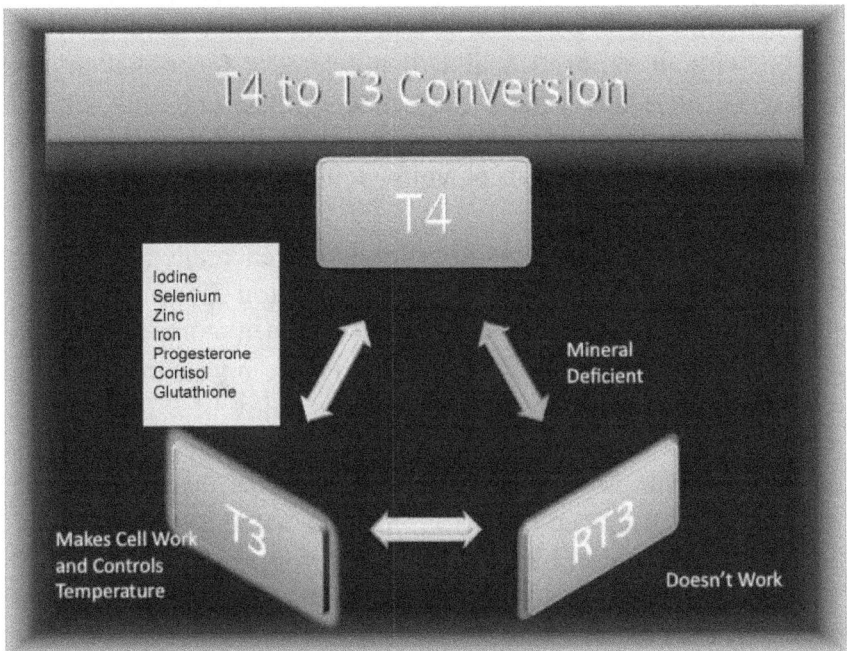

The active form of thyroid hormone is T-3. For a consistent thyroid function throughout the day, mammals normally make eighty percent T-4 and almost twenty percent T-3. (We also make a small amount of T-1 and T-2). Thus the T-4 must be converted to the active form of T-3. This conversion requires iodine, selenium, zinc, iron, progesterone, cortisol, and glutathione. If you are missing one of these, you can't convert T-4 to T-3 but instead convert it to a fake hormone called RT-3 or Reverse T-3. RT-3 blocks a receptor site but doesn't work. Thus you have normal levels of TSH and T-4 (and perhaps normal levels of T-3), but the thyroid isn't functioning at the cell level!

In addition, glutathione is necessary to move the T-3 from the cell membrane to the mitochondria inside the cell. If everything else is fine but you don't have glutathione, your thyroid system can't work at the power station (mitochondria) that needs it!

You can't absorb glutathione if you eat it. You must make it from three amino acids. You can't make amino acids if you don't have

289

stomach acid to break your proteins into amino acids. Thus a person without stomach acid will not have a functional thyroid system because that person can't make glutathione, and without glutathione, the thyroid doesn't work in the mitochondrial power station where it is used to keep voltages adequate.

This clearly explains a major problem I encounter. I tell my patients to get off antacids and drugs that stop the production of stomach acid. They see no connection between stomach acid and why they are chronically tired, so they ignore my instructions and can't figure out why they are too tired to enjoy life. Their doctor tells them that it is okay to block stomach acid and so it goes—a nation of people too tired to care and depressed because without stomach acid, they can't absorb zinc, and without zinc you can't make neurochemicals like serotonin and you can't convert T-4 to T-3. Thus we have a nation of people fat, tired, and depressed—all with normal blood tests!

Iodine is a halogen. The halogens are a series of nonmetal elements from the periodic table, comprising:
1. Fluorine, F
2. Chlorine, Cl
3. Bromine, Br
4. Iodine, I
5. Astatine, At

Here are the halogens in the periodic table:

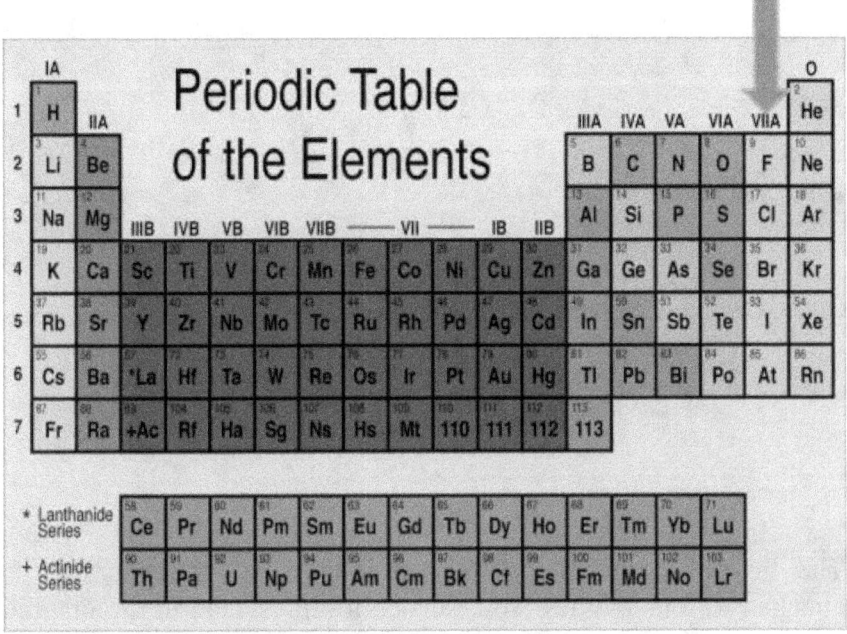

As you can see, the halogens are in a column in the periodic table of elements.

The problem is that fluoride is a "bully." Any time an atom of fluoride and an atom of any other halogen are in the same vicinity, the fluoride will displace the other halogen and take its place.

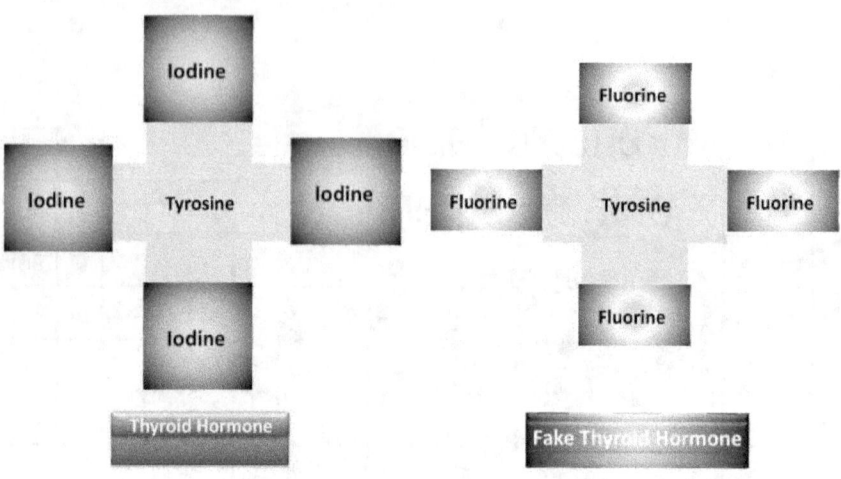

The thyroid hormone T-4 is a protein called tyrosine that is attached to four iodines. You can see it represented in the graphic as "thyroid hormone." However, when you consume fluoride, it displaces the iodine and you get the fake thyroid hormone noted in the right of the graphic.

One problem is that our blood tests can't tell the difference between the real and the fake hormone. Another problem is that the fake one doesn't work. Thus your blood tests are normal but your body is really deficient of functional thyroid hormone. This is called type II hypothyroidism. This form of type II hypothyroidism is often due to glutathione deficiency.

Type II hypothyroidism can also be due to a failure of the hormone to work at the cell membrane or mitochondrial level.

Because most Americans consume fluoride in water, toothpaste, visits to the dentist, etc., most Americans have type II hypothyroidism!

A great book that discusses the medical literature about this subject is Hypothyroidism Type II by Mark Starr, MD. Dr. Starr has made a major contribution to the health epidemics that are ravishing our country!

Another book you should read on this subject is Hypothyroidism, The Unsuspected Illness by Broda Barnes, MD.

Damage to Thyroid Gland from Fluoride

Many assume that if you stop consuming fluoride and take iodine, the thyroid function will return to normal. This is rarely the case. In 1996, Mahmood investigated the effects of low doses of sodium fluoride on the thyroid glands of guinea pigs.

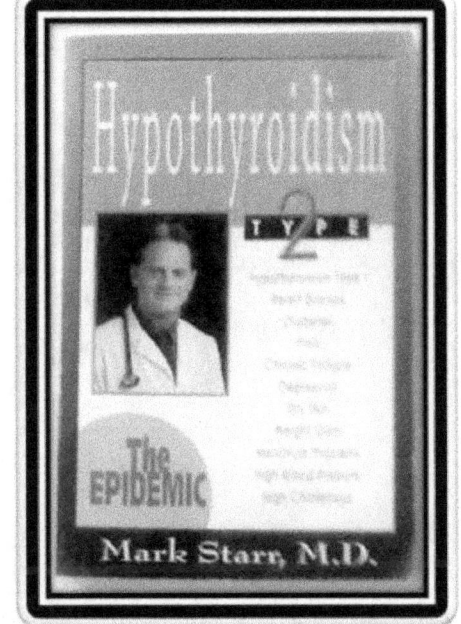

Findings were:
1. Depletion of colloid from the follicles
2. Shrinkage of follicles
3. Disruption of follicular basement membrane associated with edema and degeneration of the follicular epithelial cells
4. Increased follicular vascularity
5. Fatty degeneration in the inter-follicular connective tissue.

There is a condition of the thyroid gland called Hashimoto's disease. It is assumed it is an autoimmune disease. However, the description of Hashimoto's disease is the same as damage from fluoride. It is possible that Hashimoto's disease is simply fluoride damage.

Hashimoto's Disease

High power view of Hashimoto's thyroiditis showing lymphoid follicles within thyroid tissue. The arrow points to a germinal center. Note the small lymphocytes infiltrating between the follicular cells. The thyroid follicles are small, with no colloid, and the follicular cells have eosinophilic cytoplasm (Hürthle cells).

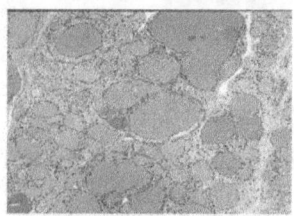

Normal Thyroid Hormone

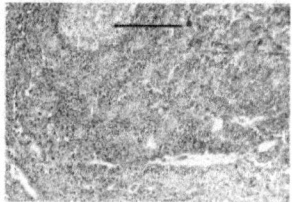

Hashimoto's Thyroid (Fluoride ?)

In the graphic, the upper image is of a normal thyroid gland. The lower one is Hashimoto's disease (fluoride damage?).

Since fluoride permanently damages the thyroid gland, most people require both iodine for its anti-infective effects and thyroid hormone to have normal thyroid function.

We are seeing an increase in the number of people with Hashimoto's disease. Remember that it is characterized by having antibodies to the thyroid gland. These antibodies will attack desiccated thyroid such as Armour and Nature-Throid. There is controversy about whether this matters. Even though the antibodies attack the proteins in the desiccated thyroid pills, it appears they do not attack the actual hormones since the blood tests of patients on desiccated thyroid with antibodies are still altered as you change the dosage of hormone.

We are also seeing a relationship between Hashimoto's disease and gluten sensitivity.

Other Causes of Hypothyroidism

Although fluoride is perhaps the major cause of hypothyroidism, there are other things that cause/contribute to it. A major issue is estrogen dominance.

Estrogen dominance means that you have effectively more estrogen than you do progesterone. That is true for female and males. Estrogen dominance shuts down the thyroid as well as often being associated with other issues such as breast and prostate cancer.

Estrogen dominance can be caused by soy, petrochemicals, fuel exhaust we breathe, estrogenic hormones in meat and chicken, plastics, propylene glycol (deodorants), sodium laurel sulfate in toothpaste and ointments, herbicides, and pesticides. These potent estrogenic substances block the production of thyroid hormone and greatly magnify the incidence of estrogen-dependent cancers. All males and females in developed nations have estrogen dominance. Obviously you should attempt to avoid these things:

1. Antibiotics
2. Chlorine from our water purification systems
3. Fluoride
4. NSAID drugs used for arthritis all kill the healthy bacteria in the intestinal tract. This results in overgrowth in the intestines of Candida, fungi, mycoplasma, and anaerobic bacteria (yeast syndrome). These dangerous organisms release powerful neurotoxic substances into the blood stream that damage the hypothalamus, often resulting in multiple endocrine disorders including under-activity of the thyroid gland.
5. Mercury released from our dental amalgams is toxic to the thyroid gland.
6. Selenium deficiency is related to lack of trace minerals in our soil. The proper conversion of precursors into thyroid hormone depends on a selenium-containing enzyme which is lacking.

7. Lack of iodine in our soil and diet leads to decreased thyroid hormone production.
8. Diagnostic x-rays injure the thyroid gland (dental, neck, spine).
9. Perchlorates widely found in drinking water inhibit the production of thyroid hormone by blocking the re-uptake of iodine.
10. Another cause of hypothyroidism is lack of vitamin C. The body uses vitamin C to make hydrogen peroxide. Hydrogen peroxide is necessary to convert T-4 to T-3.

How Can We Diagnose Hypothyroidism?

Thyroid hormone affects body temperature in a major way. Extensive research by Broda Barnes, MD, had shown that basal body temperature was a reliable way of diagnosing thyroid function. He did most of his work in the 1970s and much of Dr. Mark Starr's recommendations are based on the writings of Dr. Barnes.

The body keeps its core temperature constant at about 37 C by physiological adjustments controlled by the hypothalamus (Thermostat Center) where there are neurons sensitive to changes in skin and blood temperatures. The temperature-regulating centers are found in the Preoptic Area (the anterior portion of the hypothalamus). This area receives input from temperature receptors in the skin and mucous membranes (Peripheral Thermoreceptors) and from internal structures (Central Thermoreceptors), which include the hypothalamus itself. The temperature sensory signals from the preoptic area and those from the periphery are combined in the posterior hypothalamus to control the heat producing and conserving reactions of the body.

The activation of Sympathetic Centers results in several responses including:
1. Norepinephrine release from sympathetic fibers constricts skin vessels.

2. Brown fat (found in infants and some animals) oxidation increases causing thermogenesis.
3. Piloerection ("chilly bumps"), occurs when hairs stand up which traps air close to skin.
4. Adrenalin (epinephrine = adrenalin) secretion from adrenal medulla increases thermogenesis.
5. Shivering Center in the hypothalamus is also activated which activates the Brainstem Motor Centers to initiate involuntary contraction of skeletal muscles causing shivering, which generates heat.

Note that one of the mechanisms that controls temperature is adrenalin from the adrenal medulla. About 90% of the people I see in my office are deficient in adrenalin.

Vitamin A also has a role in temperature control. Since vitamin A is fat-soluble, if you don't have a functioning gall bladder, it can affect your temperature.

Many doctors including me have attempted to follow the teachings of Drs. Barnes and Starr by using temperature to diagnose hypothyroidism because of our lack of satisfaction with the TSH test commonly used to diagnose hypothyroidism. Using the TSH test as currently used by most physicians ignores and does not deal with the hypothyroid symptoms so many people have.

Over the last few years, I have encountered many patients that have low basal temperature but no matter how much thyroid I give them, their temperature remains low. It has become obvious that

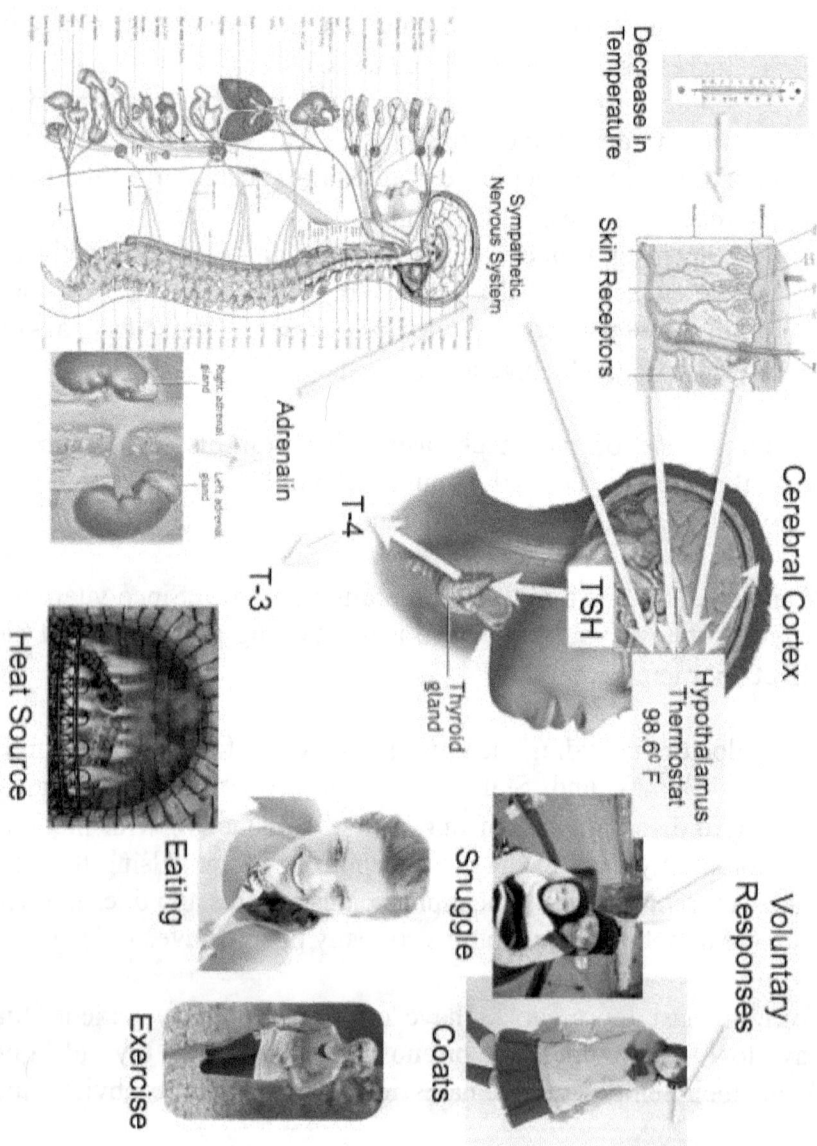

for about 20% of my patients, basal temperature does not work to identify and correct hypothyroidism.

I then took another look at the TSH test. It was invented in the late 1960s and put in place in 1971. They used only 29 patients (not a statistically adequate sample) to develop the normal. Normal was set as 1-10 and doctors were told to adjust their patients dose so that the TSH test was in this range. To get the test above 1, most patients had to have their dose of thyroid medication cut in half! Their symptoms returned but were ignored in order to get the blood test into the "normal" range. To this date, no study has ever compared symptoms to the TSH test.

Eventually it was noted that the 1-10 range wasn't working and it was gradually changed. In addition, more sensitive procedures were developed so that levels below 1 could be recognized. Currently most labs use 0.4 - 4.6 as normal.

Here is an excerpt from a January 2003 American Academy of Clinical Endocrinology press release:

"Until November 2002, doctors had relied on a normal TSH level ranging from 0.5 to 5.0 to diagnose and treat patients with a thyroid disorder who tested outside the boundaries of that range. Now AACE encourages doctors to consider treatment for patients who test outside the boundaries of a narrower margin based on a target TSH level of 0.3 to 3.0. AACE believes the new range will result in proper diagnosis for millions of Americans who suffer from a mild thyroid disorder, but have gone untreated until now."

In 2002, the National Academy of Clinical Biochemistry and the Academy of the American Association for Clinical Chemistry also made recommendations that normals for the TSH test be modified:

"NACB: Laboratory Support for the Diagnosis and Monitoring of Thyroid Disease: Published Guidelines" (US, 2002)
...given the high prevalence of mild (subclinical) hypothyroidism in the general population, it is likely that the current upper limit of the population reference range is skewed by the inclusion of persons with occult thyroid dysfunction....
...In the future, it is likely that the upper limit of the serum TSH euthyroid reference range will be reduced to 2.5 mIU/L

because >95% of rigorously screened normal euthyroid volunteers have serum TSH values between 0.4 and 2.5 mIU/L....

A serum TSH result between 0.5 and 2.0 mIU/L is generally considered the therapeutic target for a standard L-T-4 replacement dose for primary hypothyroidism.

Demers LM, Spencer CA. NACB. Laboratory Support for the Diagnosis and Monitoring of Thyroid Disease. Published guidelines. Online at The National Academy of Clinical Biochemistry (NACB) / The Academy of the American Association for Clinical Chemistry (AACC) (accessed 2003/09/08).

Thus our labs are about ten years late in updating their normal range for the TSH test. Assume your test comes back 4.0. The lab report says that normal is 0.4-4.6 and thus your doctor will tell you that your thyroid is working normally. However, with the updated normal of 0.3-2.0, you are very hypothyroid!

There are other problems with the TSH. It is unreliable while undergoing chemotherapy and with fever. The amount of TSH produced by the pituitary is controlled primarily by the amount of T-4 made by your thyroid gland. Thus the feedback mechanism of TSH/T-4 can be balanced so that the levels of TSH and T-4 are normal with current normal values. However, T-3 is the active form of hormone. So even with a normal TSH/T-4 balance, if you can't convert T-4 to T-3, you are still hypothyroid.

The conversion of T-4 to T-3 requires iodine, selenium, zinc, iron, progesterone, glutathione, cortisol, and hydrogen peroxide. In addition, the thyroid is under the control of the parasympathetic nervous system. If you are missing one of these vitamins/minerals, you will be deficient in T-3 even if your TSH/T-4 are normal.

In correcting hypothyroidism, one must first give enough T-4 to get the TSH below 1 but above 0.3. Then one must be sure to correct the vitamins/minerals to allow for conversion and add enough T-3 to get it close to 4.0.

The following is quoted from the LabCorp website:

Spurious increase from antibovine TSH antibodies by double-antibody technique has been reported. TSH may be affected by glucocorticoids, dopamine, and by severe illness, and these remain limitations even for the new, sensitive TSH assays. TSH suppression in hypothyroidism with severe illness has been reported with TSH increase with recovery. Normal TSH levels in the presence of hypothyroidism have been reported with head injury. Iopanoic acid, ipodate, and an antiarrhythmic drug, amiodarone, cause changes in thyroid test results including increases in T4, free T4, and TSH and decreases of T3. TSH is not elevated in secondary hypothyroidism.

Probably no single test, even the sensitive immunoassays, can be expected to adequately reflect thyroid status under all circumstances. Among possible problems are the recovery phase of nonthyroidal illness, states of resistance to thyroid hormone, thyrotropin-producing tumors, thyroid status in acute psychiatric illness, early in thyrotoxicosis and in subacute thyroiditis.

In patients who are receiving replacement therapy, the dose should be adjusted so serum TSH values range from 0.3-3.0 µIU/mL. An exception is thyroid hormone replacement treatment after thyroidectomy for differentiated thyroid cancer, in which case, a mildly to moderately suppressed TSH level is generally desirable. It is reasonable to consider serum TSH measurement for pregnant women or women planning to become pregnant with a family history of thyroid disease, prior thyroid dysfunction, symptoms or physical findings suggestive of hypo- or hyper-thyroidism, an abnormal thyroid gland on examination, type 1 diabetes mellitus, or a personal history of autoimmune disorder. Suggested upper limit for the TSH reference range for pregnant women and preconception is: first trimester is <2.5 µIU/mL, and 3.0 µIU/mL in the second and third trimesters.

It is of interest that this information never appears on lab reports. Lab reports list normal as 0.4-4.6. This leads to the majority of physicians under-diagnosing and under correcting most hypothyroid patients!

Traditionally, desiccated thyroid hormone has been the best choice for hormone replacement. It is dried (desiccated) thyroid gland from hogs. Thus it contains the hormone plus the proteins of the gland itself. If you don't have enough stomach acid to break these proteins into amino acids, you will develop antibodies to these proteins.

There is also a cross-reaction between gluten antibodies and anti-thyroid antibodies. We are seeing more and more people with both of these antibodies. When they are present, you may need to take a synthetic hormone that does not contain the proteins from the thyroid gland if you wish your hormone replacement to work. Thus a compounded T-4/ T-3 may be the best choice although some continue to do well on desiccated thyroid.

Some doctors recommend synthetic T-4 (levothyroxine, Synthroid) and synthetic T-3 (liothyronine, Cytomel). However the short half-life of T-3 sometimes results in one having too much effect during one part of the day and too little effect later as the effects of the hormone dissipate. Using a T-4/T-3 combination allows a smoother effect throughout the day as T-4 is converted by the body to T-3.

Giving T-3 by itself solves the problem of not being able to convert, but T-3 has very little suppression of TSH. Thus patients often feel good on sustained release T-3 but their TSH test can soar very high giving great alarm to many physicians when they see the test so high.

As we will discuss, one must be sure there is enough adrenal function to support the increased metabolism caused by correcting the thyroid function or the patient will feel worse as the thyroid is corrected.

Local Control of Thyroid Function

Cellular control of thyroid hormone (and thus cellular voltage) is primarily mediated by enzymes called deiodinase enzymes. There are three types of these enzymes:

1. Type I (D1): converts inactive T-4 to the active form T-3 throughout the body.
2. Type II (D2): converts inactive T-4 to the active form T-3 in the pituitary gland.
3. Type III (D3): reduces cellular thyroid activity by converting T-4 into Reverse T-3 (rT-3).

D1 (and thus conversion of the inactive T-4 to the active T-3 is suppressed by the following:

1. Physiological stress
2. Emotional stress
3. Depression
4. Dieting
5. Weight gain
6. Leptin resistance
7. Insulin resistance
8. Obesity
9. Diabetes
10. Inflammation
11. Autoimmune diseases (dental and other infections)
12. Systemic illness
13. Chronic fatigue
14. Fibromyalgia
15. Chronic pain
16. Exposure to toxins

17. Plastics

When any of the above are present, D1 activity is suppressed resulting in decreased thyroid function in the tissues but normal or increase thyroid function in the pituitary.

D1 activity is lower in females than in males making them more susceptible to these problems.

Some studies state that the amount of TSH produced by the pituitary is controlled by the amount of intra-pituitary T-3. Most doctors believe that it is controlled by the systemic level of T-4. Generally when you find a high TSH level and give supplemental T-4, the TSH decreases.

The pituitary contains little D1 (converts T-4 to T-3) and no D3 (converts T-4 to rT-3) so pituitary levels of T-3 are controlled by D2 (converts T-4 to T-3 in the pituitary). D2 is 1000 times more efficient at converting T-4 to T-3 than D1 is in the rest of the body. Because of this 80-90% of T-4 is converted to T-3 by D2 in the pituitary whereas only 30-50% of T-4 is converted to T-3 by D1 in the periphery. Because of this, giving supplemental T-4 gives a relatively higher amount of T-3 in the pituitary than in the periphery and suppresses TSH production greater than it increases cellular activity. This makes TSH levels much less reliable as an indicator of cellular activity than is recognized by most physicians.

There is another problem. Remember that D1 is suppressed from the illnesses/events listed above. This results in less T-3 being available to the cells. However, D2 is increased by the same list of illnesses/events resulting in increased T-3 in the pituitary with a lowering of TSH. Thus as tissues have less active T-3, the TSH actually drops. The lower TSH causes the thyroid to make less hormone and causes the physician to lower instead of raise the dose of thyroid hormone given to support thyroid function!

Since pituitary thyroid levels are controlled independently from the cellular thyroid levels (D1 versus D2), pituitary T-3 levels will always be higher than anywhere else in the body. Therefore even a mild elevation of TSH means that many of the body tissues will be deficient in T-3! Also a normal TSH cannot be a reliable indicator that there are normal levels of T-3 in the rest of the body. You must also look at Free T-3 (FT-3) and Reverse T-3 (rT-3) levels.

Remember that as T-4 levels drop in hypothyroidism, D2 increases and thus increases the levels of T-3 in the pituitary with a compensatory suppression of TSH even as tissue levels of T-3 are falling due to decreased T-4 to convert and a drop in efficiency of D1 to do the conversion. While serum T-3 may drop by 30%, tissue T-3 may drop 70-80%! One may end up with a normal serum TSH, T-4, and T-3 with a profound tissue hypothyroidism.

Chronic stress suppresses D1 (conversion of T-4 to T-3) with less cellular T-3 and increases D3 (converts T-4 to rT-3) so that rT-3 blocks receptors for T-3 resulting in diminished voltage in the cells. This may play a more important role in weight gain, fatigue, and depression than the elevated cortisol that is commonly associated with stress. Along with the decreased voltage of diminished T-3 at the cellular level one gets decreased oxygen, pain, decreased ATP, and infections.

Remember that stress commonly results in very low levels of adrenalin. This can be diagnosed with the Ragland Test. Take the blood pressure laying down and immediately on standing. The systolic (upper number) blood pressure should go up 10 points. If it doesn't, you are adrenalin depleted. Correct it with tyrosine, vitamin C, and vitamin B6. Also remember that lack of adrenalin makes your temperature low, another sign of hypothyroidism.

Lack of stomach acid to break proteins into amino acids including tyrosine means that you don't have the amino acid necessary to make adrenalin and thyroid hormone (tyrosine).

Almost all the autistic children/adults I have evaluated are hypothyroid. Studies also show that undiagnosed hypothyroidism is basic to depression and bipolar disorders. In the Journal of Affective Disorders 2009: 116:222-226, Kelly describes his study of bipolar disorder in those that had failed to respond to an average of 14 medications. Giving from 13-188 micrograms of T-3 with an average dose of 90.4 micrograms, 84% improved and 33% had a full remission of their bipolar symptoms!

One word of caution: when you give large doses of T-3 without any T-4, the TSH often rises to dramatic levels. I have seen them in the 80's. This makes many internists, family practitioners, and pediatricians spastic even if the patient feels good.

In Am J Psychiatry 2006; 163:1519-1530, Nierenberg reports on the use of T-3 in those that failed to respond to medication for depression. Using T-3 was found to be 50% more effective than antidepressant drugs even with the small dose of 50 micrograms.

Remember that chronic pain depletes adrenal function (both cortex production of cortisol and medulla production of adrenalin). It also down-regulates D1 and up-regulates D2 with the resultant normal to decreased TSH but low cellular T-3. Many of these patients are given narcotics and this further down-regulates D1. Almost all chronic pain patients need their tissue levels of T-3 and rT-3 evaluated and corrected.

Horm Metab Res. 2011 Feb;43(2):130-4. Epub 2010 Nov 22.
T3/rT-3-ratio is associated with insulin resistance independent of TSH.

Ruhla S, Arafat AM, Weickert MO, Osterhoff M, Isken F, Spranger J, Schöfl C, Pfeiffer AF, Möhlig M. Source
Department of Endocrinology, Diabetes and Nutrition, Charité-University Medicine Berlin,
Campus Benjamin Franklin, Berlin, Germany.
Abstract

Thyroid dysfunction has been shown to be associated with insulin resistance (IR). This may involve peripheral thyroid hormone metabolism, which is assumed to be reflected by the ratio triiodothyronine/reverse triiodothyronine (T3/rT-3-ratio). To explore a potential association between theT3/rT-3-ratio and IR we investigated pairs which differed in IR, but were matched by sex, age, body mass index (BMI), and thyroid stimulating hormone (TSH). For this purpose, matched pair analyses were embedded into a cross sectional study group.

22 pairs were matched from either the first or the third tertile of HOMA%S of a cohort of 353 euthyroid subjects with normal glucose metabolism who did not take any medication. The T3/rT-3-ratio was compared in the matched pairs. The T3/ rT-3-ratio was significantly increased in the insulin resistant subjects compared to their insulin sensitive partners (8.78 ± 0.47 versus 7.33 ± 0.33, p=0.019). Furthermore the T3/rT-3-ratio was lower in men compared to women (p for the within-subject effect=0.046) both in the insulin sensitive and the insulin resistant subjects. Here we show that theT3/rT-3-ratio, which is supposed to reflect the tissue thyroid hormone metabolism, is significantly increased in insulin resistant subjects. This further supports a link between thyroid function and IR.

The problem is we want to know how much FT-3 we have relative to the amount of rT-3. To be in best health, we want at least twenty times as much T-3 as rT-3, so a ratio greater than 20.

Labs report both FT-3 and rT-3 in two different ways, so we often have to do some conversion to make sure we are comparing apples to apples. Free T3 is sometimes reported as a number that is in the hundreds, like 332, and other times it is a number with only one digit before the decimal, like 3.3. Reverse T3 is reported differently also. Sometimes it is a number that is in the hundreds, like 240, and other times it is a two digit number like 24.

We have to make adjustments when the labs don't do it the way we like! So this is how to calculate the FT-3: Rt-3 ratio:

~take the FT-3 result

~multiply it by 100 if it's not in the hundreds
~multiply it by 10 if the rT-3 is in the hundreds

~divide by the rT-3 result

Example #1

Free T3 - 476

RT3 - 24

The FT3 is in the hundreds and the RT3 is a two digit number, so this is the simplest example.

This ratio is 476 / 24 = 19.8 (under 20, this means you have an RT3 issue although a very slight one)

Example #2

FreeT3 - 3.89

RT3 - 12

The FT3 is not in the hundreds so we have to multiply by 100.

This ratio is 3.89 * 100 / 12 = 32.4 (over 20, good)

Example #3

Free T3 - 389

RT3 - 312

The RT3 is in the hundreds so we have to multiply by 10. This ratio is 389 * 10 / 312 = 12.5 (well under 20, definite RT3 problem)

Example #4

Free T3 - 3.9 rT3 - 220

The FT3 is not in the hundreds, so we have to multiply by 100 AND the RT3 is in the hundreds so we have to multiply by 10, so we have to multiply by 1000 overall.

This ratio is 3.9 x 1000 / 220 = 17.7 (under 20, not good)

Just remember that you need the FT-3 to have one more digit to the left of the decimal place than the rT3 before you divide the FT-3 by the rT-3. So look at the rT-3 and see how many digits are to the left of the decimal. Move the decimal of the FT-3 to the right to give it one more digit to the left of the decimal than the rT-3. Now do the math. Example: FT-3 is 2.6. The rT-3 is 465. The rT-3 has 3 digits to the left of the decimal so we will move the FT-3 decimal to the right so it has one more digit or 2600. Then 2600/465 = 5.59. Since this is less than 20, you have a problem.

If you only have a T-3 reading rather than an FT-3 reading then the ratio of T-3 to rT-3 needs to be 10 or greater.

For a more thorough explanation of these enzymes and the references that support these comments, see www.nahypothyroidism.org. Click on the deiodinases tab.

Physicians that understand these issues have a dilemma. At a recent conference of the American Association for Anti-Aging Medicine, it was stated that the primary reason that physicians lose their license is to prescribe thyroid hormone when the TSH is normal. Lab values for "normal" are ten years out of date. As we have been discussing, you can have a normal TSH, T-4 and even T-3 and still have a 70-80% reduction of T-3 at the cellular level. Without looking at the FT-3 and rT-3 levels and treating those, patients suffer.

So what's a doctor to do? The best advice I can give is to push the TSH down to 0.3 with T-4 and push the FT-3 up to 4.0 with T-3. Look at the FT-3/rT-3 ratio and correct if necessary. Be sure to supplement with the vitamins and minerals necessary to convert T-4 to T-3.

This approach may not be optimal but it is defensible when the state medical board challenges whether you are practicing "standard of care" medicine.

The other problem is finding a doctor that understands any of this.

Special Signs of Hypothyroidism

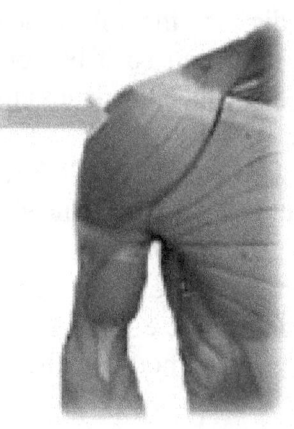

Mucin is like clear Karo syrup. It is deposited into the tissue in hypothyroid patients. It is mistaken for fat in metabolic syndrome X. People with hypothyroidism and metabolic syndrome X have a combination of fat and mucin in their tissue. If you pinch over your deltoid muscle, you should be able to almost put your fingers together. Any bulk you feel is mucin. When you make mucin, it begins to fill your whole body with "goo." However, it tends to collect in a special pattern. The face becomes round. There is a pouch under the chin. The shoulders appear that you were wearing shoulder pads. The area over the deltoid becomes rounded. The chest becomes shaped like a barrel. Breasts become pendulous. You become bigger around the waist than the hips ("beer belly"). The buttocks become large and wide. The thighs touch in the middle of the legs.

Although there is a long list of symptoms from hypothyroidism, common complaints are weight you cannot lose, insomnia, dry skin, poor memory, bouts of anger, constipation, and hair loss.

Remember that metabolic syndrome X has the following features:
1. Fasting hyperglycemia – diabetes mellitus type 2 or impaired fasting glucose, impaired glucose tolerance, or insulin resistance
2. High blood pressure

3. Central obesity (also known as visceral, male-pattern, or apple-shaped adiposity), overweight with fat deposits mainly around the waist
4. Decreased HDL cholesterol and elevated triglycerides – when mucin is inserted into the tissues, the cells are surrounded by goo. This makes it more difficult for insulin to be able to access the cell membrane. You develop "insulin resistance" and type II diabetes. One of the problems with using medication to lower the blood sugar is that it also lowers the amount of glucose getting into the cells.

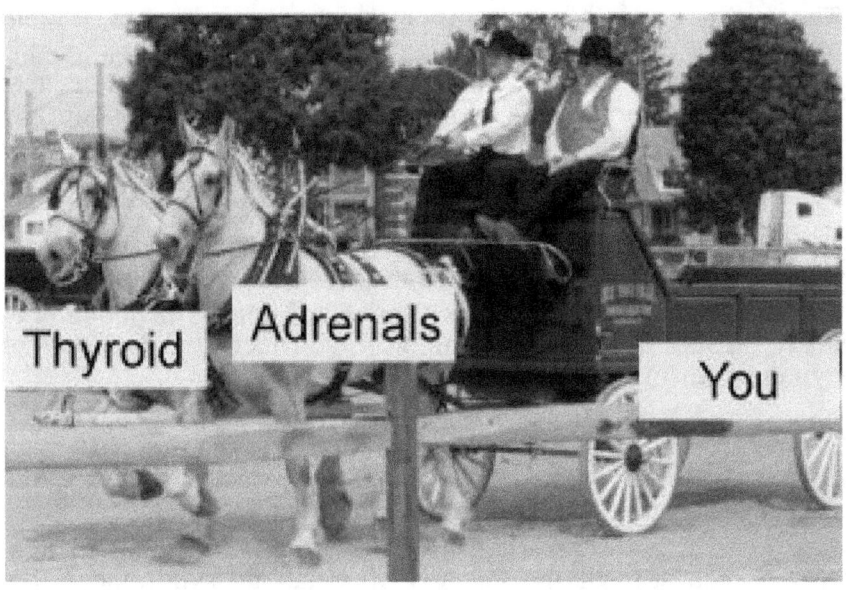

Think of thyroid and adrenals as two horses in a team that are pulling your wagon (the thyroid and adrenals are making the rest of you work). The first horse to lie down is the thyroid horse. When that happens, the adrenal horse tries to keep pulling. Thus as you become hypothyroid, your adrenals "keep pushing through." You keep trying to do what you need to do with sheer willpower even though your voltage is low because you don't have enough thyroid hormone that works. However, eventually the adrenal horse wears out too. Now your wagon isn't going anywhere!

Blood pressure, voltage, and symptoms are good guides of where you are on this spectrum. As you fill your body with mucin and

311

your adrenals make more adrenalin, your blood pressure tends to go up to push through the mucin and, in response, to the adrenalin. However, as your adrenals fail, your diastolic blood pressure tends to drop below normal. You will also notice that you feel dizzy as you first stand up from lying down because you don't have the adrenalin to compensate for your change in position and gravity.

When you are making mucin and depositing it into the omentum and the parts of the body described above, you appear to be obese. In addition, when you are hypothyroid, you crave sugar and caffeine to give you a little "spark." This extra sugar does add fat to the mix, particularly if you drink high fructose sodas.

The entire endocrine system depends upon adequate thyroid hormone to function and make other hormones. Most of the hormones are made from cholesterol. When the liver notices that you are hormone deficient, it makes more cholesterol to help you make more hormones. Suppressing the liver's ability to make cholesterol further reduces your hormone levels.

In addition, the brain is fifty percent cholesterol by weight. It replaces itself every eight months. If there isn't enough cholesterol available, one cannot make hormones and repair the brain. For many years, high cholesterol was considered diagnostic of hypothyroidism.

A careful review of the medical literature shows that high cholesterol levels of any kind do not increase the risk of dying from a heart attack. This will be discussed in another chapter.

As you can see, all the features of metabolic syndrome X are features of hypothyroidism. This explains the epidemics of hypertension, diabetes, obesity, high cholesterol, heart attacks, strokes, depression, ADHD, anxiety, chronic fatigue, and cancer that plague Americans.

More about Fluoride and Hypothyroidism

It has been known since 1917 that fluoride causes goiters. F.S.McKay, DDS, noted that people in Colorado Springs, Colorado, had mottled teeth. He also noticed that they didn't get cavities. In 1918, Professor Greves in Utrecht, Holland, noted that people who drank the local water got both mottled teeth and goiters (goiters are usually associated with hypothyroidism). It was later determined that the water in Colorado and Holland had high levels of naturally occurring fluoride. McKay is credited with the idea of supplementing fluoride to prevent cavities. Unfortunately, trading a few cavities for heart attacks, strokes, diabetes, cancer, etc., is not a good trade.

In 1919, Goldemberg in Argentina also noted that people who drank the local water with high levels of fluoride developed goiters. He reviewed the literature and concluded that hypothyroidism was caused more by high levels of fluoride than low levels of iodine. In 1926 he reported on his use of fluoride to treat hyperthyroidism (overactive thyroids).

In 1932, Machoro (Italy) used sodium fluoride in the successful treatment of hyperthyroidism. In 1932, Wilhelm May (Germany) also started fluoride therapy in the treatment of hyperthyroidism, and in 1933, Gorlitzer von Mundy (Austria) reported more on fluoride's effect on the thyroid.

The amount of fluoride they used to combat an overactive thyroid is the same amount we put in our city water supply. Thus we are treating almost our entire population with a therapy known since 1926 to shut down thyroid function.

In 1934, Purjesz and colleagues (Poland) gave chicken eggs high in fluoride to hyperthyroid patients and achieved lowering of body temperature, of pulse and BMR, as well as weight gain. They reported that most of the fluoride is found in the liver; no fluoride is found in the blood of healthy people.

1937 – Kraft (Knoll AG, Germany) investigates inorganic sodium fluoride and organic fluoride compounds fluorobenzoic acid and fluorotyrosine and reports that all fluoride compounds inhibit thyroid hormones. It is a matter of amplification—the fluoride component is essential.

1941 – Wilson (UK) reports in the Lancet on his findings that mottling of teeth is prevalent in the same areas in the UK that had previously been prevalent with goiter.
1941 – Schwarz (Germany) prepares fluoride/iodide anti-thyroid medications and combines with sedatives.

1946 – The Atomic Energy Commission (Department of Pharmacology & Toxicology—headed by Harold Carpenter Hodge, incomprehensibly at the same time also head of the International Association for Dental Research)— acknowledges the German findings that all fluoride compounds—organic or inorganic—inhibit thyroid hormone activity and declares this issue a research priority. No further research into this issue is conducted, however.

1952 – In the court case Reynolds Metals Corp. versus Paul Martin hypothyroidism caused by fluoride is documented.

1953 – Wadwhani (India) reports that fluoride is concentrated in the thyroid glands of rats consuming 0.9mg fluoride per day.

1957 – Galetti et al. treat hyperthyroid patients with fluoride at daily doses lower than those estimated being the current average intake in the United States and documents a significant reduction in protein-bound iodine, as well as an overall reduction of iodine and a reduction of iodine uptake by the thyroid gland.

1959 – Jentzer again shows reduced iodine levels in the pituitary gland under the influence of fluorides.

1960 – Gordinoff and Minder describe the results of experiments with radioactive iodine (I131) which show that fluorides remove an iodine atom during the conversion process (T-4 to T-3). Effects are dose-responsive, meaning the higher the fluoride intake the lower the iodine measurements.

1962 – Steyn (Africa) reports that drinking water containing "as little as 1 to 2 ppm of fluorine can cause serious disturbances of general health and especially in normal thyroid gland function and in the normal processes of calcium-phosphate metabolism (parathyroid function)."

1962 – Spira reports on the fluorine-induced endocrine disturbances in mental illness.

1963 – Gorlitzer von Mundy reports on the [then] current knowledge gained from experiments by Gordonoff with I131 as to how the effects of the enzymes responsible for the T-4 to T-3 conversion were inhibited if a fluorine ion was absorbed before the conversion from T-4 to T-3 occurs.

1969 – Siddiqui shows small visible goiters in persons fourteen to seventeen years of age in India to be connected directly to high fluoride concentrations in drinking water.

1991 – Lin Fa-Fu et al. reports that a low iodine intake coupled with "high" (0.88ppm) fluoride intake exacerbates the central nervous lesions and the somatic developmental disturbance of iodine deficiency. The authors consider the possibility that "excess" fluoride ions affected normal de-iodination. Fluorides caused increase of reverse T-3 (rT-3) and elevated TSH levels, as well as increased I131 uptake (see: Bachinskii et al., 1985).

2008 – Remember that fluoride damages collagen anywhere in the body. This is one of the reasons it is a major cause of heart attacks, back pain, weak knees, etc. I will discuss this in the chapter on heart disease.

Some people's Achilles tendons rupture after only one dose of an antibiotic made with fluoride. On July 8, 2008, the FDA announced that a so-called "black-box" warning would be added to the package insert, or label, to strengthen existing warnings about the increased risk of developing tendonitis and tendon rupture associated with the following fluoroquinolones:
1. Ciprofloxacin (marketed as Cipro and generic ciprofloxacin)
2. Ciprofloxacin extended release (marketed as Cipro XR and Proquin XR)
3. Gemifloxacin (marketed as Factive)
4. Levofloxacin (marketed as Levaquin)
5. Moxifloxacin (marketed as Avelox)
6. Norfloxacin (marketed as Noroxin)
7. Ofloxacin (marketed as Floxin and generic ofloxacin)

This is a very small sample of the medical literature on the toxicity of fluoride. For more information, see http:// poisonfluoride.com/ pfpc/html/thyroid_history.html.

The point is that you must avoid fluoride if you are to be healthy. Don't sacrifice your health to avoid a few cavities.

One thing that will help detoxify the fluoride is boron. Boron is also present in turmeric.

Paradoxical Hypothyroidism

A minority of people with hypothyroidism are skinny, have a rapid heartbeat, and suffer tremors and anxiety. The only way to diagnose hypothyroidism in them is the temperature and the fact that their symptoms disappear with thyroid therapy. Thyroid is one of the few diseases where too little hormone or too much hormone can give you exactly the same symptoms! The temperature is the key to figuring out what is happening.

TSH and Osteoporosis

In the early 1990s it was suggested that very low levels of TSH (and thus too high levels of thyroid hormone) were associated with osteoporosis. For this reason, doctors are currently taught to lower the amount of thyroid hormone taken if the TSH is lower than "normal." Remember that the TSH and T-3-4 labs are made incorrect by fluoride!

A December 2003 medical journal review article conducted a systematic review of the effects of TSH-suppressive (such as in thyroid cancer) and replacement levothyroxine therapy (Synthroid) on bone mineral density to determine the main causes of the conflicting results and their implications. The goal of the review was to evaluate existing studies in order to provide guidance for patient management and to recommend the directions that future studies of this question should take.

Included in the review were sixty-three separate English-language studies published from 1990 to 2001 that were identified by a

Medline search. Many of these studies were designed to determine whether the patients taking thyroid hormone replacement had a reduction in bone mineral density. What the reviewers found was of interest to patients and practitioners: All studies provided results that were considered by the reviewers to be either limited and/ or controversial.

Of the sixty-three studies reviewed:
1. Thirty-one reported no effects of levothyroxine on bone mineral density
2. Twenty-three studies found partial beneficial or adverse effects
3. Nine studies showed overall adverse effects.

It is quite common for patients to feel great on their thyroid hormones until their doctor does blood tests. The tests show a low TSH suggesting they are taking too much thyroid hormone. The TSH is low because both the real hormone they are taking and the fake fluoride hormone reduce the TSH. Their doctor tells them to reduce or stop their thyroid pills because the TSH is low. They feel terrible, but their doctor pays attention to the faulty blood test and not to the patients' symptoms!

Treating Hypothyroidism

You will need to take thyroid hormone as well as correct your iodine levels as discussed above. There is some argument about whether to use synthetic thyroid hormones like Synthroid (levothyroxine) or take a naturally occurring hormone like desiccated thyroid hormone. The best known brand name for desiccated thyroid hormone is Armour Thyroid. It is desiccated pork thyroid. (After over one hundred years, Forest Labs quit making Armour Thyroid in 2009 and reformulated it later. However, desiccated thyroid is available from RLC Labs under the trade names Nature-Throid and Westhroid.)

Synthetic thyroid hormones can cost two to five times as much as desiccated hormone. There is a strong pressure on doctors from medical boards and the FDA to prescribe synthetic drugs instead of bioidentical hormones. The question is, "Which works the best?"

Desiccated thyroid hormone contains T1, T2, T-3, and T-4 in the natural balance. Synthroid contains only synthetic T-4. Remember that the active form of thyroid is T-3. Also remember that fluoride inhibits the conversion of T-4 to T-3. Thus it can be difficult to find the right dose of Synthroid, especially since doctors are trained to find the correct dose using blood tests that are inactivated by fluoride and have outdated normal values.

There are synthetic T-3 hormones available like Cytomel. The problem with giving just T-3 is that it is short lived. If you take enough of it to correct your needs for hormones, you will often have spells during the day in which you feel hyper and jittery and other times when you are exhausted. One of the advantages of desiccated thyroid hormone is that it can slowly convert T1, T2, and T-4 to T-3 as needed. Many patients have been converted from Synthroid to desiccated thyroid hormone and feel much better.

Drug salespeople tend to say that desiccated thyroid hormone has inconsistent hormone amounts where synthetics are always the same. The opposite appears to be true. There have been recalls for the synthetics because they contained wrong amounts of hormones. The following is from the Armour Thyroid website:

"To ensure that Armour Thyroid tablets are consistently potent from tablet to tablet and lot to lot, analytical tests are performed on the thyroid powder (raw material) and on the actual tablets (finished product) to measure actual T-4 and T-3 activity. Different lots of thyroid powder are mixed together and analyzed to achieve the desired ratio of T-4 to T-3 in each lot of tablets."

Synthroid has been recalled by the FDA multiple times for containing an amount of thyroid hormone different from the label. The FDA also posted that it cannot recommend Synthroid since it has never been tested! (See letter from FDA to Synthroid manufacturer)

318

DEPARTMENT OF HEALTH & HUMAN SERVICES   Public Health Service

---

Food and Drug Administration
Rockville MD 20857

AUG - 1 1997

TRANSMITTED VIA FACSIMILE

Robert Ashworth, Ph.D.
Director, Regulatory Affairs
Knoll Pharmaceuticals
199 Cherry Hill Road
Parsippany, NJ   07054

RE: Synthroid
MACMIS ID # 5632

Dear Dr. Ashworth:

Reference is made to Knoll Pharmaceutical Company (Knoll's)
advertisements for Synthroid.   These advertisements contain the
claims "Synthroid The Measure of Excellence in Thyroid Hormone
Replacement Therapy" and "The Rule in Dispensing Thyroid Hormone
Replacement."   The Division of Drug Marketing, Advertising and
Communications (DDMAC) has reviewed these advertisements and
finds them to be in violation of the Federal Food, Drug, and
Cosmetic Act and the applicable regulations.

Specifically, DDMAC objects to the following claims and
representations:

- The headlines "Synthroid, The Measure of Excellence in
  Thyroid Hormone Replacement Therapy" and "The Rule in
  dispensing Thyroid Hormone Replacement," and the graphic of
  a large ruler are misleading because they suggest that
  Synthroid is the reference standard by which levothyroxine
  products are measured.   These ads also contain reference to
  FDA determinations in bulleted statements under these
  headlines, suggesting that this standard or "measure" was a
  determination made by the agency.   However, neither
  Synthroid nor any other levothyroxine product is currently
  recognized by the FDA as a reference product or standard for
  levothyroxine products.

Dr. Robert Ashworth   Page 2
Knoll Pharmaceuticals
Synthroid

- The claims "There is no substitute for Synthroid," "FDA has
  not determined bioequivalence among levothyroxine sodium
  products," "No AB rating according to the FDA Orange.Book,"
  and "No proven bioequivalent product" are misleading. These
  claims suggest that Synthroid is the standard for
  levothyroxine products; that it is superior to other
  levothyroxine products; and that no other levothyroxine
  product is equivalent to or useful in place of Synthroid.
  However, Knoll fails to reveal facts material to such
  representations. For example, such facts material to
  Knoll's representations include information that such
  determinations have not been made by FDA because the
  information and applications necessary to make such a
  determinations have not been submitted to the agency. We
  also note that at least some data comparing the
  bioequivalence of Synthroid and other levothyroxine products
  is under the control of Knoll, but that Knoll has not made
  the data available for independent review by FDA.

Accordingly, DDMAC has determined that the dissemination of these
misleading advertisements by Knoll causes Knoll's product,
Synthroid, to be misbranded. Knoll should immediately
discontinue these advertisements and all other promotional
materials that contain similar issues or themes. DDMAC requests
that Knoll submit a written response by August 15, 1997 and
include a list of all materials that have been discontinued.

If Knoll has any questions or comments, please contact me by
facsimile at (301) 594-6771, or at the Food and Drug
Administration, Division of Drug Marketing, Advertising and
Communications, HFD-40, Rm 17B-20, 5600 Fishers Lane,
Rockville, MD 20857. In all future correspondence regarding the
materials discussed in this letter, please refer to MACMIS ID
#5632 in addition to the NDA number.

                         Sincerely,

                         Anne M. Reb, NP
                         Regulatory Review Officer
                         Division of Drug Marketing,
                             Advertising and Communications

Synthetic hormones are usually dosed in micrograms. Desiccated
thyroid hormone is measured in grains or milligrams. One grain is
approximately 60 mg. In many cultures, a grain is a unit of
measurement of mass that is based upon the mass of a single seed
of a typical cereal. Historically in Europe, the average masses of
wheat and barley grain were used to define units of mass. Since
1958, the grain or troy grain (Symbol: gr.) measure has been

defined in the International System of Units as precisely 64.79891 milligrams. However, it is common to round it off to 60 milligrams

Correct Thyroid Slowly

If you put new tires, battery, and gas in an old car and drive it 90 miles per hour, it will blow a gasket. One must start slowly at first. The same will happen to you if we give too much thyroid too quickly. We must work up slowly so we don't aggravate your system, particularly your heart.

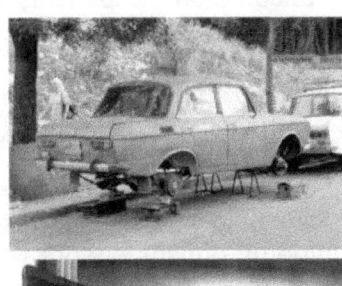

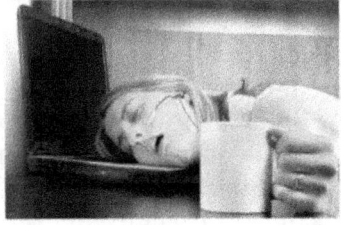

instead of 65 milligrams.

Most adults who have been consuming fluoride will need to take about three grains (180 milligrams) of desiccated thyroid hormone per day. However, if you start with that much, you will "blow a gasket." By that I mean that you will feel jittery, have a fast heartbeat, an increase in blood pressure, and just feel terrible. Thus you must start slowly and work up, giving your body time to make new mitochondria to use the hormone. Start with one-quarter grain (15 mg) in the morning and again at about 3:00 p.m. for a total of one-half grain (30 mg/day). After 2-4 weeks, repeat the TSH, FT-3 and rT-3 and adjust as necessary.

As you continue increasing the dose, nothing much will happen for the first two months, so don't be discouraged. After about two months, your energy will start to rise. Notice that it often takes about six months to achieve the correct dose.

The mucin does not tend to leave the body until the thyroid dose is normal. That is about six months. Most of the weight loss happens between the six and twelfth month. Generally speaking, you will be at your ideal weight at the end of a year if you are simultaneously correcting stomach acid production, avoiding foods you are allergic to, and stop consuming high fructose corn syrup and white foods. However, you will likely not lose weight unless you exercis. You will have to correct any adrenal insufficiency and correct mineral, vitamin, and glutathione levels as well.

It is not uncommon for patients to require up to five grains (300 mg) of desiccated thyroid per day or the equivalent of compounded T-4/T-3 to achieve normal values and feel good. However, I don't give more than 180 mg/day without carefully reviewing whether there is compliance for the other things mentioned above.

Remember that thyroid hormone requires a prescription in the United States, so you will need to find a doctor that understands type II hypothyroidism to work with you.

WARNING!
Many are tempted to ramp up the dose of thyroid hormone too fast. They are impatient to get rid of the fatigue and extra pounds and do not pay attention to not increasing the dose by more than one-half grain (30 mg) (T-4/T-3 25/6.2) per month. This can be dangerous or even fatal! Don't do it! The common symptoms that you are taking too much thyroid hormone are:

1. Anxiety
2. Confusion or disorientation
3. Heart palpitations
4. An irregular heart rhythm (arrhythmia)
5. High blood pressure (hypertension)
6. A rapid heart rate (tachycardia)
7. Seizures
8. Strokes
9. Coma
10. Death

If you develop any of these symptoms while you are taking thyroid hormone, reduce your dose or stop taking it until you can talk to your doctor or see an emergency room doctor. You can have problems if you just stop taking it altogether as well. Let your doctor help you adjust the dosage.

Summary

Thyroid hormone is pivotal in good health. Cells cannot perform correctly without having -20 to -25 millivolts. Neither can they perform their chemical reactions correctly if the temperature is too low. Forty percent of T-3 is used by the cell to maintain body temperature and sixty percent is used to maintain body voltage. Thus without enough functional thyroid hormone, your cells can't work correctly and you will be fatigued and sick.

Unfortunately, doctors are trained to only look at lab tests with outdated normals and ignore your symptoms. Fluoride, soy, and other toxins shut down your thyroid gland and make fake thyroid hormone.

Lab normals are created by looking at the results in a few people considered normal. If most of those tested have been consuming fluoride and soy, the lab "normals" will be "normal" for sick people!

It is very hard to feel normal unless you get the thyroid and adrenal levels normal.

7 Cholesterol and Heart Disease

Because understanding how medical studies are manipulated to confuse doctors and others on the efficacy of drugs, I am repeating the information about absolute risks versus relative risks in this chapter. It is also discussed in another chapter.

Understanding Medical Studies

Besides publishing only positive studies and hiding negative ones, publishing fake studies, and only indexing twenty percent of the studies, another deceit has come into prominence. It is the difference between absolute risk and relative risk.

A good explanation of this problem is described in the book *The Illusion of Certainty: Health Benefits and Risks* by Ed Bouwer and Eric Rivkin, from Johns Hopkins University.

Absolute risk is your risk of developing a disease over a specified time. Absolute risk reflects the number of people who will be harmed compared to the total number of people being considered.

If six out of one hundred get a disease and die, the AR (absolute risk) is 6/100 or 0.06 or 6 percent.

Absolute risk reduction is the difference between two absolute risks in two groups. In the above example, if people take a drug and only four out of one hundred get the disease and die, the ARR is 6% - 4% = 2% (0.02). Two lives are saved out of one hundred.

ARR compares the number of people who will benefit from intervention to the total number of people being considered.

Relative risks are based on the ratio of two absolute risk numbers. When using relative risks, the absolute risk levels for the experimental and control groups may not be known. If taking a new drug reduces the number of disease deaths from six out of one hundred (6%) to four out of one hundred (4%), then the relative risk difference is 33 percent (0.33) because 4 percent is 33 percent less than 6 percent. The absolute risk difference is 2 percent (6% - 4%). However, 33 percent sounds much better than 2 percent.

Let's say we looked at ten thousand people, five thousand of whom chewed bubble gum and five thousand who did not. If one of five thousand who chewed bubble gum had a heart attack and two out of the five thousand who did not chew bubble gum had a heart attack, we could report that only half as many people developed a heart attack if they chewed bubble gum. The FDA would then allow us to market bubble gum as preventing fifty percent of heart attacks because the relative risk is 0.50. It would be reported in our study as RR 0.50 (95% CI) 0.40-0.60.

This ignores the fact that 0.02 percent of those who chewed bubble gum had a heart attack while 0.04 percent of those that did not have the same event. Certainly one case different between the two groups is not significant. However, it can be reported as a relative risk of fifty percent.

This is a significant problem in that almost all medical studies are now reported with relative risk instead of absolute risk. This sleight-of-hand reporting is the primary way that physicians are tricked into believing that drugs work.

This graph is from the MRFIT study and shows deaths versus cholesterol levels. It assumes a current benchmark of 200 mg/100 milliliters.

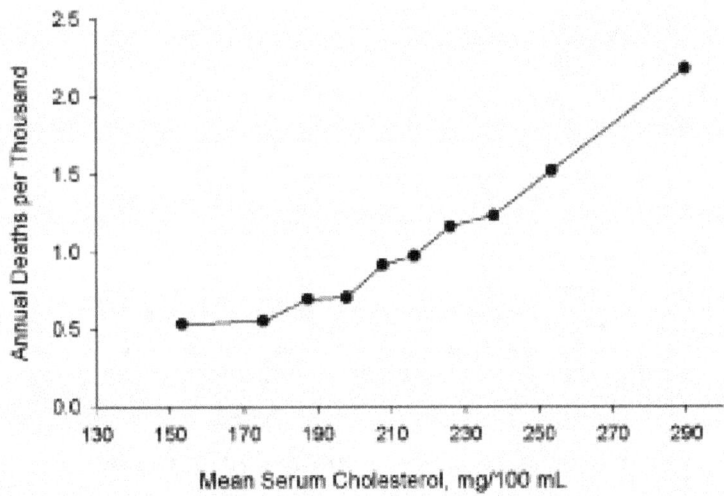

Mean Serum Cholesterol, mg/100 mL

"Is Relationship Between Serum Cholesterol and Risk of Premature Death from Coronary Heart Disease Continuous and Graded? Findings in 356,222 Primary Screenees of the Multiple Risk Factor Intervention Trial (MRFIT)," Stamler, J., Wentworth, D., and Neaton, J.D., *JAMA* (1986 Nov 28), 256(20): 2823–8, ISSN: 0098-7484.

Out of two thousand people with cholesterol over 200 mg/100 milliliters, there will be one additional death each year from CHD as compared to two thousand people with "normal cholesterol." This means that 99.95 percent of the population would not benefit from efforts (diet and/or drugs) to reduce blood serum cholesterol levels.

This graph is the same data as above except the data line has been trended and the y-axis extended to make it more visual how little difference cholesterol makes in deaths per

327

thousand.

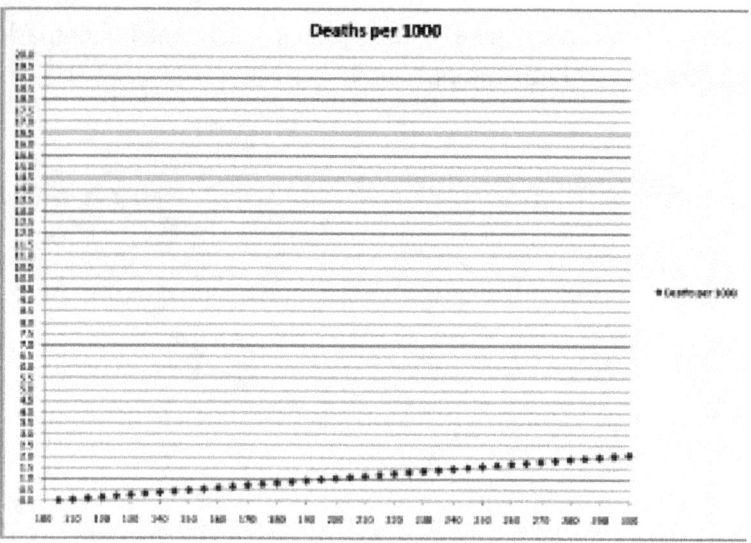

To put it another way, for 1,999 out of 2,000 individuals each year, it makes no difference whether they have elevated cholesterol or normal cholesterol in terms of whether they develop coronary heart disease!

Clearly it doesn't make much sense to focus so much time, energy, and money on the subject of cholesterol. Despite the science, the politics of medicine says that doctors should lose their license if they don't put patients with "elevated" cholesterol on statin drugs. The American Heart Association states that you are at high risk of coronary heart disease if your cholesterol level is above 240. However, the study showed that the cholesterol of 240 is only 0.5percent more likely to have a heart attack than those with the cholesterol of 200! Economics versus Science at work again!

Current guidelines suggest that anyone with cholesterol over 180 should be put on statin drugs. If you have a heart attack, you are put on statins no matter how low your cholesterol already is.

Statin drugs cost between $900 and $1,400 per year per person. This means that we waste about $12.5 billion per year in therapies that are not supported by science for cholesterol treatment alone. Now expand this into all areas of medicine. It then becomes easy to see why Americans spend more money on health care than anyone in the world and yet have outcomes equivalent to Third World countries.

Cholesterol is one of the most critical chemicals needed by the body. However, it has been characterized as a pest that must be stamped out at all costs. Cholesterol is necessary for the following reasons:

1. Serves to waterproof each cell
2. Repair of injuries: all scars, including those we call plaque in arteries, contain large amounts of cholesterol
3. Making Vitamin D
4. Making bile
5. Mineral metabolism
6. Cholesterol is an antioxidant (electron donor)
7. Memory
8. Uptake of serotonin in the brain
9. One-half of the dry weight of the brain is cholesterol
10. Making adrenal hormones that control all sugar metabolism
11. Making adrenalin so we can deal with stress
12. Making sexual hormones
13. Control of allergies

We physicians have another great burden—the legal and insurance systems. When we determine that we have been mislead by our peers with fictitious studies or by the FDA, CDC, etc., as in the case of mercury, we want to change the way we treat our patients. However, the insurance industry has set up "standards of practice" that tells doctors how they must treat patients. If we don't follow those guidelines, we can be charged with malpractice.

Often we are caught between doing what we know is right and being sued for malpractice. Doctors often choose doing what we know is wrong to enable us to keep our license and our reputation for integrity, our homes, money, etc., that we have worked years to achieve. Only a few states offer physicians the ability to let their patients choose "standard of practice" care or "scientifically proven" care.

I am going to prove to you that the medical literature does not support the theory that cholesterol has anything significant to do with coronary artery disease. To do so, I must first talk about why we doctors became confused about the role of cholesterol and fats in causing heart attacks and strokes.

It is known that heart attacks and strokes happen when a substance made primarily of calcium and cholesterol is found in the wall of an artery. This is called "plaque." Over time, the plaque can enlarge and cause turbulence in the flow of blood over it. When a blood clot forms suddenly on the plaque, blood can no longer flow and the tissue beyond the plaque/clot dies for lack of blood and oxygen.

Because the plaque contains cholesterol, it was theorized that high levels of cholesterol in the blood leak through the walls of the arteries causing the plaques. It was assumed that consuming cholesterol would raise the levels of cholesterol in the blood. This theory was confirmed (fraudulently, it turns out) with the prolific work of a physiologist named Ancel Keys. (Note: Dr. Keys' name is spelled various ways on the Internet such as Ansel, Ancel, Keys, Keyes, but in *Time* magazine and in his published articles, it is spelled "Ancel Keys.")

In 1956, Dr. Keys said, "In the adult man the serum cholesterol level is essentially independent of the cholesterol intake over the whole range of human diets."

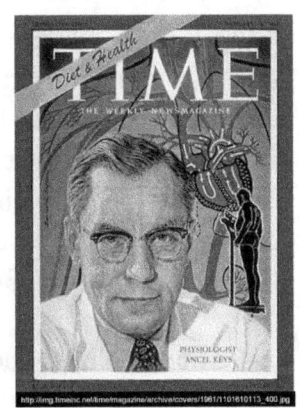

http://img.timeinc.net/time/magazine/archive/covers/1961/1101610113_400.jpg

He published nearly one hundred papers from 1985 to 1995 while he was at the University of Minnesota and was instrumental in convincing doctors that cholesterol causes heart disease. One of his papers stated, "It can be concluded that this study suggests that mean serum cholesterol is the major risk factor in explaining cross-cultural differences in coronary heart disease." 1993.

After stopping his work in Minnesota, he said, "…There's no connection whatsoever between cholesterol in food and cholesterol in the blood. None. And we've known that all along." 1997

Dr. Keys was instrumental in doctors beginning to believe that cholesterol causes heart attacks. His article that became known as the "Seven Country Study" was the one that started most doctors believing that the more fat you eat, the more likely you are to have a heart attack.

"Sixteen cohorts of men aged 40–59 years at entry were examined with the measurement of some risk factors and then followed up for mortality and causes of death for 25 years. These cohorts were located in the USA (1), Finland (2), the Netherlands (1), Italy (3), the former Yugoslavia (5), Greece (2), and Japan (2), and included a total of 12,763 subjects. Large differences in age-adjusted coronary heart disease death rates were found, with extremes of 45 per 1,000 in 25 years in Tanushimaru, Japan, to 288 per 1,000 in 25 years in East Finland.

Changes in mean serum cholesterol between year 0 and 10 helped in explaining differences in coronary heart disease death rates from year 10 onward. It can be concluded that this study suggests that mean serum cholesterol is the major risk factor in explaining cross-cultural differences in coronary heart disease." Ancel Keys, *Eur J Epidemiol* (1993 Sep) 9(5): 527–36.

This article included the graphic. It shows that the more fat you eat, the more heart attacks occur. It shows that people in the United States eat the most fat and have the most heart attacks. (It does differentiate between good fat and plastic trans fats. (Since Americans eat more processed foods with trans fats, one could explain the findings on that alone.)

However, Keys hid the data that did not support his intention to prove that eating fat causes heart attacks. On the right you see all the data. Here you see that those who ate the most fat had *fewer* heart attacks.

Data That Keys Published   Data That Keys Hid

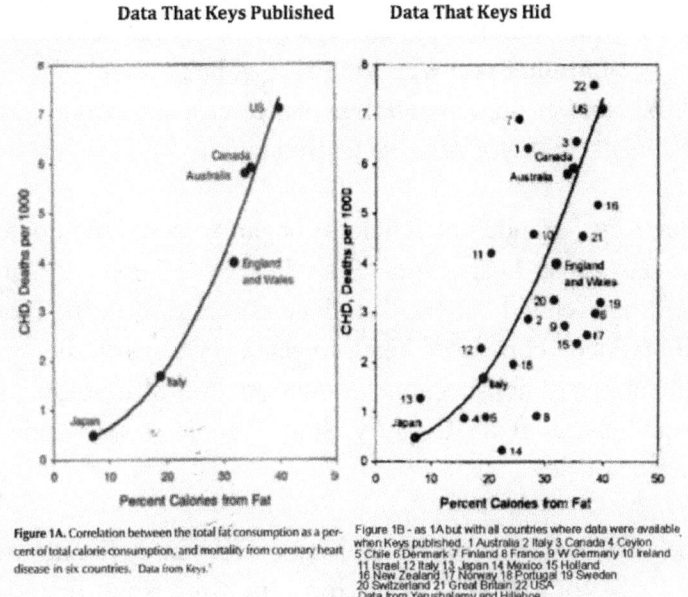

Figure 1A. Correlation between the total fat consumption as a per-cent of total calorie consumption, and mortality from coronary heart disease in six countries. Data from Keys.'

Figure 1B - as 1A but with all countries where data were available when Keys published. 1 Australia 2 Italy 3 Canada 4 Ceylon 5 Chile 6 Denmark 7 Finland 8 France 9 W Germany 10 Ireland 11 Israel 12 Italy 13 Japan 14 Mexico 15 Holland 16 New Zealand 17 Norway 18 Portugal 19 Sweden 20 Switzerland 21 Great Britain 22 USA
Data from Yerushalamy and Hilleboe

From *The Cholesterol Myth* by Uffe Ravnskow, MD, PhD, New Trends Publishing

Thus the article that induced doctors to believe that eating fat causes heart attacks is fraudulent! That also draws suspicion on the integrity of Dr. Keys' eighty-plus other articles. His prolific publications while he was at the University of Minnesota versus what he said in 1997 after he left that position makes one wonder.

As I will show you, multiple studies on thousands of patients show that Keys was incorrect. The medical literature does not support the theory that fats have anything to do with coronary heart disease. What the medical literature does show is:

1. The amount of cholesterol you eat has nothing to do with the levels of cholesterol in your blood.
2. The amount of saturated fat (red meat, animal fat, coconut oil, palm oil, etc.) you eat has nothing to

do with the amount of cholesterol in your blood.

3. The amount of cholesterol in your blood has nothing to do with your risk of heart attack.

4. Neither LDL nor HDL cholesterol has anything to do with your risk of heart attack.

After Keys' fraudulent article(s) began to convince doctors that fats cause heart disease, studies were begun to show that drugs (called "statins") reduce cholesterol in the blood and reduce coronary heart disease. One of the first influential studies became known as the "4S Study" for "Four Scandinavian Country Study" since it was done in those countries.

"Risk Factors for a Major Coronary Event after Myocardial Infarction in the Scandinavian Simvastatin Survival Study (4S). Impact of Predicted Risk on the Benefit of Cholesterol-lowering Treatment," Wilhelmsen, L., Pyorala, K., Wedel, H., Cook, T., Pedersen, T., and Kjekshus, J., *Eur Heart J* (2001 Jul), 22(13): 1119–27

Abstract:
AIMS: To analyze (1) the prognostic importance of clinical findings and lipids in patients with a previous myocardial infarction and (2) the relative and absolute benefit of simvastatin (Zocor) in patients at low, medium, and high predicted risk.

METHODS: The 4S was a double-blind, randomized, clinical trial of long-term treatment with simvastatin or matching placebo in patients with myocardial infarction or angina pectoris, serum total cholesterol 5.5–8.0 mmol x l(-1), and serum triglycerides <or=2.5 mmol x l(-1). The present study only deals with those 3,525 patients

who had a previous myocardial infarction. End points comprised coronary death, definite and probable hospital verified myocardial infarction, and resuscitated cardiac arrest. Because there were few women, the primary analyses were performed among men.

RESULTS: A Cox model analysis in the placebo group identified the following independent predictors of coronary events: a history of hypertension (P=0.023), diabetes (P=0.0001), smoking after the myocardial infarction (P=0.010), total cholesterol (P=0.020), and HDL cholesterol (P=0.062). The relative reduction of risk by simvastatin treatment in patients at low, medium, and high predicted risk was 38%, 39%, and 42%, respectively, but the corresponding absolute benefit per 100 patients treated for 6 years increased from 7.9 to 16.2.

CONCLUSION: In addition to serum lipids, clinical variables contributed significantly to prediction. The relative benefit from simvastatin treatment was independent of predicted risk, but the absolute benefit increased from low to high risk. The primary endpoint was total mortality. During the double-blind study period 438 patients died, 256 (12%) in the placebo group and 182 (8%) in the simvastatin group (table 2); the relative risk was 0.70 (95% CI 0.58-0.85, p=0.0003) with simvastatin.

The Kaplan-Meier 6-year (70 months) probability of survival (fig. 1) was 87.7% in the placebo group and 91.3% in the simvastatin group. Adjustment for the baseline covariates made no material difference

335

to the results for survival or the other endpoints. There were 189 coronary deaths in the placebo group (74% of all deaths in this group), compared with 111 in the simvastatin group. The relative risk of coronary death was 0.58 (95% CI 0.46-0.73) with simvastatin. This 42% reduction in the risk of coronary death accounts for the improvement in survival.

There was no statistically significant difference between the two groups in the number of deaths from non-cardiovascular causes. There were similar numbers of violent deaths (suicide plus trauma) in the two groups, 7 versus 6. Of the fatal cancers, 12/35 in the placebo group and 9/33 in the simvastatin group arose in the gastrointestinal system. There were similar numbers of cerebrovascular deaths in the two groups, and the difference (6 vs. 11) in deaths from other cardiovascular diseases is not significant.

Doctors latched onto the authors' conclusion that treating patients with simvastatin (Zocor) to lower cholesterol reduced the risk of having a heart attack by forty-two percent! But wait a minute—look at what the results actually are:

"During the double-blind study period 438 patients died, 256 (12%) in the placebo group and 182 (8%) in the simvastatin group. ... This 42% reduction in the risk of coronary death accounts for the improvement in survival."

They first say that the difference in survival was 12% - 8% = 4%. They then call this a "42% reduction in risk" because they are reporting relative risk and not absolute risk (8/12 = 0.67 = 67%). Thus they call this a "42% reduction."

Then the article says, "The Kaplan-Meier 6-year (70 months) probability of survival was 87.7% in the placebo group and 91.3% in the simvastatin group." Thus the absolute risk is 91.3 - 87.7 = 3.6%. Thus again we see that it is more impressive to say there is a 42% reduction in heart attacks with the drug than to say that there is a 3.6% reduction. One can argue that both are true. Even though it is misleading, the authors tried (successfully, I might add) to convince doctors that using the drug Zocor significantly reduces the risk of heart attack.

The problem is that doctors are busy and tend to read the authors' conclusions instead of reading the fine print in the article. In addition, doctors don't understand the statistical terms used in analyzing medical studies.

"The relative reduction of risk by simvastatin treatment in patients at low, medium, and high predicted risk was 38%, 39%, and 42%, respectively."

Another way to look at the data is to take the RR number and divide it by one plus that number. That gives you the odds that the drug worked.

What this means is that the odds that Zocor reduced deaths from heart attacks in the low-risk group were a 27 percent chance it was helpful and a 73 percent chance Zocor didn't work. In the medium-risk group, the odds that Zocor helped were 28 percent and the odds it didn't work were 78 percent. In the high-risk group, the odds that Zocor helped were 30 percent and the odds it didn't were 70 percent.

"During the double-blind study period 438 patients died, 256 (12%) in the placebo group and 182 (8%) in the simvastatin group (table 2); the relative risk was 0.70 (95%

CI 0.58-0.85, p=0.0003) with simvastatin."

What this means is that the odds that Zocor reduced the risk of dying from a heart attack were 42 percent and the odds that Zocor didn't reduce the risk of dying from a heart attack were 58 percent. This is because 0.7 / 1 + 0.7 = 0.7/1.7 = 0.42. You calculate the *odds* that the drug worked by dividing the relative risk by one plus the relative risk.

The authors' conclusion that there was a 42 percent reduction in the risk of coronary death is not what the study really says. However, drug salespeople convinced doctors that if they put their patients on Zocor, 42 percent fewer would have a heart attack. Doctors quickly started prescribing statin drugs believing that 42 percent of their patients wouldn't get heart attacks instead of a 3.6 percent reduction.

With Keys' fraudulent Seven Country Study and a faulty conclusion by the authors of the 4S study combined with aggressive marketing by the pharmaceutical companies, doctors became convinced that cholesterol was the cause of coronary artery disease and must be lowered in almost all people. What do other studies show?

Additional Studies Prove no Relationship between Cholesterol and Coronary Artery Disease

In 1948, the Framingham Heart Study—under the direction of the National Heart Institute (now known as the National Heart, Lung, and Blood Institute—embarked on an ambitious project in health research. Since 1971, the Framingham Heart Study has been conducted in collaboration with Boston University. The objective of the Framingham Heart Study was to identify the common factors or characteristics that contribute to cardiovascular disease by following its development over a long time in a large group of participants who had not yet developed overt symptoms of cardiovascular disease or suffered a heart attack or stroke.

The researchers recruited 5,209 men and women between the ages of thirty and sixty-two from the town of Framingham, Massachusetts, and began the first round of extensive physical examinations and lifestyle interviews that they would later analyze for common patterns related to cardiovascular disease development. Since 1948, the subjects have continued to return to the study every two years for a detailed medical history, physical examination, and laboratory tests.
Http:// www.nhlbi.nih.gov/about/framingham/

The graph appears to suggest that coronary artery disease increases steadily from twenty percent at a cholesterol level of 200 to ninety percent at a cholesterol level of 300. One should realize that those with cholesterol levels around the level of 300 have a genetic defect called "familial hypercholesterolemia" and should be removed from consideration because of it. Next, it should be noted that the death rates are unchanged from cholesterol levels of 205 to 264.

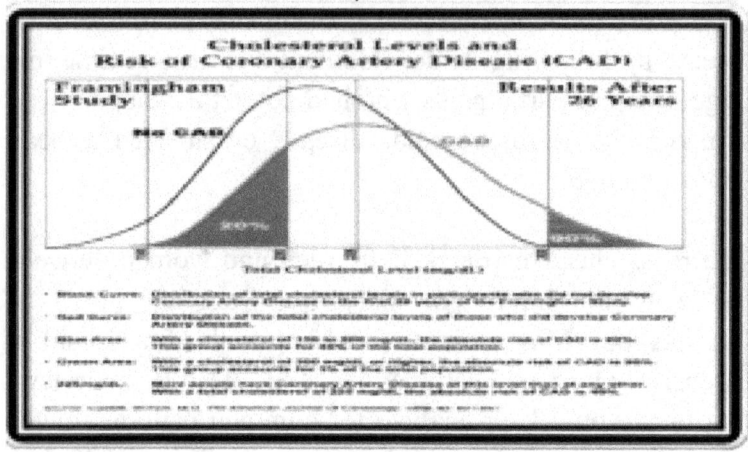

This chart shows that the level of blood cholesterol was completely independent of the amount of cholesterol consumed. No matter whether they ate, only 43 mg of cholesterol or 925 mg of cholesterol or anywhere in between, the average blood cholesterol did not change.

	Cholesterol Intake	Blood Cholesterol Low Intake	Blood Cholesterol High Intake
Men	43–925 mg	231 mg/dl	231 mg/dl
Women	322–662 mg	251 mg/dl	235 mg/dl

Today, after forty years, the current director of this study admits:

"In Framingham, Mass., the more saturated fat one ate, the more cholesterol one ate, the more calories one ate, the lower the person's serum cholesterol. ... [W]e found that the people who ate the most cholesterol, ate the most saturated fat, and ate the most calories weighed the least and were the most physically active."

Thus we see that eating fat doesn't make you fat (unless it's trans fats). Eating enough good fat to make functional new cells and hormones makes you healthy.

In 1976, a large study done in Tecumseh, Michigan, was published:

"Independence of Serum Lipid Levels and Dietary Habits, The Tecumseh Study," Nichols, A.B., Ravenscroft, C., Lamphiear, D.E., and Ostrander, L.D., *JAMA* (1976 Oct 25), 236(17): 1948–53

"Serum cholesterol and triglyceride levels were correlated with dietary habits of 4,057 adult participants in a prospective epidemiologic survey of cardiovascular disease in Tecumseh, Mich. Frequency of consumption of 110 different food items was determined for each participant and average weekly consumption rates of foods high in fat, sugar, starch, and alcohol content were calculated. Frequency of consumption of these nutrients was then correlated with serum cholesterol and triglyceride levels of individual subjects. Serum cholesterol and triglyceride values were not positively correlated with selection of dietary constituents. Positive correlations between serum lipid levels and adiposity were statistically significant. These findings suggest that serum cholesterol and triglyceride levels among Americans are more dependent on degree of adiposity than on frequency of consumption of fat, sugar, starch, or alcohol."

This study of over four thousand patients clearly shows the following:
1. There is no relationship whatsoever between the amount of cholesterol eaten and the levels of blood cholesterol.
2. There is no relationship whatsoever between the

amount of saturated fat (animal fat, coconut oil, palm oil, etc.) eaten and the levels of blood cholesterol.

3. There is no relationship whatsoever between the amount of total fat eaten and the levels of blood cholesterol.

4. "Serum cholesterol and triglyceride values were not positively correlated with selection of dietary constituents."

So the five thousand-plus patients in the Framingham Study and the four thousand patients in the Tecumseh Study show that you can eat as much or little cholesterol, animal fat, or saturated fats as you like and it will have no effect on your blood cholesterol levels. Note that these studies do not address the consumption of "plastic" trans fats.

Saturated Fat

Okay, so I've been misled about whether eating fat affects my cholesterol level. Does it affect whether I will have a heart attack? I could only find two studies that considered the effect of eating saturated fats on coronary artery disease.

"Design of Practical Fat-controlled Diets, Foods, Fat Composition, and Serum Cholesterol Content," Brown, H.B., Farrand, M., and Page, I.H., *JAMA* (1966 Apr 18), 196 (3): 205–13.

The Anti-Coronary Club Project, launched in 1957 and published in 1966 in the *Journal of the American Medical Association*, compared two groups of New York businessmen, aged forty to fifty-nine years. One group followed the so-called "Prudent Diet" consisting of corn oil and margarine instead of butter, cold breakfast cereals instead of eggs, and chicken and fish instead of beef; a control group ate eggs for breakfast and meat three times per day.

The final report noted that the "Prudent Dieters" had average serum cholesterol of 220 mg/l compared to 250 mg/l in the eggs-and-meat group. There were eight deaths from heart disease among the "Prudent Dieters" group, and none among those who ate meat three times a day. http://www.westonaprice.org/modern diseases/

This study shows that you are less likely to die from heart disease if you eat saturated fat like butter, eggs, and beef instead of corn oil, margarine, cereal, chicken, and fish.

"Corn Oil in Treatment of Ischaemic Heart Disease," Rose, G.A., Thomson, W.B., and Williams, R.T., *BR MED J* (1965 Jun 12), 544: 1531–3.

In this study published in the *British Medical Journal*, 1965, patients who had already had a heart attack were divided into three groups:

1.   One group got polyunsaturated corn oil.
2.   The second got monounsaturated olive oil.
3.   The third group was told to eat animal fat.

After two years, the corn oil group had thirty percent lower cholesterol, but only fifty-two percent of them were still alive. The olive oil groups fared little better—only fifty-seven percent were alive after two years. Of the group that ate mostly animal fat, seventy-five percent were still alive after two years. In patients who had already had a heart attack, eating animal fat instead of polyunsaturated corn oil cut the risk of death from 24 percent per year to 12.5 percent per year.

Spread	Breakfast	Meat	Cholesterol	Deaths/9 Years
Corn Oil & Margarine	Cereal	Chicken/Fish	220 mg/dl	8
Butter	Eggs	Beef	250 mg/dl	0

These two studies support the concept that you are less likely to have a heart attack if you eat beef and eggs than if you eat chicken and fish! Combine that with the certainty of the Framingham and Tecumseh studies that your diet has nothing to do with your cholesterol level and it begins to make the cholesterol theory of heart attacks fall apart!

When we talk about "blood cholesterol," that really isn't accurate. Since cholesterol is insoluble in water, it cannot be suspended in blood but must be carried by a protein. These proteins that carry cholesterol are called "lipoproteins" and vary in size from large to small. Along with cholesterol, these proteins carry other fats. These various fats are attached to glycerol, and this unit is called a triglyceride because the fats are in units of three.

When you eat any fat except cholesterol, it is attached to a glycerol to make triglycerides. Cholesterol remains unchanged as it and triglycerides are put into packages called *chylomicrons* within the intestinal wall. Chylomicrons transport triglycerides (fats attached to glycerol) and cholesterol to the liver. The fats are released there and reconstructed by the liver in very low density lipoproteins (VLDL). These carry the fats and cholesterol to the body where they are used and become smaller and smaller units called low density lipoproteins (LDL).

The fats carried to the cells as VLDL are used by the cells and leave some LDL behind to be recycled to the liver to be made back into VLDL. Saturated fats never become cholesterol. They are entirely separate substances. The only connection between saturated fats and cholesterol is that they both ride around the body in a lipoprotein since both are insoluble in water. Thus eating red meat cannot possibly influence your cholesterol level!

LDLs (low density lipoproteins) are called "bad cholesterol." It is assumed that when a blood test is done for cholesterol, LDL is measured. It is not. Your LDL level is calculated by the formula LDL = Total Cholesterol – (HDL + Triglycerides/5). This is important because if you raise your triglyceride level by eating more carbohydrates, it will appear that your LDL has elevated when in reality it hasn't changed at all.

If you want to lower your LDL, you can just eat fewer carbohydrates. Again, what you eat has absolutely no effect on your blood cholesterol. However, you can change the *calculations* of the percentages of LDL or HDL by changing your triglyceride level. Triglyceride levels change with the amount of carbohydrates you eat.

The liver doesn't make LDL—it is a metabolic residue of VLDL. When VLDL loses a triglyceride, it is normally called LDL.

HDLs (alpha lipoproteins, "good cholesterol") are mainly protein with a small amount of cholesterol. Their primary purpose is to remove cholesterol from the periphery and transport it back to the liver.

1. The liver synthesizes 1,500–2,000 mg of new cholesterol each day.
2. A raised VLDL level is normally called an elevated triglyceride level.
3. A raised LDL level is normally called an

elevated cholesterol level.

The widely believed concept in coronary heart disease is that the portion of cholesterol called low density lipoprotein (LDL), when elevated, goes through the wall of the arteries and begins to build up as a cholesterol plaque. It is believed that using medications (statin drugs) to keep the liver from making cholesterol and thus lowering your blood cholesterol reduces the risk of heart attacks by fifty percent. This theory is simply wrong. A convincing argument against the current belief that cholesterol causes heart attacks is made in the article:

"Why the Cholesterol-Heart Disease Theory Is Wrong," by Malcolm Kendrick, Mbchb, Mrcgp:

1. Fact one: The liver does not use fats, saturated or otherwise to make cholesterol.
2. Fact two: The liver does not make LDL; it makes VLDL.
3. Fact three: VLDL is converted into LDL through triglyceride loss.
4. Fact four: VLDL levels and LDL levels are totally unrelated – totally.

This means that: saturated fat intake has no affect on LDL levels.

There are several things wrong with the idea that LDL cholesterol goes through the artery wall and causes a plaque leading to a heart attack:

1. If LDL is the primary cause of heart attacks, then almost everyone who has a heart attack should have a high LDL level. They don't. Fifty percent of heart attack victims have a low LDL.

346

2. LDL can't get through the wall of the artery.
3. If LDL goes from the blood into the wall of the artery, you should find plaques evenly distributed throughout the artery walls. You don't. Plaques are usually where arteries branch.

If LDL or any portion of cholesterol is the cause of heart disease, its levels should correspond to the amount of plaque seen in coronary angiography. It doesn't!

"The Relationship of Oxidized Lipids to Coronary Artery Stenosis," Kummerow, F.A., Olinescu, R.M., Fleischer, L., Handler, B., and Shinkareva, S.V., *Atherosclerosis* (2000 Mar), 149(1): 181–90 ISSN: 0021-9150

Abstract: A total of 1,200 patients with angina were cardiac catheterized establishing that 63% had 70%-100% stenosis, 12% had 0%-69% stenosis of one or more of their coronary arteries, and 25% had microvascular angina listed as 0% stenosis. Prior to catheterization, 10 ml of blood was drawn and the plasma subjected to analysis for the concentration of cholesterol, lipid peroxides (LPX), total antioxidant capacity (TA OC), fibrinogen (FB), ceruloplasmin (CP), and activation of polymorphonuclear leukocytes (PMNLs). Comparisons were made to non-smoking controls without angina.

Significant differences in LPX were found between the patients with 0 and 10%-69% stenosis (P<0.001), with 10%-69% and 70%-100% stenosis (P<0.001), and with 0% and 70%-100% stenosis (P< 0.001). Under 70 years of age there was a significant difference in LPX between patients with all levels of stenosis and age and sex matched controls (P< 0.001). Differences in the mean plasma cholesterol concentration for different levels in the degree of stenosis were not significant, indicating that lipid peroxides provided consistent data on the severity of stenosis while the plasma cholesterol concentration did not.

Compared with controls, an increase in activation of PMNLs (P< 0.01), an increase in concentration of both fibrinogen and ceruloplasm (P< 0.01), and a decrease in total antioxidant capacity were noted in the plasma of catheterized patients. In summary the concentration of oxidation products (electron-stealers, JLT) rather than the concentration of cholesterol in the plasma identified stenosis in cardiac catheterized patients.

Statins Drugs to Lower Cholesterol and Heart Attacks

Now let's see what the other studies say about cholesterol levels lowered with drugs and whether that reduces heart attacks.

Note: Simvastatin is marketed under the trade names Zocor, Simlup, Simcard, Simvaco

"The MRC/BHF Heart Protection Study: Preliminary Results," Collins, R., Peto, R., and Armitage, J., *Int J Clin Pract* (2002 Jan-Feb), 56(1): 53–6 ISSN: 1368-5031

Published Abstract:
The Heart Protection Study (HPS), with over

20,500 subjects, is the largest trial of statin therapy ever conducted. It provides important and definitive new information on women, the elderly, diabetics, and people with low baseline cholesterol pretreatment and those with prior occlusive non-coronary vascular disease. It is a prospective double blind randomized controlled trial with a 2 x 2 factorial design investigating prolonged use (>5 years) of simvastatin 40 mg and a cocktail of antioxidant vitamins (650 mg vitamin E, 250 mg vitamin C, and 20 mg beta-carotene).

The HPS specifically included patients with high risk for coronary heart disease (CHD) but characteristics that excluded them from participation in previous statin trials. Simvastatin 40 mg treatment showed benefit across all patient groups regardless of age, gender, or baseline cholesterol value and proved safe and well tolerated. Results show a 12% reduction in total mortality, a 17% reduction in vascular mortality, a 24% reduction in CHD events, a 27% reduction in all strokes, and a 16% reduction in non-coronary revascularizations.

Among high-risk patients in this western population (with a minimum total cholesterol [TC] > or = 3.5 mmol/l at entry) there appears to be no threshold cholesterol value below which statin therapy is not associated with benefit; even among those with pretreatment cholesterol levels below current national recommended targets. Over the 5.5-year study period patients and their doctors were encouraged to add an active non-study statin to the study regimen if they wished to do so. Thus the trial eventually had only two-thirds complying with the original intention-to-treat design. Nevertheless, results were highly significant for the study statin— simvastatin 40 mg once daily. Preliminary results of the HPS are negative for the antioxidant vitamin cocktail but provide reassurance that vitamins do no harm."

A follow-up analysis of this study was published:

"Treatment with Statins: Further Data from the Heart Protection Study," [Article in Norwegian] Tonstad, S., and Holme, I. Avdeling for preventiv kardiologi, Klinikk for Forebyggende Medisin Tidsskr Nor Laegeforen, (2002 Nov 30), 122(29): 2777–80, Medisinsk Divisjon Ulleval Universitetssykehus 0407 Oslo

Abstract:

BACKGROUND: Statins have been shown to reduce cardiovascular disease in subjects with coronary heart disease, in men with high cholesterol levels, and in men and postmenopausal women with low high-density lipoprotein cholesterol levels. In meta-analysis, reduction in events is associated with reduction in serum low-density lipoprotein (LDL) cholesterol levels; however, some studies have proposed a threshold level for the effect.

MATERIAL AND METHODS: A clinician and a statistician reviewed the Heart Protection Study in the context of previous similar studies.

RESULTS: High-risk men and women (n = 20,536) aged 40-80 years with coronary heart disease, peripheral artery disease, or diabetes and a cholesterol level of at least 3.5 mmol/l (137 mg/dl) were randomized to simvastatin 40 mg or placebo.

After 5.5 years, the incidence of nonfatal myocardial infarction or coronary death was reduced from 11.8% in the placebo group to 8.7% in the simvastatin group, and a similar reduction was seen in subjects with diabetes but no cardiovascular disease. There was no threshold of LDL cholesterol below which lowering it did not reduce risk.

INTERPRETATION: The study adds to the body of evidence indicating that cholesterol lowering with statins is indicated for subjects with high risk and that LDL cholesterol reduction explains the reduction in events.

It is interesting to note the difference in these two reports on the same data. In the first one, relative risk is used to say there was a twenty-four percent reduction in heart attacks. The second report tells us the absolute risk reduction. It is 11.8 - 8.7 = 3.1 percent. Thus the drug simvastatin (Zocor) reduced heart attacks by 3.1 percent, not 24 percent.

Remember that statin drugs reduce inflammation as well as cholesterol. It has become clear that any beneficial effect they have is due to reduction of inflammation, not the reduction of cholesterol. As you will see, they also increase the risk of dying from cancer and other diseases.

This study of atorvastatin (Lipitor) again shows that Lipitor has very little effect in reducing heart attacks.

"Effects of Atorvastatin (Lipitor) on Early Recurrent Ischemic Events in Acute Coronary Syndromes: The MIRACL Study: a Randomized Controlled Trial," Schwartz, G.G., Olsson, A.G., Ezekowitz, M.D., Ganz, P., Oliver, M.F., Waters, D., Zeiher, A., Chaitman, B.R., Leslie, S., and Stern, T.,

351

JAMA (2001 Apr 4), 285 (13): 1711–8

Published Abstract:

CONTEXT: Patients experience the highest rate of death and recurrent ischemic events during the early period after an acute coronary syndrome, but it is not known whether early initiation of treatment with a statin can reduce the occurrence of these early events.

OBJECTIVE: To determine whether treatment with atorvastatin, 80 mg/d, initiated 24 to 96 hours after an acute coronary syndrome, reduces death and nonfatal ischemic events.

DESIGN AND SETTING: A randomized, double-blind trial conducted from May 1997 to September 1999, with follow-up through 16 weeks at 122 clinical centers in Europe, North America, South Africa, and Australasia.

PATIENTS: A total of 3,086 adults aged 18 years or older with unstable angina or non-Q-wave acute myocardial infarction.

INTERVENTIONS: Patients were stratified by center and randomly assigned to receive treatment with atorvastatin (80 mg/d) or matching placebo between 24 and 96 hours after hospital admission.

MAIN OUTCOME MEASURES:
Primary end point event defined as death, nonfatal acute myocardial infarction, cardiac arrest with resuscitation, or recurrent symptomatic myocardial ischemia with objective evidence and requiring emergency re-hospitalization.

RESULTS: A primary end point event occurred in 228 patients (14.8%) in the atorvastatin (Lipitor) group and 269 patients (17.4%) in the placebo group (relative risk [RR], 0.84; 95% confidence interval [CI], 0. 70-1.00; P =.048). There were no significant differences in risk of death, nonfatal myocardial infarction, or cardiac arrest between the atorvastatin (Lipitor) group and the placebo group, although the atorvastatin group had a lower risk of symptomatic ischemia with objective evidence and requiring emergency re-hospitalization (6.2% vs.. 8.4%; RR, 0.74; 95% CI, 0.57-0.95; P =.02).

Likewise, there were no significant differences between the atorvastatin (Lipitor) group and the placebo group in the incidence of secondary outcomes of coronary revascularization procedures, worsening heart failure, or worsening angina, although there were fewer strokes in the atorvastatin group than in the placebo group (12 vs. 24 events; P =.045).

In the atorvastatin group, mean low-density lipoprotein cholesterol level declined from 124 mg/ dL (3.2 mmol/L) to 72 mg/dL (1.9 mmol/L). Abnormal liver transaminases (>3 times upper limit of normal) were more common in the atorvastatin (Lipitor) group than in the placebo group (2.5% vs. 0.6%; P<.001).

The conclusions of these authors match the study in saying that Lipitor has no effect on decreasing death from heart attacks. (Relative risk [RR], 0.84; 95% Confidence Interval [CI], 0. 70-1.00; P =.048). There were no significant differences in risk of death, nonfatal myocardial infarction, or cardiac arrest between the atorvastatin (Lipitor) group and the placebo group.

This means that the odds that Lipitor prevented death from heart attack were forty-six percent and the odds that Lipitor didn't work were fifty-four percent.

Thus in over three thousand patients, there were no significant differences in risk of death, nonfatal myocardial infarction, or cardiac arrest between the atorvastatin (Lipitor) group and the placebo group. However, those who took the drug were four times more likely to have liver damage (2.5% vs. 0.6%; P<.001).

Another large study was published in 2002 about the use of the statin drug pravastatin (Pravachol).

> "Major Outcomes in Moderately Hypercholesterolemic, Hypertensive Patients Randomized to Pravastatin (Pravachol) vs. Usual Care: The Antihypertensive and Lipid-Lowering Treatment to Prevent Heart Attack Trial (ALLHAT-LLT)," *JAMA* (2002 Dec 18), 288(23): 2998–300
>
> CONTEXT: Studies have demonstrated that statins administered to individuals with risk factors for coronary heart disease (CHD) reduce CHD events. However, many of these studies were too small to assess all-cause mortality or outcomes in important subgroups.
>
> OBJECTIVE: To determine whether pravastatin (Pravachol) compared with usual care reduces all-cause mortality in older, moderately hypercholesterolemic, hypertensive participants with at least one additional CHD risk factor.

DESIGN AND SETTING: Multicenter (513 primarily community-based North American clinical centers), randomized, non-blinded trial conducted from 1994 through March 2002 in a subset of participants from the Antihypertensive and Lipid-Lowering Treatment to Prevent Heart Attack Trial (ALLHAT).

PARTICIPANTS: Ambulatory persons (n =10,355), aged 55 years or older, with low-density lipoprotein cholesterol (LDL-C) of 120 to 189 mg/dL (100 to 129 mg./dL if known CHD) and triglycerides lower than 350 mg/dL, were randomized to pravastatin (n = 5,170) or to usual care (n = 5,185). Baseline mean total cholesterol was 224 mg/dL; LDL-C, 146 mg/dL; high-density lipoprotein cholesterol, 48 mg/dL; and triglycerides, 152 mg/dL. Mean age was 66 years, 49% were women, 38% black and 23% Hispanic, 14% had a history of CHD, and 35% had type II diabetes.

INTERVENTION: Pravastatin, 40 mg/d, vs. usual care

MAIN OUTCOME MEASURES: The primary outcome was all-cause mortality, with follow-up for up to 8 years. Secondary outcomes included nonfatal myocardial infarction or fatal CHD (CHD events) combined, cause-specific mortality, and cancer.

RESULTS: Mean follow-up was 4.8 years. During the trial, 32% of usual care participants with and 29% without CHD started taking lipid-lowering drugs. At year 4, total cholesterol levels were reduced by 17% with pravastatin vs. 8% with usual care; among the random sample who had LDL-C levels assessed, levels were reduced by 28% with pravastatin vs. 11% with usual care. All-cause mortality was similar for the 2 groups (relative risk [RR], 0.99; 95% confidence interval [CI], 0.89-1.11; P =.88), with 6-year mortality rates of 14.9% for pravastatin (Pravachol) vs. 15.3% with usual care. CHD event rates were not significantly different between the groups (RR, 0.91; 95% CI, 0.79-1.04; P =.16), with 6-year CHD event rates of 9.3% for pravastatin and 10.4% for usual care.

CONCLUSIONS: Pravastatin did not reduce either all-cause mortality or CHD significantly when compared with usual care in older participants with well-controlled hypertension and moderately elevated LDL-C. The results may be due to the modest differential in total cholesterol (9.6%) and LDL-C (16.7%) between pravastatin and usual care compared with prior statin trials supporting cardiovascular disease prevention."

This study of 10,355 patients with an average follow-up of nearly five years showed that the odds that Pravachol reduced the risk of death from all causes were 15.3 - 14.9 = 0.4% difference in the treated vs. untreated groups.

Cardiac deaths were 10.4 - 9.3 = 1.1% difference in the treated vs. untreated groups.

The odds calculation shows that the odds the drug worked were 49.7% and the odds that Pravachol did not change the risk of death were 50.3%. The odds that Pravachol reduced the changes of having a heart attack were 47.6 percent and the odds that the drug didn't work were 52.4 percent.

When studies are done and there is no apparent benefit in taking the drug, one can attempt to manipulate the data to try to show a benefit. Such an attempt is called a "meta analysis."

"Statin-related Adverse Events: A Meta-analysis," Silva, M.A., Swanson, A.C., Gandhi, P.J., and Tataronis, G.R., *Clin Ther* (2006 Jan), 28(1): 26–35

Published Abstract:

BACKGROUND: The absolute frequencies of adverse events (AEs) between statins and placebo are very low in clinical trials, making clinical interpretation and application difficult.

OBJECTIVES: This meta-analysis was intended to synthesize the collective AE data observed in prospective randomized clinical trials to facilitate clinical interpretation.

METHODS: Using the search terms atorvastatin, simvastatin, pravastatin, rosuvastatin, fluvastatin, lovastatin, prospective trial, and randomized trial, the MEDLINE/EMBASE and the Cochrane Collaboration databases were reviewed for prospective randomized primary and secondary prevention trials of statin monotherapy. Non-randomized uncontrolled studies and those missing AE data were excluded. The Mantel-Haenszel test for fixed and random effects was used to calculate odds ratios (ORs) and log ORs.

RESULTS: Eighteen trials including 71,108 persons, and 301,374 person-years of follow-up were represented in this analysis. There were 36,062 persons receiving a statin and 35,046 receiving a placebo. Statin therapy increased the risk of any Adverse Event by 39% (OR = 1.4; 95% CI, 1.09- 1. 80; P = 0. 008; NNH [number needed to harm] = 197) compared with placebo. Statins were associated with a 26% reduction in the risk of a clinical cardiovascular event (OR = 0.74; 95% CI, 0. 69-0.80; P < 0.001; number needed to treat = 27).

This is a meta-analysis. That means that they took many studies and tried to combine them into one set of data. The odds that cholesterol-lowering statin drugs caused damage to patients were 58.3 percent, and the odds they didn't damage patients were 41.7 percent. The odds that the drugs reduced heart attacks/death were 42.5 percent and the odds they didn't help were 57.5 percent.

It should now be apparent that we doctors, and thus our patients, have been manipulated to believe that cholesterol is the critical factor controlling coronary artery disease when it is not. It has only minor effects that may not be significant. We have also been manipulated into believing that lowering cholesterol and/or LDL cholesterol reduces heart attacks.

Doctors, and thus their patients, have been misled into believing:

1. Eating cholesterol raises your blood cholesterol.

2. Eating saturated fat (e.g., animal fats) raises your blood cholesterol and causes coronary heart disease.

3. Elevated blood cholesterol increases your risk of coronary heart disease (heart attacks) and strokes.

4. The portion of cholesterol called LDL ("bad cholesterol") increases your risk of coronary heart disease.

5. Labs actually measure LDL cholesterol when you order cholesterol tests.

6. The portion of cholesterol called HDL ("good cholesterol") protects against heart attacks.

7. Using medications (statin drugs) to keep the liver from making cholesterol and thus lowering your blood cholesterol reduces the risk of heart attacks by 50 percent.

A careful reading of the medical literature shows that *none of this is true*. The medical literature does not support the theory that cholesterol has anything major to do with coronary heart disease. It would be one thing if the billions of dollars wasted on statin drugs did no harm. However, that is not true.

Low Cholesterol Increases Your Risk of Dying

There are many studies that show that lowering total cholesterol levels and/or LDL levels have very little effect on the likelihood that you will die of a heart attack. Studies do show that lowering your cholesterol levels significantly will increase your risk of dying of cancer.

"Cholesterol and All-cause Mortality in Elderly

People from the Honolulu Heart Program: A Cohort Study," Schatz, I.J., Masaki, K., Yano, K., Chen, R., Rodriguez, B.L., and Curb, J.D., *Lancet* (2001 Aug 4), 358(9279): 351–5

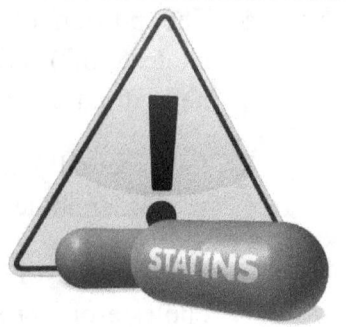

Published Abstract:

BACKGROUND: A generally held belief is that cholesterol concentrations should be kept low to lessen the risk of cardiovascular disease. However, studies of the relation between serum cholesterol and all-cause mortality in elderly people have shown contrasting results. To investigate these discrepancies, we did a longitudinal assessment of changes in both lipid and serum cholesterol concentrations over 20 years and compared them with mortality.

METHODS: Lipid and serum cholesterol concentrations were measured in 3,572 Japanese/ American men (aged 71-93 years) as part of the Honolulu Heart Program. We compared changes in these concentrations over 20 years with all-cause mortality using three different Cox proportional hazards models.

FINDINGS: Mean cholesterol fell significantly with increasing age. Age-adjusted mortality rates were 68.3, 48.9, 41.1, and 43.3 for the first to fourth quartiles of cholesterol concentrations, respectively. Relative risks for mortality were 0.72 (95% CI 0.60-0.87), 0.60 (0.49-0. 74), and 0.65 (0.53-0.80), in the second, third, and fourth quartiles, respectively, with quartile 1 as reference.

INTERPRETATION: We have been unable to explain our results. These data cast doubt on the scientific justification for lowering cholesterol to very low concentrations (<4.65 mmol/L) in elderly people. Our data accords with previous findings of increased mortality in elderly people with low serum cholesterol and show that long-term persistence of low cholesterol concentration actually increases risk of death. Thus, the earlier that patients start to have lower cholesterol concentrations, the greater the risk of death. ... The most striking findings were related to changes in cholesterol between examination three (1971-74) and examination four (1991-93). There are few studies that have cholesterol concentrations from the same patients at both middle age and old age.

Although our results lend support to previous findings that low serum cholesterol imparts a poor outlook when compared with higher concentrations of cholesterol in elderly people, our data also suggest that those individuals with a low serum cholesterol maintained over a 20-year period will have the worst outlook for all-cause mortality.

This study shows that the lower your cholesterol is, the higher your risk of dying from all causes! It also shows that the earlier you have lower cholesterol, the greater the risk of death.

In a study by H.E. Sartori, it was found that the cholesterol level present when cancer is diagnosed is a good indicator of how long that patient will live. This makes sense since

361

the more disabled the liver is (and thus unable to make enough cholesterol to heal), the more likely the patient is to die. This should have some meaning to the cardiologists who are insisting on getting cholesterol levels down below 100!

Statins Cause Diabetes

The following is from www.fda.gov

If you're one of the millions of Americans who take statins to prevent heart disease, the Food and Drug Administration (FDA) has important new safety information on these cholesterol-lowering medications. FDA is advising consumers and health care professionals that:

1. Routine monitoring of liver enzymes in the blood, once considered standard procedure for statin users, is no longer needed. Such monitoring has not been found to be effective in predicting or preventing the rare occurrences of serious liver injury associated with statin use.

2. Cognitive (brain-related) impairment, such as memory loss, forgetfulness and confusion, has been reported by some statin users.

3. People being treated with statins may have an increased risk of raised blood sugar levels and the development of Type 2 diabetes.

4. Some medications interact with lovastatin (brand names include Mevacor) and can increase the risk of muscle damage.

5. This new information should not scare people off statins, says Amy G. Egan, M.D., M.P.H., deputy director for safety in FDA's Division of Metabolism and Endocrinology Products (DMEP). "The value of statins in preventing

heart disease has been clearly established," she says. "Their benefit is indisputable, but they need to be taken with care and knowledge of their side effects."

6. FDA will be changing the drug labels of popular statin products to reflect these new concerns. (These labels are not the sticker attached to a prescription drug bottle, but the package insert with details about a prescription medication, including side effects.)

Why You Need Cholesterol

Cholesterol is necessary for the nervous system to work. It is necessary for memory and for the function of serotonin.

Cholesterol is necessary for serotonin receptors to work.

Over half of the dry weight of the brain is cholesterol. Since the brain rebuilds itself every eight months, if you don't have lots of cholesterol, you can't rebuild it.

Cholesterol is the raw material used to make all the hormones produced in the adrenal cortex including glucocorticoids. They regulate blood sugar levels and mineralocorticoids, which regulate mineral balance. Balanced minerals are the on/off switches of the body.

The ability to control stress is related to corticosteroids. They are made from cholesterol. If you can't control stress, you can't heal, and chronic inflammation will be present.

Sexual hormones including testosterone, estrogen, and progesterone are made from cholesterol. Without cholesterol, sexual dysfunction occurs.

Thus low cholesterol, whether caused by liver disease or induced by statin drugs, can be expected to cause:

1. Disruption of the production of adrenal hormones
2. Blood sugar problems
3. Edema
4. Mineral deficiencies
5. Chronic inflammation
6. Difficulty in healing
7. Allergies
8. Asthma
9. Reduced libido
10. Infertility and various reproductive problems

Dangers of Statin Drugs
Sally Fallon and Mary Enig

The most common side effect of statin drugs is muscle pain (rhabdomyolysis). Golomb found that 98 percent of patients taking Lipitor and one-third of the patients taking Mevachor (a lower-dose statin) suffered from muscle problems.
Beatrice A. Golomb, MD, PhD on Statin Drugs, March 7, 2002.

Gaist and his associates found that statins cause pain in the hands and feet of 26.4 percent of those who have taken statin drugs for two or more years:

> "Statins and Risk of Polyneuropathy: A Case-control Study," Gaist, D., Jeppesen, U., Andersen, M., Garcia, Rodriguez L.A., Hallas, J., and Sindrup, S.H., *Neurology* (2002 May 14), 58(9): 1333–7; ISSN: 0028-3878

Published Abstract:

BACKGROUND: Several case reports and a single epidemiologic study indicate that use of statins occasionally may have a deleterious effect on the peripheral nervous system. The authors therefore performed a population-based study to estimate the relative risk of idiopathic polyneuropathy in users of statins.

METHOD: The authors used a population-based patient registry to identify first-time-ever cases of idiopathic polyneuropathy registered in the 5-year period 1994 to 1998. For each case, validated according to predefined criteria, 25 control subjects were randomly selected among subjects from the background population matched for age, sex, and calendar time. The authors used a prescription register to assess exposure to drugs and estimated the odds ratio of use of statins (ever and current use) in cases of idiopathic polyneuropathy compared with control subjects.

RESULTS: The authors verified a diagnosis of idiopathic polyneuropathy in 166 cases. The cases were classified as definite (35), probable (54), or possible (77). The odds ratio linking idiopathic polyneuropathy with statin use was 3.7 (95% CI 1.8 to 7. 6) for all cases and 14.2 (5.3 to 38. 0) for definite cases. The corresponding odds ratios in current users were 4.6 (2.1 to 10.0) for all cases and 16.1 (5.7 to 45.4) for definite cases. For patients treated with statins for 2 or more years the odds ratio of definite idiopathic polyneuropathy was 26.4 (7.8 to 45.4).

CONCLUSIONS: Long-term exposure to statins

may substantially increase the risk of polyneuropathy.

This study shows that the odds of cholesterol-lowering drugs causing painful/numb hands and feet were 78.7 percent and the odds they do not cause this problem were 21.3 percent. If patients are on the drugs more than two years, the odds they cause this problem were 96.3 percent and the odds they didn't cause polyneuropathy were 3.7 percent.

Statin drugs inhibit the enzyme in the liver called *HMG CoA-reductace*. This enzyme is necessary for manufacturing cholesterol and also to make the vitamin CoQ10. This vitamin is necessary for muscle contraction, including heart muscle function. It appears likely that this may contribute to the epidemic of congestive heart failure in the United States.

"The Clinical Use of HMG CoA-reductase Inhibitors and the Associated Depletion of Coenzyme Q10: A Review of Animal and Human Publications," Langsjoen, P.H., and Langsjoen, A.M., *Biofactors* (2003), 18 (1-4):101–11; ISSN: 0951-6433

Published Abstract:

The depletion of the essential nutrient CoQ10 by the increasingly popular cholesterol-lowering drugs, HMG CoA reductase inhibitors (statins), has grown from a level of concern to one of alarm. With ever higher statin potencies and dosages, and with a steadily shrinking target LDL cholesterol, the prevalence and severity of CoQ10 deficiency is increasing noticeably. An estimated 36 million

Americans are now candidates for statin drug therapy. Statin-induced CoQ10 depletion is well documented in animal and human studies with detrimental cardiac consequences in both animal models and human trials. This drug-induced nutrient deficiency is dose related and more notable in settings of preexisting CoQ10 deficiency such as in the elderly and in heart failure.

Statin-induced CoQ10 deficiency is completely preventable with supplemental CoQ10 with no adverse impact on the cholesterol lowering or anti-inflammatory properties of the statin drugs. We are currently in the midst of a congestive heart failure epidemic in the United States, the cause or causes of which are unclear. As physicians, it is our duty to be absolutely certain that we are not inadvertently doing harm to our patients by creating a wide-spread deficiency of a nutrient critically important for normal heart function.

Studies by Langsjoen support the suspicion that statins are the cause of the epidemic of congestive heart failure in the United States:

"Effect of Atorvastatin (Lipitor) on Left Ventricular Diastolic Function and Ability of Coenzyme Q10 to Reverse that Dysfunction," Silver, M.A., Langsjoen, P.H., Szabo, S., Patil, H., and Zelinger, A., *Am J Cardiol* (2004 Nov 15), 94(10): 1306–10; ISSN: 0002-9149

This study evaluated left ventricular diastolic function with Doppler echocardiography before and after statin therapy. Statin therapy worsened diastolic parameters in most patients; coenzyme

Q(10) supplementation in patients with worsening diastolic function with statin therapy improved parameters of diastolic function.

The Center for Practice Management and Outcomes Research has published an important article in the *Annals of Internal Medicine*, the conclusions of which I have written about in this chapter. Notice their conclusion is also that "current clinical evidence does not demonstrate that titrating lipid therapy to achieve proposed low LDL cholesterol levels is beneficial or safe."

"Narrative Review: Lack of Evidence for Recommended Low-Density Lipoprotein Treatment Targets: A Solvable Problem," Hayward, R.A., Hofer, T.P., and Vijan, S., *Ann Intern Med* (2006 Oct 3) 145(7): 520–30 Issn: 1539-3704, Department of Veterans Affairs VA Center for Practice Management and Outcomes, Research VA Ann Arbor Healthcare System and University of Michigan Schools of Medicine and Public Health Ann Arbor, Michigan

Abstract:
Recent national recommendations have proposed that physicians should titrate lipid therapy to achieve low-density lipoprotein (LDL) cholesterol levels less than 1.81 mmol/L (<70 mg/dL) for patients at very high cardiovascular risk and less than 2.59 mmol/L (<100 mg/dL) for patients at high cardiovascular risk. To examine the clinical evidence for these recommendations, the authors sought to review all controlled trials, cohort studies, and case-control studies that examined the independent relationship between LDL cholesterol and major cardiovascular outcomes in patients with

LDL cholesterol levels less than 3.36 mmol/L (<130 mg/dL).

For those with LDL cholesterol levels less than 3.36 mmol/L (<130 mg/dL), the authors found no clinical trial subgroup analyses or valid cohort or case-control analyses suggesting that the degree to which LDL cholesterol responds to a statin independently predicts the degree of cardiovascular risk reduction. Published studies had avoidable limitations, such as a reliance on ecological (aggregate) analyses, use of analyses that ignore statins' other proposed mechanisms of action, and failure to account for known confounders (especially healthy volunteer effects). Clear, compelling evidence supports near-universal empirical statin therapy in patients at high cardiovascular risk (regardless of their natural LDL cholesterol values), but current clinical evidence does not demonstrate that titrating lipid therapy to achieve proposed low LDL cholesterol levels is beneficial or safe.

In 2004, a National Cholesterol Education Program expert panel recommended that physicians titrate lipid therapy to reach a low-density lipoprotein (LDL) cholesterol level less than 1.81 mmol/L (<70 mg/dL) in patients at very high risk for cardiovascular events. The panel stated that consistent and compelling evidence showed a strong relationship between LDL cholesterol level and cardiovascular outcomes down to this level. However, others have reviewed the same literature and have concluded that there is no valid evidence from clinical trials supporting this conclusion.

Since the early 1900s, we have known that familial hyperlipidemia syndromes result in premature cardiovascular disease, and in the United States and northern Europe, cohort studies have usually found that LDL cholesterol is a major independent cardiovascular risk factor at levels above 3.75 mmol/L (>145 mg/dL). However, these studies had limited ability to assess whether this relationship continued at lower LDL cholesterol levels, and some suggested that this association was less marked as LDL cholesterol level approached 3.36 mmol/L (130 mg/dL), especially when high-density lipoprotein cholesterol levels were normal.

Furthermore, studies in southern Europe, where LDL cholesterol levels tend to be lower in general, have often found a less strong association than those conducted in northern Europe, even in the moderate LDL cholesterol range (3.36 to 4.14 mmol/L [130 to 160 mg/dL]). In addition, studies in Asia and in elderly persons have often found no decrease or even an increase in cardiovascular risk when LDL cholesterol level drops below 3.36 mmol/L (130 mg/dL).

These results raised questions about whether the strong association found at higher levels of LDL cholesterol could be extended to lower LDL cholesterol levels; they also raised concerns that total LDL cholesterol is an unreliable marker of benefit and may be confounded by dietary factors or LDL subparticles that are the true causal factors.

These concerns seemed to be allayed when multiple clinical trials showed that statin therapy dramatically decreased cardiovascular events in almost all groups at high risk and that this benefit extended to those with pretreatment LDL cholesterol levels of 2.33 to 2.59 mmol/L (90 to 100 mg/dL). Several recent trials have also shown greater benefits for high-dose statin therapy compared with low to moderate doses for those with acute coronary syndromes and known coronary artery disease (although the results in the IDEAL [Incremental Decrease in Endpoints Through Aggressive Lipid Lowering] study, in which participants had stable coronary artery disease, did not reach statistical significance). However, these studies generally used fixed doses of statins (placebo vs. statin or low-dose vs. high-dose statin) and therefore cannot directly shed light on whether clinicians should prescribe the doses used in the studies or titrate lipid therapy to achieve recommended LDL cholesterol goals.

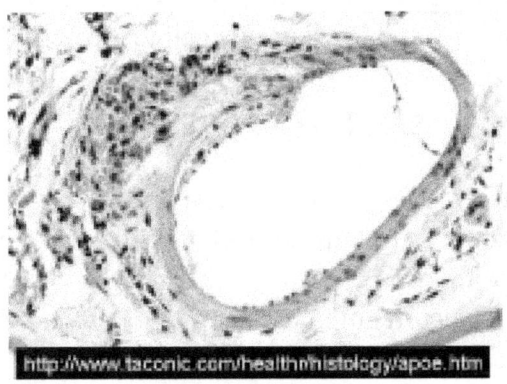

http://www.taconic.com/health/histology/apoe.htm

This is particularly relevant because statins do much more than decrease LDL cholesterol levels. Although strong mechanistic evidence supports the LDL hypothesis, strong basic science evidence also suggests that the effects of statins on inflammation, thrombosis, and oxidation are plausible mechanisms for mediating the benefits of statin therapy (often

371

referred to as "pleiotropic effects"). Indeed, some statin trials seem to run counter to the LDL hypothesis. For example, trials have found that statins substantially reduce the risk for stroke, which is more consistent with their hypothesized antithrombotic effects than with their LDL-lowering effects (high LDL levels are not a major independent risk factor for stroke). In addition, a recent large statin trial conducted in patients receiving dialysis found no substantial benefit despite reductions of 42% in LDL cholesterol levels, suggesting that even dramatic reductions are not always associated with clinically significant lowering of cardiovascular risk.

It has become apparent that the real cause of coronary artery disease is inflammation in the wall of the arteries. When the wall of the artery becomes weak, the body uses a "putty" made of cholesterol and calcium to strengthen the wall so it won't blow out. We call that patch a "plaque."

Tennant Theory of Coronary Artery Disease

The current theory of coronary artery disease teaches that the plaque that leads to a clot inside the coronary artery starts with high levels of fractions of cholesterol in the blood. The current theory states that coronary artery disease progresses in these steps:

1. Oxidative stress: Free radicals (electron stealers) from cigarettes, radiation, heavy metals, antioxidant deficiencies, etc.

2. Oxidation of LDL

3. Increased endothelial permeability

372

4. Promotes pro-thrombotic state

5. Modification of lipids

6. Up-regulation of WBC (white blood cells) and endothelial adhesion molecules

7. Fatty streak formation

8. Smooth muscle migration

9. Plaque formation

10. Sticky platelets cause clot on plaque, obstruction flow of blood through artery

The following things are considered to be the significant risk factors for having a heart attack:

1. High cholesterol

2. Hypertension

3. Diabetes

4. Smoking

"Factors of Antecedents of Fatal and Nonfatal Coronary Heart Disease Events," *JAMA* 2003, 290(7): 891–904

The Framingham Heart Study suggests that eighty-seven to one hundred percent of those with fatal CHD had at least one of these four major risk factors.

Note: 1,2, and 3 above are all symptoms of hypothyroidism! Thus we see that hypothyroidism and smoking are the major risk factors for having a heart attack.

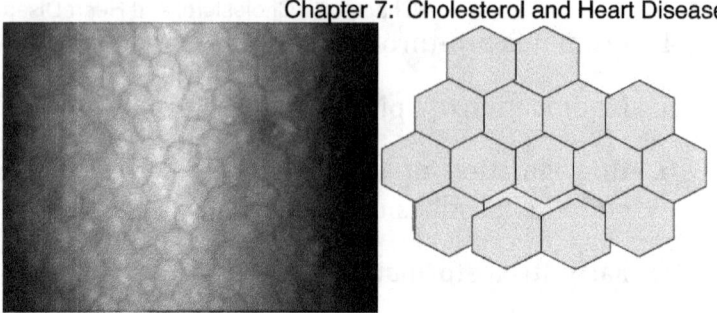

Arteries are lined on the inside with a single-cell-thick layer called the endothelium. As you can see in the photo, it looks like a cobblestone walkway. This fragile structure cannot tolerate being stretched very far.

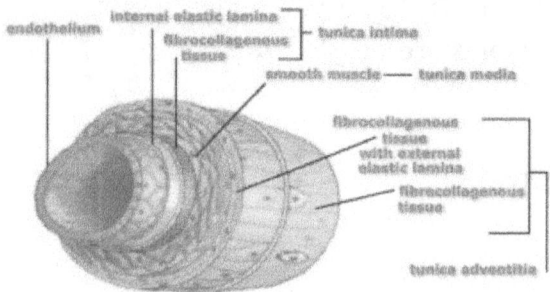

Surrounding this endothelial layer is a layer of smooth muscle. The function of the smooth muscle is to control the blood pressure. If it contracts, it makes the lumen of the artery smaller and thus raises blood pressure. If it dilates, the blood pressure lowers.

Like the endothelium, the smooth muscle is weak and does not tolerate being overstretched.

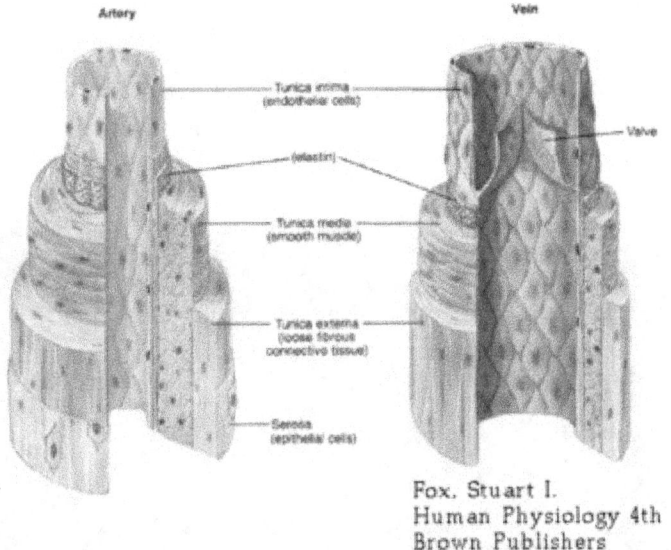

Fox, Stuart I.
Human Physiology 4th
Brown Publishers

To protect the fragile endothelium and smooth muscle, they are surrounded by a sheath made of a combination of elastin and collagen. It is called the *adventitia*. This mixture gives it the ability to stretch just a little to accommodate dilation of the smooth muscle to lower blood pressure but not enough to allow the smooth muscle and endothelium to be damaged. It functions like a bungee cord or cargo netting.

It is my theory that coronary artery disease starts with failure of the cargo netting, not with the endothelium!

When the adventitia becomes weak, it allows the artery to overstretch. This damages the smooth muscle, but what is more important, it opens a wound in the endothelium. Wounds always stimulate the formation of a scar. All scars are made from cholesterol, calcium, and fibrous strands. The scar that fills this wound in the artery is called a "plaque."

In this photo you can see the swollen endothelial cells that surround the wound. In the wound you can see the beginnings of the scar. It is called a "fatty streak."

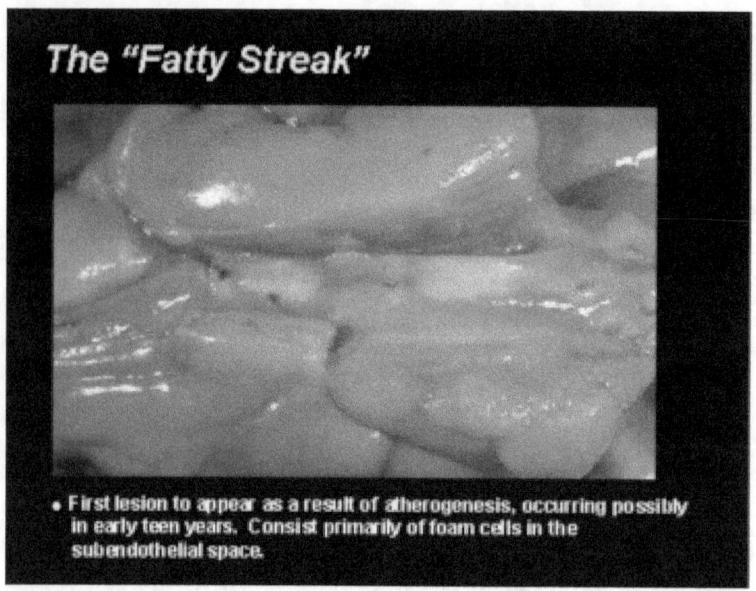

The "Fatty Streak"

• First lesion to appear as a result of atherogenesis, occurring possibly in early teen years. Consist primarily of foam cells in the subendothelial space.

If we want to stop coronary artery disease, we must look at the things that weaken the cargo netting (tunica adventitia).

The collagen in the cargo netting requires the following to be strong and repair itself:

1. Vitamin C

2. Vitamin B6

3. Vitamin B12

4. Copper

5. Folic acid

6. Voltage

Many Americans are deficient in these nutrients. However, the voltage is one of the more important items. It is controlled primarily by thyroid hormone and the fats in the cell membranes. If the fats are plastic trans fats, they can't hold the charge.

Remember that the leading risks for heart attacks are high cholesterol (a sign of hypothyroidism), diabetes (a symptom of hypothyroidism), hypertension (a symptom of hypothyroidism), and smoking.

The iodine/fluoride problem is a major issue. Iodine is necessary for thyroid hormone production and function. Iodine is displaced by fluoride, so consuming fluoride causes hypothyroidism that reduces the voltage available for the adventitia to be strong.

Perhaps just as important is that fluoride damages all collagen! A perfect example of this is the number of people whose Achilles tendon or shoulder tendons rupture when taking as little as one capsule of an antibiotic made from fluoride. Examples are Levaquin and Cipro.

When you consume fluoride, it damages the collagen in your arteries, allowing them to overstretch. This opens the wound in the endothelium leading to a scar. This sets you up for a heart attack.

In 1972, Broda Barnes published an important study about thyroid and heart attacks. He showed that if thyroid function was normalized using body temperature instead of blood tests as a guide, the incidence of heart attacks was 0.25 percent. Of course this was before fluoride was placed in our water supply and our toothpaste and mouthwash and dentists started flushing our teeth with fluoride when they cleaned our teeth.

Sex	Classification	# patients Rx	Patient Years	Expected cases Framingham	Actual in Hypothyroid RX Patients
F	Age 30-59	490	2705	7.6	0
F	High-risk Cholesterol or BP High or Both	172	1086	7.3	0
F	> Age 60	182	955	7.8	0
M	Age 30-59	382	2192	12.8	1
M	High-risk Cholesterol or BP High or Both	186	1070	18.5	2
M	> Age 60	157	816	18	1
	Totals Overall Percentage	1569	8824	72 4.59%	4 0.25%
	High Risk Females Percentage	172	1086	7.3 4.24%	0 0.00%
	Males Percentage	186	1070	18.5 9.95%	2 1.08%
	Overall Percentage of Anticipated CHD That Actually Had Heart Attack			5.56%	
	Thus Rx to Normal Thyroid Levels Prevents 94% of Expected Heart Attacks				

Barnes, Broda O; Heart Attack Rareness in Thyroid Treated Patients; Charles Thomas, Springfield, Illinois, 1972, p. 30.

Zeta potential is an abbreviation for electrokinetic potential in colloidal systems. Zeta potential is the potential difference between the dispersion medium and the stationary layer of fluid attached to the dispersed particle.

What this means is that when there are particles in a solution, the magnetic field around the particles pushes the other particles away so they don't form a clump. For example, paint is made with pigment particles suspended in a fluid. If the zeta potential is high, the paint goes on smoothly without clumping. However, if the magnetic field around the pigments (zeta potential) is diminished, they clump together.

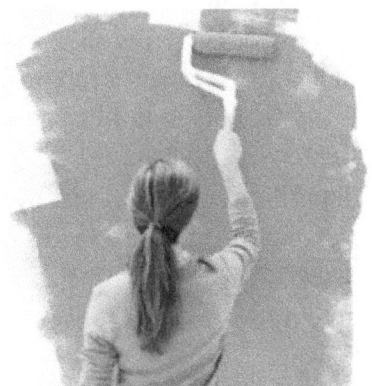

The same is true for blood. If the body voltage is low, the magnetic field around the RBC will be low, allowing clumping/clotting to occur.

Of course if the magnetic field around the red blood cells and in the endothelium of the artery is low (low zeta potential), the cells and platelets will clump, causing a heart attack.

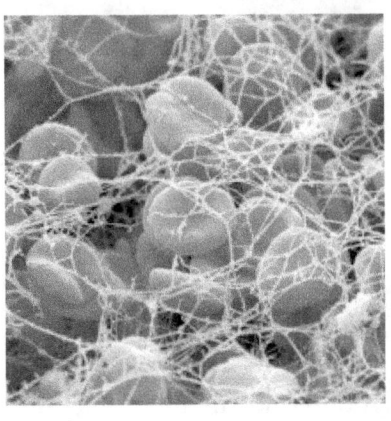

What controls the magnetic field of cells? The voltage, of course.

Remember that diabetes is primarily a vascular disease. The high blood sugar, blindness, kidney failure, etc., are the result of obstruction of the fine blood vessels. These small vessels react to the fluoride and lack of voltage the same way as the coronary artery vessels.

High blood pressure increases plaque formation because it

presses against the cargo netting. The higher the blood pressure and the weaker the cargo netting, the more plaque you will make.

Consuming omega-3 fats instead of trans fats improves the ability of cells to hold a charge.

The inflammation caused by the rupture of the endothelium and smooth muscle creates inflammation. This is detected by tests that look for inflammation including the C-reactive protein test.

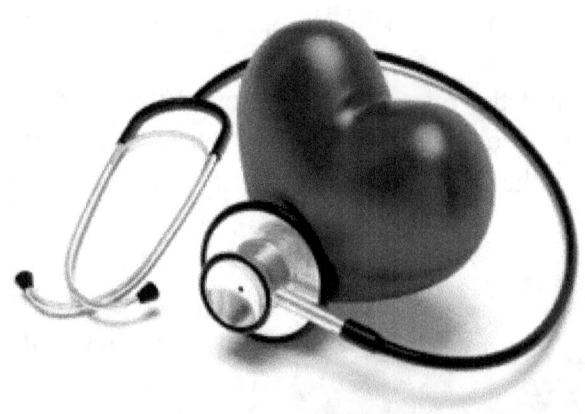

Dilation of blood vessels is controlled by nitric oxide. I have devoted an entire chapter to it.

To avoid a heart attack:
1. Correct your hypothyroidism
2. Correct your adrenal function to reduce your blood pressure
3. Correct your iodine levels.
4. Avoid fluoride.
5. Correct your vitamin and mineral levels.

6.   Correct vitamin C levels in particular.

7.   Take omega-3 fats and natural fats.

8.   Avoid trans fats.

9.   Correct stomach acid to avoid allergies.

10. Look for and remove heavy metals, particularly lead.

11. Remove toxins.

12. Be sure to maintain the voltage in your chest BioTerminal by monitoring it regularly with the Tennant BioModulator.

13. Eat leafy green vegetables to correct your nitric oxide levels so you avoid hypertension.

8 Infections

Most people think of infections as something you "catch". "I caught MRSA staph infection" or "I caught strep throat from my sister." Infections such as this are found to be bacteria with cell membranes like the photo of Staphylococcus aureus seen here.

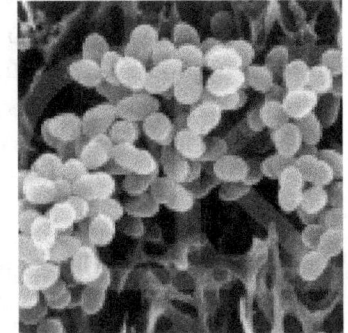

Most antibiotics work by interfering with the cell membrane and prevent bacteria from duplication. Obviously if the bacteria doesn't have a cell membrane, antibiotics have no effect.

One significant problem with antibiotics is that they cause antibiotic-resistant forms such as MRSA (Methicillin Resistant Staphylococcus aureus), Clostridium difficile, etc. Clostridium difficile is a species of Gram-positive bacteria of the genus Clostridium that causes diarrhea and other intestinal disease when competing bacteria are wiped out by antibiotics.

Clostridia are anaerobic, spore-forming rods (bacilli). C. difficile is the most serious cause of antibiotic-associated diarrhea (AAD) and can lead to pseudomembranous colitis, a severe infection of the colon, often resulting from eradication of the normal gut flora by antibiotics. The C. difficile bacteria, which naturally reside in the body, become overpopulated: The overpopulation is harmful because the bacterium releases toxins that can cause bloating, constipation, and diarrhea with abdominal pain, which may become severe.

The increasing incidence of infections and deaths from antibiotic resistant Staph and Clostridium are major concerns for anyone going to a hospital.

There are also side effects of antibiotics relating to killing of the good bacteria in the gut. Also, the need for the body to remove antibiotics (they can't be used to make cells, so the body has to find a way to get rid of them) places stress on the liver and kidneys and often damages them.
A little recognized effect of antibiotics is the formation of bacteria without cell membranes call L-forms or pleomorphic forms.

Bacteria without cell membranes are largely ignored by medical doctors because they do not grow in a standard culture plate. If a doctor takes a swab of fluid from a wound or a drop of blood and sends it to the lab for culture, it will often come back as "No Growth". Doctors believe this means that there are no bacteria present. However, bacteria without cell membranes are almost always present.

Cell Wall Deficient Organism

L-form bacteria also known as L-phase bacteria, L-phase variants or cell wall deficient (CWD) bacteria, are strains of bacteria that lack cell walls They were first isolated in 1935 by Emmy Klieneberger-Nobel, who named them "L-forms" after the Lister Institute in London where she was working. Two types of L-forms are distinguished: unstable L-forms, spheroplasts which are capable of dividing, but can revert to the original morphology and stable L-forms, L-forms which are unable to revert to the original bacteria.

These forms were apparently first described by Antoine Béchamp in 1857. Considering early work of Bechamp,

Günther Enderlein, who was an opponent of Louis Pasteur, and based on a point of view of contemporary Wilhelm von Brehmer (1883-1958), and based on his own microscopic observation, developed his own complicated pleomorphism hypothesis. He was convinced that every microorganism would pass through a

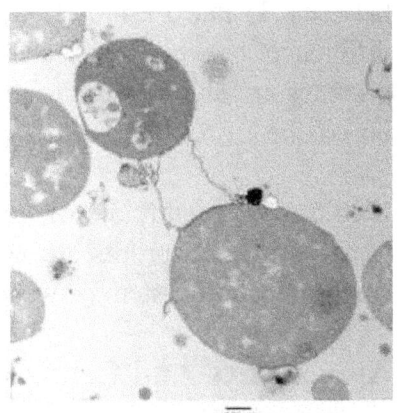

Transmission electron micrograph of L-form Bacillus subtilis, showing a range of sizes. Scale bar is 10 micrometers.

particular development-cycle, that he called cyclode (bacterial cyclode). Bechamp had issued earlier the opinion that in every animal or plant cell there were small particles, that he called microzymas or granulations moleculaires. These particles were able to transform into pathogen bacteries, under certain circumstances. Pasteur and the scientific community did not accept this opinion.

At that time it was also known that plasmodia (causing agents of malaria) were able to change form during the different development stages.

In 1925 Enderlein published his main work: Bakterien-Cyklogenie. He developed not only a complex hypothesis, but at the same time he created also his own terminology that makes reading of his papers difficult or even impossible. He stated that small harmless and beneficial herbal particles were present in every animal or plant and may transform into larger and pathogen bacteria or fungi under certain circumstances. The smallest particles are called protit, symbionts or endobionts. Protits are, according to Enderlein, small colloids of proteins, sized between 1 and 10 nm. Enderlein believed there was a difference between acid and alkaline symbionts. These particles are able to be transmitted by way of the placenta before the birth.

It has been recently shown that these small particles that Enderlein called protits are actually microcysts that are a communication system between cells.

Appearance And Cell Division

Bacterial morphology is determined by the cell wall. As L-forms have no cell wall, their morphology is different from the strain of bacteria from which they are derived. Typically L-form cells are spheres or spheroids. For example, L-forms of the rod shaped bacterium Bacillus subtilis appear round when viewed by phase contrast microscopy or by transmission electron microscopy.

Although L-forms can develop from Gram-positive as well as from Gram-negative bacteria, in a Gram stain preparation the L-forms always color Gram-negative, due to the lack of a cell wall.

The cell wall is important for cell division which, in most bacteria, occurs by binary fission. The lack of cell walls in L-forms means that division is disorganized, creating a variety of cell sizes, from very tiny to very big.

In bacteria, cell division usually requires a cell wall and components of the bacterial cytoskeleton. The ability of L-form bacteria to grow and divide in the absence of both of these structures is highly unusual, and may represent a form of cell division that was important in early forms of life. This novel mode of division seems to involve the extension of thin protrusions from the cell's surface and these protrusions then pinching off to form new cells.

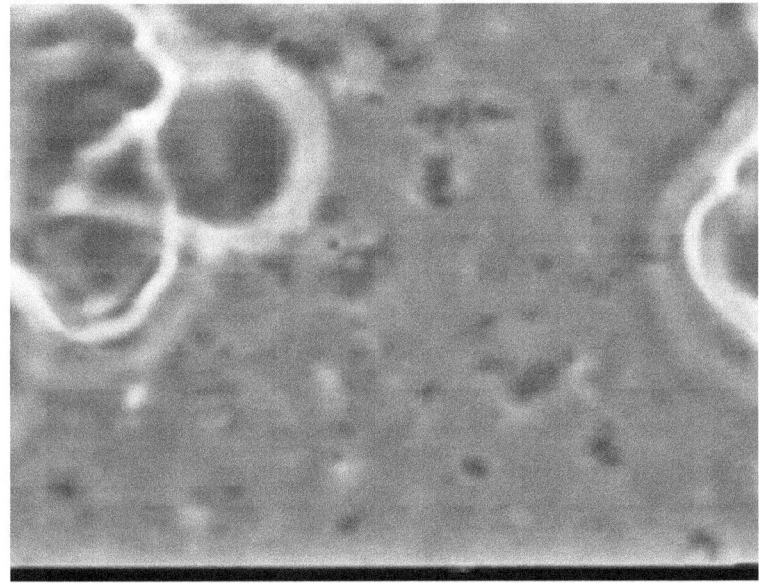

The photo here shows fungal forms that have been named Mucor racemos fresens and are associated with cancer. This phase contrast microscope photo is from a patient with leukemia.

Generation In Cultures

L-forms can be generated in the laboratory from many bacterial species that usually have cell walls, such as Bacillus subtilis or Escherichia coli. This is done by inhibiting peptidoglycan synthesis with antibiotics or treating the cells with lysozyme, an enzyme which digests cell walls. The L-forms are generated in a culture medium that is the same osmolarity as the bacterial cytosol (an isotonic solution), which prevents cell lysis by osmotic shock. L-form strains can be unstable, tending to revert to the normal form of the bacteria by regrowing a cell wall, but this can be prevented by long-term culture of the cells under the same conditions that were used to produce them. Some studies have identified mutations that occur as these strains are derived from normal bacteria. One such point mutation is in an enzyme involved in the mevalonate pathway of lipid metabolism that increased the frequency of L-form formation 1,000-fold. The reason for this effect is not known, but may relate to this enzyme's role in making a lipid that is important in peptidoglycan synthesis. www.wikipedia.com

Note the statement that the formation of L-forms is accomplished by the use of antibiotics!

Koch's Postulates

Heinrich Hermann Robert Koch (11 December 1843 – 27 May 1910) was a German physician. He became famous for isolating Bacillus anthracis (1877), the Tuberculosis bacillus (1882) and the Vibrio cholerae (1883) and for his development of Koch's postulates

Koch's postulates are:

1. The microorganism must be found in abundance in all organisms suffering from the disease, but should not be found in healthy animals.
2. The microorganism must be isolated from a diseased organism and grown in pure culture.
3. The cultured microorganism should cause disease when introduced into a healthy organism.

4. The microorganism must be re-isolated from the inoculated, diseased experimental host and identified as being identical to the original specific causative agent.

Koch's postulates say that you find bacteria in someone that is ill and that these bacteria are not normally found in healthy people. You collect the bacteria from the person that is ill and grow them in a culture. You then take the cultured bacteria and put them into a healthy person where it causes the same disease as the person from which it came originally.

Koch's postulates are still considered the way to prove or disprove infectious diseases. However, they ignore cell-wall-deficient organisms because they cannot be cultured in the absence of antibiotics or lysozyme! We will discuss shortly the likelihood that they play a role in what is considered autoimmune diseases.

Many scientists and physicians ignore L-forms since they are not part of the usual paradigm of bacteriology.

Most of the time, slides of bacteria are observed with a bright light microscope at a reasonability low power, e.g. 40x and with a stain. However, L-forms are difficult to see unless you use a phase contrast microscope or a dark-field microscope at 1000 x power. When blood is observed under these conditions, you will always find L-forms present!

As the voltage and oxygen levels drop in the blood, the L-forms change from spherical to rod-shaped to yeast-shaped to fungal-shaped forms.

A relatively new microscope has been developed in Germany called the Ergonom microscope. Most microscopes can only achieve 1000 power. This amazing microscope can achieve 40,000 power and see living microorganisms in 3D and color and watch them change from one kind to another! See videos at www.grayfieldoptical.com.

Koch's postulates are still considered the way to prove or disprove infectious diseases. However, they ignore cell-wall-deficient organisms because they cannot be cultured in the absence of antibiotics or lysozyme!

According to Beauchamp and others, L-forms cannot be killed by the heat of a volcano, radiation, freezing, or any known method except by changing the energy (voltage) of the environment. When the environment changes for the better, they change to nonpathogenic forms. As the environment changes for the worse, they change to increasingly pathogenic forms.

What does all this mean? What is the difference between a sore throat caused by a streptococcus bacteria and illness caused by L-forms? First, the immune system functions by surrounding the body with a shield of iodine. It places 30x as much iodine in the parts of the body as in the blood. Since iodine kills all microorganisms, it is the body's first line of defense against regular bacteria entering the body. If bacteria get past this shield (usually because you are iodine deficient), they are consumed by white blood cells and killed with ozone or hydrogen peroxide made by the white blood cells.

Now assume you take antibiotics. They kill the streptococcus but some of them morph into L-forms. Since these L-forms are not affected by antibiotics, they assume the form dictated by their environment. If the environment is low voltage, low oxygen, etc., they will assume a pathological form. They can only exist in a pathological form if the conditions allow it. However, as long as the conditions in the body allow it, they will continue to duplicate themselves and morph to the form that matches their environment. The only way you can alter that is to change the environment or change the voltage.

The Consequences of Low Voltage

The amount of oxygen that will dissolve in water is dictated by the voltage of the water. As the voltage increases, more oxygen dissolves in it. As the voltage drops, the oxygen leaves solution and escapes.

Cells are 70% water. As their voltage drops, the oxygen levels drop. When oxygen levels drop, many bacteria (called anaerobic bacteria) can grow. This allows regular bacteria to grow and L-forms to become more pathogenic. Thus whenever we have low voltage, we always have infections taking advantage of us.

Some examples of facultative anaerobic bacteria are the Staphylococci (Gram positive), Escherichia coli (Gram negative), Corynebacterium (Gram positive), and Listeria (Gram positive). Organisms in the Kingdom Fungi can also be facultative anaerobic, such as yeasts.

When bacteria are active in our bodies, they want to have lunch. Since they don't have teeth, they must dissolve our cells to get the nutrients. These digestive enzymes get into our bloodstream and go throughout the body. They attack cells distant from where the bacteria or L-forms exist. The damage caused by these toxins is often diagnosed as an autoimmune disease.

391

Along with lack of voltage adequate for the cells to function, chronic pain, decreased oxygen, and bugs having lunch, a reduction in voltage causes poor metabolism. Remember that voltage determines the amounts of oxygen available. When oxygen is available, for each unit of fatty acids one metabolizes, you get 36-38 molecules of ATP (charged batteries). When oxygen is decreased, you get two molecules of ATP. It's like your car going from 38 miles to the gallon to 2 miles to the gallon!

Remember: every time your voltage drops, you get
1. Chronic pain
2. Inability of cells to do their job or take trash to the curb
3. Waste buildup
4. Diminished oxygen
5. Inefficient metabolism
6. Bugs having lunch--> autoimmune symptoms
7. Infections like strep throat, bladder infections, etc.

Treating such problems with antibiotics may be necessary for serious problems like meningitis, but the side-effect is always an increase in L-forms and formation of bacteria resistant to the antibiotic.

Oxidative Therapy

The terminology can be confusing when you talk about oxidation. We all know that oxygen is good for us and not breathing for a few minutes is disastrous. However, oxidation is bad for us. It is unfortunate that the term "oxidation" was chosen for this process. What oxidation means is that an electron stealer is "mugging you" and stealing your electrons. In the process, the mugger hurts or kills you.

Oxidation describes the loss of electrons / hydrogen or gain of oxygen / increase in oxidation state by a molecule, atom or ion.

Reduction describes the gain of electrons / hydrogen or a loss of oxygen / decrease in oxidation state by a molecule, atom or ion.

Oxidants are highly electronegative substances that can gain one or two extra electrons by oxidizing a substance (O, F, Cl, Br). $O2 --> 2\ O^{-2}$ - 4 e-   (electron stealer needs four electrons). Ozone $O3 --> 3\ O^{-2} - 6$ e-

The Reductant transfers electrons to another substance, and is thus oxidized itself. Because it "donates" electrons it is also called an electron donor. (Li, Na, Mg, Fe, Zn, Al). These metals donate or give away electrons readily. Fe (s) $----> Fe^{3+} + 3$ e- (electron donor of three electrons).

Oxidation refers to the loss of electrons, while reduction refers to the gain of electrons.

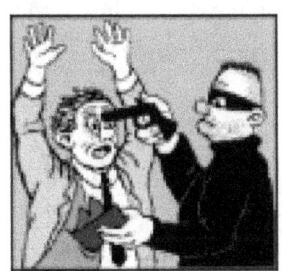

The way the body kills bacteria is with a white blood cell called a **neutrophil**.   The neutrophil surrounds the bacteria and then kills it by stealing its electrons (oxidation).   It uses an electron stealer ("mugger") called ozone or hydrogen peroxide.

This photo from Wikipedia shows a neutrophil engulfing an anthrax bacteria.   After it finishes swallowing it, the bacteria will be killed with ozone or hydrogen peroxide by the process of oxidation or stealing its electrons.

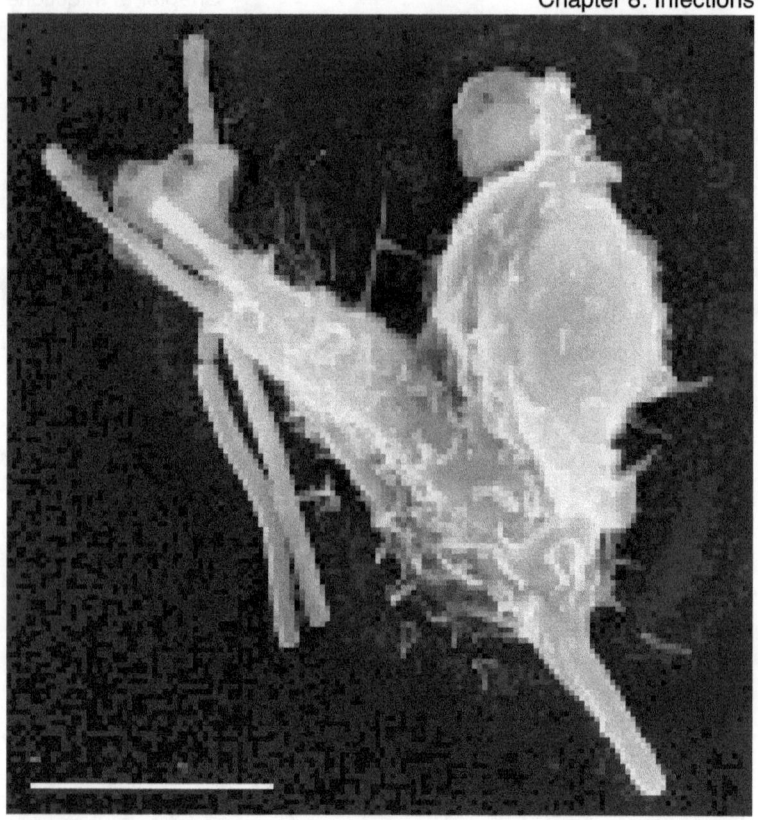

Contrast this with the way antibiotics work. They stop bacteria by interfering with the cell membranes so they cannot reproduce.

One can simulate the normal way the body kills bacteria by consuming or getting IV hydrogen peroxide or ozone. Ozone is rarely given orally but is often given rectally or vaginally. More commonly it is given intravenously.

Such oxidative therapies are extremely effective. It should be no surprise since that is the body's normal mechanism. No microorganism can withstand oxidative therapy, so it is ideal for any infection, but it is amazing for MRSA (Methicillin-resistant staph), Clostridium difficile, Anthrax, etc.

You must remember, however, that you are consuming electron stealers. Taken over the long term, they can lower your body voltage and causes all the problems listed above. If you start using oxidative therapy when your total body voltage is already low, your body may not be able to deal with all the dead bugs and it can make you feel terrible. Always check your total body voltage before you start treatment with oxidative therapy like ozone or hydrogen peroxide.

An oxidative therapy that is considered to be a nutrient is sodium chlorite. It is sold under the trade name MMS (miracle mineral solution). The free acid, chlorous acid, $HClO_2$, is only stable at low concentrations. Since it cannot be concentrated, it is not a commercial product. However, the corresponding sodium salt, **sodium chlorite, $NaClO_2$** is stable and inexpensive enough to be commercially available.

When sodium chlorite is mixed with a weak organic acid like citric acid, it changes to chlorine dioxide. As you can see, chlorine dioxide is two oxygens attached to a chloride. Chlorine dioxide (ClO_2) is highly reactive with thiols (RSH), polyamines, purines, certain amino acids and iron, all of which are necessary for the growth and survival of pathogenic microbes. Whenever it finds a microorganism, it releases the chloride. That steals electrons from the organism, killing it immediately. All that is left is that the two oxygens make water and the dead bug.

An application of sodium chlorite is the generation of chlorine dioxide for bleaching and stripping of textiles, pulp, and paper. It is also used for disinfection of a few municipal water treatment plants after conversion to chlorine dioxide. An advantage in this application, as compared to the more commonly used chlorine, is that trihalomethanes (such as chloroform) are not produced from organic contaminants. Sodium chlorite, $NaClO_2$ also finds application as a component in therapeutic rinses, mouthwashes, toothpastes and gels, mouth sprays, chewing gums and lozenges, and in contact lens cleaning solution under the trade name purite. Under the brand name Oxine it is used for sanitizing air ducts and HVAC/R systems and animal containment areas (walls, floors, and other surfaces). Wikipedia

I have yet to find any virus, bacteria, yeast, fungus, parasite, or poison it will not destroy. I have seen the fever and fatigue/muscle aches of flu disappear in 2-3 hours using it.

There's only one human case in the medical literature of chlorite poisoning. Theoretically it could cause life threatening hemolysis in Glucose-6-Phosphate Dehydrogenase deficient persons.

Gallium

Gallium is a chemical element with symbol Ga and atomic number 31. Elemental gallium does not occur in nature, but as the gallium(III) compounds in trace amounts in bauxite and zinc ores. Gallium has no known role in biology. Because gallium(III) and ferric salts behave similarly in biological systems, gallium ions often mimic iron ions in medical applications. Gallium-containing pharmaceuticals and radio-pharmaceuticals have been developed. Gallium attacks most other metals by diffusing into their metal lattice. Gallium must not be put into metal containers. Only glass should be used.

Although gallium has no known role in biology, it mimics iron(III), the gallium ion localizes to and interacts with many processes in the body in which iron(III) is manipulated. As these processes include inflammation, which is a marker for many disease states, several gallium salts are used, or are in development, as both pharmaceuticals and radio-pharmaceuticals in medicine. When gallium ions are mistakenly taken up by bacteria such as Pseudomonas, the bacteria's ability to respire is interfered with and the bacteria die. The mechanism behind this is that iron is redox active, which allows for the transfer of electrons during respiration, but gallium is redox inactive.

Gallium nitrate (brand name Ganite) has been used as an intravenous pharmaceutical to treat hypercalcemia associated with tumor metastasis to bones. Gallium is thought to interfere with osteoclast function. It may be effective when other treatments for maligancy-associated hypercalcemia are not. Gallium maltolate an orally absorbable form of gallium(III) ion, is in clinical and preclinical trials as a potential treatment for a number of types of cancer, infectious disease, and inflammatory disease. A complex amine-phenol Ga(III) compound MR045 was found to be selectively toxic to parasites that have developed resistance to chloroquine, a common drug against malaria. Both the Ga(III) complex and chloroquine act by inhibiting crystallization of hemozoin, a disposal product formed from the digestion of blood by the parasites.

The Ga(III) ion of soluble gallium salts tends to form the insoluble hydroxide when injected in large amounts, and in animals precipitation of this has resulted in renal toxicity.

In lower doses, soluble gallium is tolerated well, and does not accumulate as a poison.
Wikipedia

Gallium has antibiotic properties to iron-dependent bacteria and has potent anti-inflammatory, anticancer and anti-hypercalcemic properties, and it readily reverses osteoporosis. Eby reported that a single topical application of a gallium nitrate solution was immediately effective in eliminating pimples, acne, boils, folliculitis and carbuncles and other bacterial skin infections. Eby also reported that a 1% gallium nitrate isotonic saline ocular solution used each several hours for a day eliminated overnight two treatment-resistant bacterial eye infections in humans.

> Eby GA. Elimination of arthritis pain and inflammation for over 2 years with a single 90 min, topical 14% gallium nitrate treatment: case reports and review of actions of Gallium-III. Med Hypotheses 2005;65:1136–41.

Rasmussen et al. in 2002 provided electron microscopic and immunological evidence of nanobacteria-like structures in calcified carotid arteries, aortic aneurysms, and cardiac valves. Others have found nanobacteria in over 90% of kidney stones.

> Rasmussen TE, Kirkland BL, Chalesworth J, et al. Electron microscopic and immunological evidence of nanobacterial-like structures in calcified carotid arteries, aortic aneurysms, and cardiac valves. JACC 2002;39:206A. (Suppl. 1).

Perhaps the most important question is how much oral gallium should be administered in treating atherosclerosis and kidney stones without the risk of side effects. The answer is unknown at this time, although some people, not being treated directly for atherosclerosis – but of an age group likely to have atherosclerosis – have taken 120– 240 mg of oral gallium (as gallium nitrate) daily for several months without evident side effects in the treatment of arthritis. On several occasions much larger oral doses were taken, with one case ten times larger resulting in diarrhea without further sequela. The LD50 oral dose for mice of gallium nitrate is 2.15 g per kilogram (equivalent to 0.59 g per kilogram elemental gallium). Ten milligrams per kilogram oral dose produced no visible toxicity in dogs despite monitoring bone marrow, kidneys and liver. Oral daily doses of 200–400 mg per kilogram of gallium chloride for 20–40 days in rats and mice induced no visible signs of toxicity. Dosages and toxicity of various gallium compounds are discussed in detail by Collery et al. The mode of delivery should be oral and not intravenous, since mainlining gallium has repeatedly been shown to cause reversible kidney damage, requiring substantial rehydration.

Collery P, Keppler B, Madoulet C, Desoize B. Gallium in cancer treatment. Crit Rev Oncol Hematol 2002;42:283–96.

Medical Hypotheses (2008) 71, 584–590

Iron-dependent pathogenic microorganisms treatable with Ga comprise:

Acinetobacter,	Escherichia,	Porphyromonas gingivalis,
Aeromonas,	Eubacterium sulci,	Proteus,
Alcaligenes,	Exophiala werneckii,	Pseudomonas,

Aspergillus spp.;	Francisella,	Salmonella,
Atopobium parvulum,	Fusarium spp.	Sporothrix schenckii,
Bacillus,	Helicobacter,	ß-hemolytic streptococci,
Brucella,	Klebsiella,	Staphylococcus aureus,
Campylobacter,	Legionella,	Staphylococcus,
Capnocytophaga,	Listeria,	Streptococcus gordonii,
Chlamydia,	Malassezia furfur,	Streptococcus mutans,
Clostridium,	Microsporum audouinii,	Streptococcus pneumoniae,
Corynebacterium minutissimum,	Microsporum canis,	Streptococcus sanguis,
Corynebacterium,	Microsporum canis,	Streptococcus,
Coxilla,	Microsporum gypseum,	Trichophyton mentagrophytes,
Ehrlichia,	Mycobacterium,	Trichophyton rubrum,
Enterobacter,	Pasteurella,	Trichosporon beigelii,
Erysipelothrix,	Pityriasis versicolor,	Tropheryma,
		Yersinia,

Microorganisms that are known to have become resistant to first-line antibiotics but are sensitive to gallium include:

Enterococcus faecalis (a causative organism for endocarditis, urinary tract infections, and wound infections),
Escherichia coli O157 (a causative organism for gastroenteritis, haemorrhagic colitis or urinary and genital tract infections),
Methicillin-resistant Staphylococcus aureus (MRSA; a causative organism for various skin infections, eye infection, wound, oral and other infections),
Salmonella LO typhii (the causative organism for typhoid fever)
Vancomycin-resistant

Fungi sensitive to gallium:

Aspergillus fumigatus,	Microsporum canis,
Blastomyces dermatitidis,	Mucor spp.
Candida albicans,	Pityriasis versicolor,
Coccidioides immitis,	Rhizopus spp.
Epidermophyton spp.,	Sporothrix schenckii,
Exophiala werneckii,	Trichophyton mentagrophytes,
Fusarium spp.,	Trichophyton rubrum,
Histoplama capsulatum,	Trichosporon beigelii,
Malassezia furfur,	Zygomyces spp.,

Mycobacterium avium subspecies *paratuberculosis* (MAP) , a cousin to tuberculosis, is the likely cause of Crohn's disease (CD) and ulcerative colitis (UC) in humans, and is believed to be the cause of the closely related Johne's disease in cattle. MAP, like all

401

Mycobacterium, is an iron-dependent bacterium. Gallium ion (Ga) is bacteriostatic to all iron dependent bacteria. Ga also has anti-inflammatory properties. Beneficial probiotic intestinal bacteria are not iron dependent, and are not injured by Ga. Crohn's disease and ulcerative colitis often respond to a course of gallium along with the GAPS diet.

Gallium comes concentrated as 42% or 14% and must be diluted to 1% for use. One quart of 1% solution is taken orally daily. It is important to take this amount of water to prevent kidney dysfunction.

Gallium and more information is available from:

George A. Eby III
George Eby Research Institute
14909-C Fitzhugh Road
Austin, Texas 78736
Telephone 1-512-263-0805
Email george.eby at george-eby-research.com

Rife Frequencies

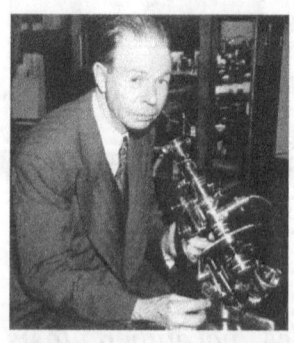

Royal Rife (1888-1971) while in medical school decided he was more interested in bacteriology than medicine. He was also interested in microscopy and studied in Germany with Zeiss. He believed that microorganisms could be killed with specific frequencies that he called the "mortal oscillatory rate" or MOR. He would place microorganisms under a microscope and expose them to frequencies from a frequency generator until they exploded. He then recorded that as their MOR.

402

He worked with Mayo Clinic physician Edward C. Rosenow, Arthur I. Kendall of Northwestern Medical School, and Milbank MD, the Medical Research Committee of the University of Southern California. He was assisted by a radio engineer named Philip Hoyland and later John Crane. When Hoyland and Rife started producing devices for use by physicians, they attempted to conceal their proprietary frequencies to protect their intellectual property.

In electronics, modulation is the process of varying one or more properties of a periodic waveform, called the carrier signal, with a modulating signal which typically contains information to be transmitted. We call that frequency modulation or FM radio.

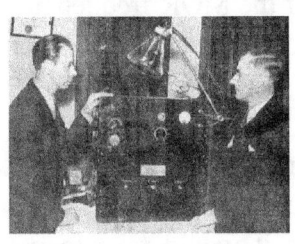 Hoyland used frequencies in the audio range (20-20,000 hertz) to modulate a radio frequency carrier of 3.30 megahertz. When you do so, it creates the actual MOR's seen in the chart below. For example, when you transmit 7,270 hertz onto a carrier wave of 3.30 megahertz, one of the frequencies created is 447,660, the frequency necessary to destroy *Staphylococcus aureus*. Since almost all devices sold by others don't have the carrier wave but simply produce the audio frequencies (7,270 in the example above), most have been unable to produce the results that Rife and those that worked with him could produce. Thus it is believed by most medical authorities that Rife technology does not work.

Medical authorities, governmental organization and courts have prosecuted many that have used or sold "Rife devices". The governmental agencies are most aggressive in prosecuting any effort to treat cancer with anything except chemotherapy, radiation and surgery. Those that claim that Rife technology can cure cancer have been imprisoned. This was true in Rife's lifetime and is still true.

I have been given videos where microorganisms on agar plates have been shielded over half the plate with aluminum foil and then exposed to Rife frequencies. The half of the plate treated grew almost nothing while the shielded half showed vigorous growth of the bacteria. I am intrigued by the technology but I am not writing about it in this book to support its use. Since awareness of Rife technology has become widespread, it is important to know that most "Rife devices" sold today do not produce Rife's frequencies and thus would not be expected to work. Most frequency generators are incapable of the MOR frequencies that Rife found to work. You should not bet your life or your current health on them.

It would be wonderful if the research would be done to reproduce Rife's work. However, that is unlikely to happen since the tens of millions of dollars it would take to get FDA approval is not likely to be given for something that can't be patented. Using $0.05 worth of electricity to replace antibiotics that can cost $10.00 per pill would not give a financial return and the pharmaceutical industry will continue to violently oppose such approval.

Organism	Frequency in Hz
Actinomycosis (Streptothrix)	191,803
Bacillus anthracis (Anthrax)	139,200

Organism	Frequency in Hz
Escherichia coli (rod form)	416,510
Escherichia coli (filterable virus)	769,035
Bacillus X or BX (carcinoma)	1,607,450
Bacillus Y or BY (sarcoma)	1,529,520
Neisseria gonorrhoeae (Gonorrhea)	233,000
Meningitis (see note below)	426,862
Staphylococcus aureus	477,660
Staphylococcus albus	549,070
Streptococcus pyogenes	719,150
Treponema pallidum (Syphilis)	788,700
Clostridium tetani (Tetanus)	234,000
Mycobacterium tuberculosis (rod)	369,433
Mycobacterium tuberculosis (virus)	769,000
Salmonella typhii (rod)	759,450
Salmonella typhii (virus)	1,445,180

Note: these frequencies are from www.rifevideos.com. There is an error in their original chart. They name organisms "*Staphylococcus Pyogenes Aureus* and *Staphylococcus Pyogenes Albus*". There are no such organisms. There are *Staphylococcus aureus* and *albus*. The term "pyogenes" is used with *Streptococcus pyogenes*. I have made this correction in the chart above.

Bacterium coli was the type species of the now invalid genus *Bacterium* when it was revealed that the former type species ("Bacterium triloculare") was missing. Following a revision of Bacteria it was reclassified as *Bacillus coli* by Migula in 1895 and later reclassified in the newly created genus *Escherichia,* named after its original discoverer.

Also note that "carcinoma" means that cancer involves the inner layers (endoderm) or outer layers (ectoderm) of the body. Sarcoma means the cancer is from the middle layers (mesoderm) of the body. Sarcomas are bone, cartilage, fat, muscle, vascular, or hematopoietic (blood) tissues. Sarcomas are relatively rare. Most cancers are carcinomas.

Meningitis is inflammation of the protective membranes covering the brain and spinal cord, known collectively as the meninges. The inflammation may be caused by infection with viruses, bacteria, or other microorganisms, and less commonly by certain drugs. *Neisseria meningitidis,* often referred to as meningococcus, is a bacterium that can cause meningitis. *Streptococcus pneumoniae* (aka pneumococcus) is the most common bacterial etiology of meningitis in children beyond 2 months of age. *Haemophilus influenzae, type B* or mumps virus infections can also cause meningitis. It is not clear which of these organisms Rife's frequency for meningitis represents.

Typhoid fever, also known simply as typhoid is a common worldwide bacterial disease, transmitted by the ingestion of food or water contaminated with the feces of an infected person, which contain the bacterium *Salmonella typhii.* Typhoid fever must not be confused with Typhus. Typhus is any of several similar diseases caused by *Rickettsia* bacteria. The causative organism *Rickettsia* is an obligate parasite bacterium that cannot survive for long outside living cells and is often spread by lice.

The term "virus" was not in general usage during Rife's work in the 1930s. Organisms that could not be cultured or seen with a microscope were called "filterable bacteria". Louis Pasteur was unable to find a causative agent for rabies and speculated about a pathogen too small to be detected using a microscope. In 1884, the French microbiologist Charles Chamberland invented a filter (known today as the Chamberland filter or Chamberland-Pasteur filter) with pores smaller than bacteria. Thus, he could pass a solution containing bacteria through the filter and completely remove them from the solution. In 1928, H. B. Maitland and M. C. Maitland grew vaccinia virus in suspensions of minced hens' kidneys. Their method was not widely adopted until the 1950s, when poliovirus was grown on a large scale for vaccine production. *Wikipedia* Remember that Rife did much of his work in the 1930s. The term virus was just becoming used during Rife's work. It is not clear whether he was working with true viruses or cell-wall-deficient organisms or both.

One of the most extensive books about Rife technology is The Rife Handbook of Frequency Therapy and Holistic Health by Nenah Sylver PhD (2011).

Malaria
Four malaria species are commonly pathogenic in humans namely: Plasmodium vivax, Plasmodium falciparum,

Plasmodium ovale and Plasmodium malariae. Just like bacteria, Plasmodia are indeed quite sensitive to oxidants. Examples of oxidants toxic to Plasmodia include: artemisinin, artemether, t-butyl hydroperoxide, xanthone, various quinones (e.g. atovaquone, lapachol, beta-lapachone, menadione) and methylene blue.

Like bacteria, fungi and tumor cells, the ability of Plasmodia to live and grow depends heavily on an internal abundance of reductants. This is especially true regarding thiol compounds also known as sulfhydryl compounds (RSH). Thiols as a class behave as reductants (electron donors). As such they are especially sensitive to oxidants (electron grabbers).

Thiols (RSH) such as glutathione and other sulfur compounds are reactive with sodium chlorite ($NaClO_2$) and with chlorine dioxide (ClO_2). These are the very agents present in MMS. Possible products of oxidation of thiols (RSH) using various oxides of chlorine are: disulfides (RSSR), disulfide monoxides (RSSOR), sulfenic acids (RSOH), sulfinic acids (RSO_2H) and sulfonic acids (RSO_3H).

None of these can support the life processes of the parasite. Upon sufficient removal of the parasite's life sustaining thiols (RSH) by oxidation, the parasite rapidly dies. A list of thiols (RSH) upon which survival of Plasmodium species heavily depend includes: dihydrolipoic acid, coenzyme-A and acyl carrier protein, glutathione, glutathione reductase, glutathione-S-transferase, peroxiredoxin, thioredoxin, glutaredoxin, plasmoredoxin, thioredoxin reductase, falcipain and ornithine decarboxylase.
http://www.bioredox.mysite.com/CLOXhtml/CLOXilus.htm

It has been claimed that over 75,000 cases of malaria have been successfully cured in Africa within 2-3 days with the use of MMS.

Rattle Snake Bite

A man was bitten by a rattle snake as he reached with his hand. The snake bit him where the thumb and index finger join the wrist. He was flown to a local trauma hospital where he received multiple vials of antitoxin.

This photo was taken two days after he was admitted to the

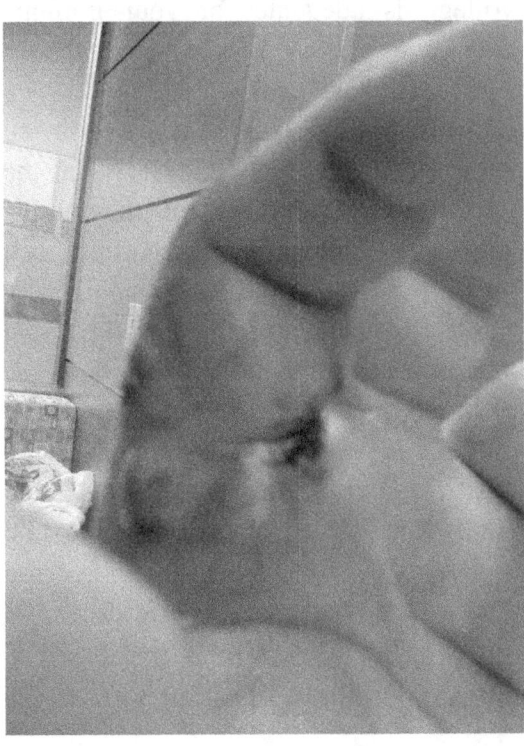

hospital. He continued to feel terrible and his arm remained swollen to the size of his leg. He couldn't move his fingers and he was in great pain.

His wife checked him out of the hospital and brought him to my office. He began to treat the arm and lesion with the Tennant BioModulator and took the malaria dose (fifteen drops twice a day) of MMS. This was a Friday. I saw him again on Monday. His arm was normal size, his pain was gone, and he could move all his fingers. This photo was taken 3 weeks after the bite.

Lyme Disease

Lyme disease is cause by a type of bacteria called a spirochete. Although it was traditionally thought to be due to a tick bite, it is now clear that Lyme disease is spread the same way as colds and flu---airborne. For this reason, almost everyone in the US is a carrier of this organism. If you do a fluorescein antibody test for the Lyme bacteria, you will find that most of us have it. The difference between whether you have symptoms or not is determined by whether you voltage is adequate for your immune system to keep it under control.

The Lyme spirochete reproduces itself, sheds its cell membrane, goes inside a cell, and lives there. When the cell duplicates, the spirochete reforms its cell membrane, makes multiple copies, and then again sheds its cell membrane and goes back inside the cell. That is why antibiotics almost never cure it. Antibiotics are effective only during the short time it has a cell membrane.

If you put a drop of blood on a coverslip and then onto a microscope slide, you will just see the blood cells. Now let the slide sit there for a few hours so that the cells consume the oxygen, you will usually see what appear to be spirochetes crawling out of the red blood cells! See the image above that I took with a phase contrast microscope in a patient known to have Lyme disease. You will find this pattern in almost all Americans if you bother to look for it.

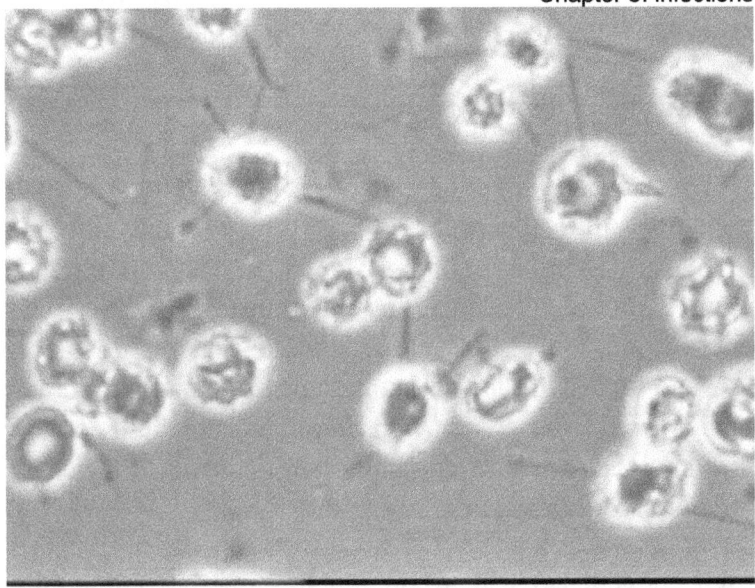

You should assume that everyone is infected with the Lyme spirochete. If their voltage is low, some of their symptoms will be due to this as well as other infections.

Lyme disease is a political disease. Doctors don't lose their license for diagnosing infectious diseases like pneumonia, strep throat, sinusitis, ear infections, etc. They do, however, lose their license for diagnosing Lyme disease. That puzzled me until I read the book Lab 257. It presents strong circumstantial evidence that Lyme disease was created as a weapon by the US government on Plum Island off the coast of Connecticut. If that is true, it would explain why the government would not want doctors to find an efficient way to treat it.

Summary

It is very difficult for the body to have an infection if there is enough iodine to form the normal shield around the body and if the voltage is normal so the immune system works.

411

Neutrophils need voltage to move about and consume the bacteria. They need voltage to make ozone or hydrogen peroxide to kill the bugs.

If you get an infection and use antibiotics, you will hopefully kill the bacteria if they haven't become antibiotic resistant. However, at the same time you will produce more L-forms. These forms will morph to match their environment. If the voltage is low and thus the oxygen is low and toxins will have accumulated, they will morph to a pathological form. As they "have lunch", they will damage distant organs and thus you will often not connect the cause to your use of antibiotics.

I am not suggesting that you should never use antibiotics. Possibly fatal infections require aggressive treatment. However, traditional antibiotics may not be as good a choice as oxidative therapy. The problem is that oxidative therapy is not "standard of care" and your physician will likely not prescribe them for you, especially if you are in a hospital setting. Fortunately, you can take your own oxidative therapy like MMS even while your doctor is giving you antibiotics. Most of the time, it is likely your oxidative therapy will kill the bugs long before the 24-48 hours it takes for antibiotics to start taking effect.

9 Dental Toxins

Much of chronic disease is caused by dental infections. Often dentists have a greater influence on your health than your physician!

Most people don't realize that dental work is *temporary*. Dental corrections don't last a lifetime but are like the tires on your car---they wear out and must be replaced. The following article shows that 71% of dental corrections are made on teeth that have been previously been filled or have crowns.

Compend Contin Educ Dent. 2000 Jan;21(1):15-8, 21-4, 26 passim; quiz 30.
Secondary caries and restoration replacement: an unresolved problem. Fontana M, González-Cabezas C.; Oral Health Research Institute, Indiana University School of Dentistry, Indianapolis, Indiana, USA.
Abstract
This article reviews the prevalence and main causes of restoration failure and replacement. It then focuses on secondary caries, its histopathology, etiology, difficulties in diagnosis, and prevention and remineralization possibilities. This article concludes that although secondary caries is still the main reason for restoration replacement, the development of new technologies for detecting and monitoring these lesions at an early stage should allow for testing new interventions to arrest or remineralize these lesions, which would delay the need for re-restoration. Seventy-one percent of all restorative treatments are performed on previously restored teeth with recurrent caries as the predominant cause.

413

Teeth are filled with tubules. Molars have up to three miles of tubules. Ralph Steinman, DDS, Loma Linda University's research showed proof of interactivity between the oral cavity and the metabolism of the body. The occurrence of decay is not due primarily to external contamination of the tooth through acid producing foods and bacteria, but through an upset of normal tooth metabolism.

Teeth are not solid, but consist of a series of dentin tubules and parallel enamel rods. Dr. Steinman proved that substances moved from within the body, through the pulp chamber, through the interstitial fluid to inside the dentin tubules, through the enamel and into the mouth. He proved this fact by injecting radioactive acriflavin hydrochloride into the abdominal cavities of rats and recovering it in the dentin tubules within six minutes and in the enamel within an hour. He believed this action to be a self-cleansing mechanism. The constant flushing of the tooth structure prevents the movement of microbes into the tooth and prevents the destructive effects of acids formed by foods. At the same time, essential nutrients are introduced into dentin tubules in order to provide a life-supporting environment for dentin, a tissue devoid of any blood supply or nerve innervations.

Roggenkamp, Clyde, PhD, Dentinal Fluid Transport, Loma Linda , Calif., Loma Linda Univ. Press, 2004.

Major problems occur when endocrine function, poor diet or stress negatively affects the hypothalamus, the regulatory gland for dentinal tubular flow. Circulatory problems, associated with ill health or aging also affect dentin tubular flow leading to flow reversal and stagnation. Odontoblasts, which lie outside dentin tubules projecting approximately one-third of the length of the associated dentin tubule, function as the pumps for the dentinal fluid. Steinman demonstrated that odontoblasts were hormonally and biochemically linked to the metabolism of the body, as well as to the health and function of the teeth. If odontoblasts cease to pump fluid, capillary action sucks bacteria and other noxious materials from the mouth or surrounding periodontium into the tooth, leading to microbial contamination and biofilm formation within the dentin tubules. Steinman produced many slides demonstrating this flow going in both directions. Since the tooth is not an isolated structure, the continued maintenance of a sterile field is impossible. This means you can never have a sterile root canal tooth.

> Note that the dentinal tubular flow is under control of the hypothalamus. The hypothalamus is under control of adrenalin. Adrenalin cannot be made if you are deficient in tyrosin, vitamin C and vitamin B6.

As part of the decay process, Steinman identified the early loss of magnesium, copper, iron and manganese, all of which are active in cellular oxidation and necessary for the metabolism of the odontoblasts. He showed that the addition of copper, iron, and manganese to a decay producing diet, almost abolished the decay rate.

415

Dr. Steinman's most dramatic discovery was that if you plot the course of dental decay: initially, function is altered, followed by the reversal of the dentinal tubular fluid flow. Next, inflammation occurs in the pulp chamber adjacent to the dentin, and finally, the disease spreads to the enamel, before the clinical appearance of the cavity.

http://www.copalite.com/Dentinal%20Tubular%20Flow%20and %20Effective%20Caries%20Treatment-%20revised.htm

If you have a computer nearby, I would like you to stop reading and watch the following videos:

Smoking Teeth at http://www.youtube.com/watch? v=9ylnQ-T7oiA

How Mercury Causes Brain Neuron Damage at http:// w w w . y o u t u b e . c o m / w a t c h ? v=XU8nSn5Ezd8&feature=related

Obviously, if you have mercury fillings in your mouth, you must get them SAFELY removed. This means that your dentist needs to give you an auxiliary air supply so you won't breath the mercury vapors coming out of your mouth as the dentist drills out the mercury. You also need a dental rubber dam. This is a piece of rubber. The dentist pokes the tooth in question through the rubber sheet. It then captures the pieces of mercury that fall into your mouth so you don't swallow them. If you don't follow these precautions, the mercury will be moved from your mouth to your brain!

416

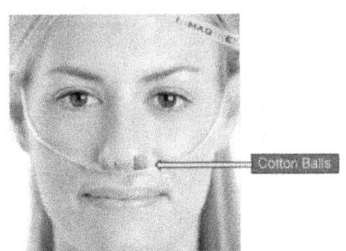 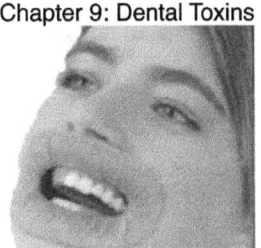

You must realize that every tooth is wired into an acupuncture meridian. Whatever happens to that tooth happens to the meridian. However, the meridians are like Christmas lights with multiple bulbs on them. Meridians are wires with multiple organs including a tooth on the same circuit. If you remove a light bulb, the circuit is still there. If you remove your gall bladder, your gall bladder circuit is still present.

As you can see from the following graphic, teeth are wired into the circuits. Notice for example, the breast wired into the stomach circuit. Another way of thinking about it is that the breast gets its voltage from the same wire or circuit as the stomach does. That means that if you have an infection in an upper molar (stomach meridian), that infection will affect the breast on that side as well as the stomach.

Loneliness, Acute Grief, Humiliated, Trapped, Inhibited, Greed, Not lovable	Anxiety, Self-Punishment, Broken Power, Hate, Low self-worth, Obsessed	Chronic Grief, Overcritical, Sadness, Controlling, Feeling trapped, Dogmatic, Compulsive, Uptight	Anger, Resentment, Frustration, Blaming, Incapable to take action, Manipulative	Fear, Shame, Guilt, Broken will, Shyness, Helpless, Deep exhaustion
Duodenum Middle Ear, Shoulder Elbow, CNS	Sinus: Maxillary Oropharynx, Larynx	Sinus: Paranasal and Ethmoid, Bronchus, Nose	Sinus: Sphenoid Palatine Tonsil Hip, Eye, Knee	Sinus: Frontal Pharyngeal Tonsil Genito-Urinary System
Heart, Small Int., Circulation/Sex, Endocrine	Pancreas Stomach	Lung Large Intestine	Liver Gallbladder	Kidney Bladder

1	2	3	4	5	6	7	8

32	31	30	29	28	27	26	25

Heart, Small Int., Circulation/Sex, Endocrine	Lung Large Intestine	Pancreas Stomach	Liver Gallbladder	Kidney Bladder
Shoulder, Elbow Ileum, Middle Ear Peripheral Nerves	Sinus: Paranasal and Ethmoid, Bronchus, Nose	Sinus: Maxillary Larynx, Lymph, Oropharynx Breast Knee	Sinus: Sphenoid Palatine Tonsil Hip, Eye Knee	Sinus: Frontal Ear, Pharyngeal Tonsil Genito-Urinary System
Loneliness, Acute Grief, Humiliated, Trapped, Inhibited, Greed, Not lovable	Chronic Grief, Overcritical, Sadness, Controlling, Feeling trapped, Dogmatic, Compulsive, Uptight	Anxiety, Self-Punishment, Broken Power, Hate, Low self-worth, Obsessed	Anger, Resentment, Frustration, Blaming, Incapable to take action, Manipulative	Fear, Shame, Guilt, Broken will, Shyness, Helpless, Deep exhaustion

Acumeridian Tooth-Organ Relationships [with Autonomic/Neurop

418

Fear, Shame, Guilt, Broken will, Shyness, Helpless, Deep exhaustion	Anger, Resentment, Frustration, Blaming, Incapable to take action, Manipulative	Chronic Grief, Overcritical, Sadness, Controlling, Feeling trapped, Dogmatic, Compulsive, Uptight	Anxiety, Self-Punishment, Broken Power, Hate, Low self-worth, Obsessed	Loneliness, Acute Grief, Humiliated, Trapped, Inhibited, Greed, Not lovable
Sinus: Frontal Pharyngeal Tonsil Genito-Urinary System	Sinus: Sphenoid Palatine Tonsil Hip, Eye, Knee	Sinus: Paranasal and Ethmoid, Bronchus, Nose	Sinus: Maxillary Oropharynx Larynx	Ileum, Jejunum Middle Ear, Shoulder Elbow, CNS
Kidney Bladder	**Liver Gallbladder**	**Lung Large Intestine**	**Stomach Spleen**	**Heart, Small Int., Circulation/Sex, Endocrine**

9	10	11	12	13	14	15	16
24	23	22	21	20	19	18	17

Kidney Bladder	**Liver Gallbladder**	**Spleen Stomach**	**Lung Large Intestine**	**Heart, Small Int., Circulation/Sex, Endocrine**
Sinus: Frontal Ear, Pharyngeal Tonsil Genito-Urinary System	Sinus: Sphenoid Palatine Tonsil Hip, Eye, Knee	Sinus: Maxillary Larynx, Lymph, Oropharynx Breast Knee	Sinus: Paranasal and Ethmoid Bronchus, Nose	Shoulder, Elbow Ileum, Jejunum, Middle Ear Peripheral Nerves
Fear, Shame, Guilt, Broken will, Shyness, Helpless, Deep exhaustion	Anger, Resentment, Frustration, Blaming, Incapable to take action, Manipulative	Anxiety, Self-Punishment, Broken Power, Hate, Low self-worth, Obsessed	Chronic Grief, Overcritical, Sadness, Controlling, Feeling trapped, Dogmatic, Compulsive, Uptight	Loneliness, Acute Grief, Humiliated, Trapped, Inhibited, Greed, Not lovable

eptide Emotion correlations] -- from various sources Dr. Ralph Wilson, N.D.

One is upper right, 16 is upper left, 17 is lower left, 32 is lower right.

The BioTerminals help you know the primary source of voltage for each circuit. In addition many organs have more than more wire that takes voltage to it.

In this chart, you see that the wire called the lung meridian also takes voltage to the nose, skin, large intestine, and shoulder. The wire called the stomach meridian takes voltage to the stomach, breast, mouth, nose, lips and upper lid.

In the following chart, you will see that some organs have multiple wires supplying voltage to them. For example, the brain gets voltage from the heart, spleen/pancreas, and bladder circuits. The eye gets voltage from the triple burner (sanjiao), liver, and bladder circuits. I have also recently discovered that the macula of the eye gets its voltage from the spleen/stomach meridians. If you study the BioTerminal circuits above, you will see that the primary BioTerminal for the eyes is in the center of the forehead. It is modulated by the Triple Burner circuit from the hand and receives voltage from the liver circuit that is

Meridians by System				
Armpit	Heart			
Adrenals	Kidney			
Body Fluids	Bladder	Spleen/Pancreas	Bladder	
Brain	Heart			
Breast	Stomach			
Cardiovascular	Pericardium	Heart	Pericardium	
Depression	Lung	Sanjaio	Gall Bladder	
Ear	Small Intestine	Kidney		
Emotions	Gall Bladder	Gall Bladder	Kidneys (adrenals)	
Endocrine	Spleen/Pancreas	Liver	Bladder	
Eye	Sanjaio		Sanjaio	
Eyelid (Upper)	Stomach	Sanjaio		
Fatigue	Heart			
Gonads	Liver			
Head	Pericardium	Gall Bladder	Gall Bladder	
Large Intestine	Lung	Small Intestine	Small Intestine	
Lips	Stomach			
Lung	Pericardium			
Lymph	Sanjaio			
Mouth	Stomach			
Mucous Membranes	Bladder			
Neck	Small Intestine			
Nervous System	Kidney	Large Intestine	Bladder	
Nose	Lung	Liver		
Parasympathetic	Pericardium			
Ribs	Spleen/Pancreas			
Shoulder	Large Intestine	Liver	Stomach	
Skin	Lung	Large Intestine	Pericardium	
Stomach	Spleen/Pancreas			Spleen/Pancreas
Sympathetic	Sanjaio			Heart
Tongue	Heart			
Tooth	Large Intestine			

attached to the top of the head.

Don't let all of this confuse you. If you want to keep it simple, just focus on the BioTerminals to provide voltage. However, when you are considering if a certain tooth is causing trouble with the organ you are interested in, look at the meridian charts. See what wires are carrying voltage to the organs you are interested in. Then look to see if you have an infection in a tooth in one of those circuits. If so, you have the reason that the voltage dropped enough in that circuit to allow the person to get sick.

There is often a recurring pattern with teeth. You get a small cavity. The dentist removes about 1/3 of the tooth with undercuts so that mercury amalgam filling won't fall out. This weakens the tooth. Soon it fractures. The dentist then puts a crown on the tooth without removing the amalgam. Now you have an open wound in the tooth with mercury leaking into it. Decay happens but the dentist cannot detect it because x-rays won't penetrate the crown

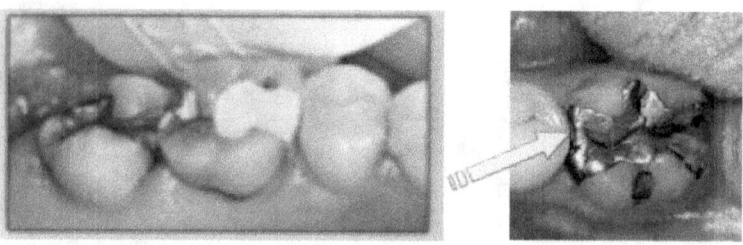

so the x-ray looks fine. Next comes pain. The dentist then recommends a root canal.

A root canal is performed by drilling a small hole into the biting surface of the tooth. An auger is then inserted into the root of the tooth and the artery and nerve are ripped out.

Everyone knows that dead tissue in the body always gets infected. That is why it is surprising that dentists

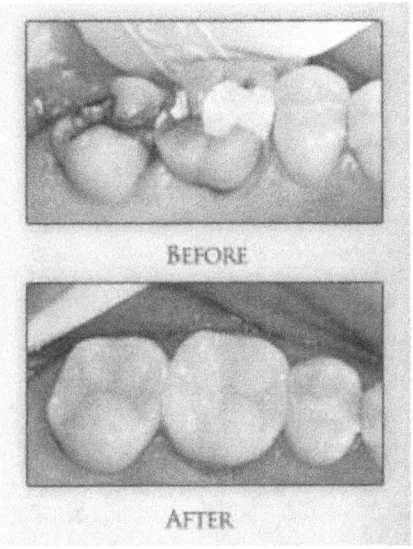

BEFORE

AFTER

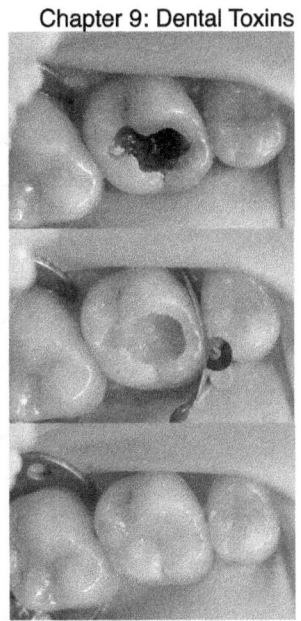

purposefully leave dead teeth in the mouth. The dentists are the only physicians that purposely leave dead tissue in the body!

Most dentists are convinced that they can seal the tooth so that infection in the tooth is impossible. Unfortunately, that is wishful thinking. This study published in the root canal doctors' own journal shows the problem clearly. They took patients that were going to have wisdom teeth removed. They did a root canal on one tooth. Then three months later they removed both teeth. What you see is that the untreated tooth had 1.1% of the tubules infected. However,

423

the tooth that had the root canal performed three months

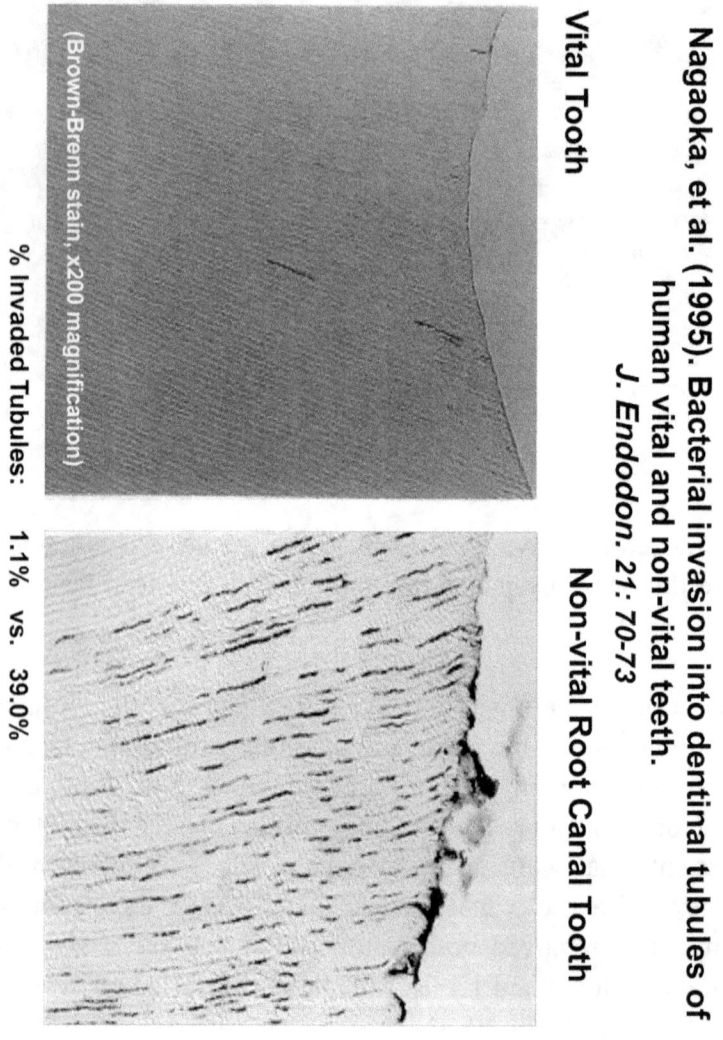

Nagaoka, et al. (1995). Bacterial invasion into dentinal tubules of human vital and non-vital teeth. *J. Endodon. 21: 70-73*

Vital Tooth

Non-vital Root Canal Tooth

(Brown-Brenn stain, x200 magnification)

% Invaded Tubules: 1.1%   vs.   39.0%

earlier had infection in 39% of the tubules!

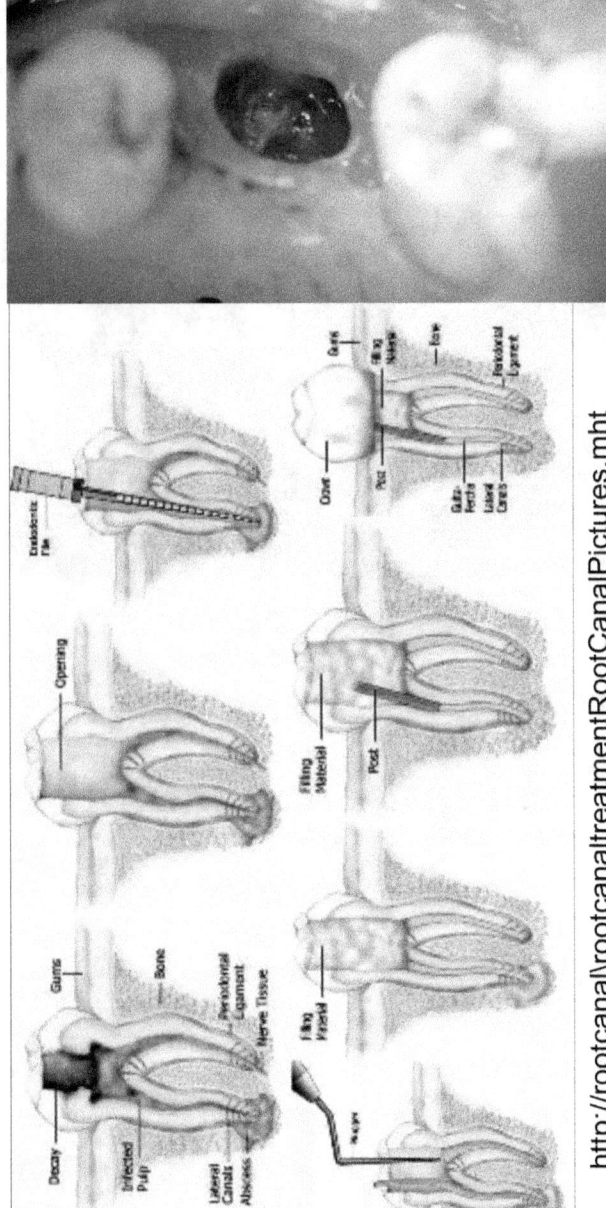

http://rootcanal\rootcanaltreatmentRootCanalPictures.mht

A study done at the University of Kentucky looked at the effects of root canal toxins on the immune system. When the teeth are infected with bacteria, they produce a toxin called thio-ethers. When the infection is caused by fungus, it produces glio-toxins.

Adriaens et al., (1988). *J. Clin. Periodontol.*59-493-503.

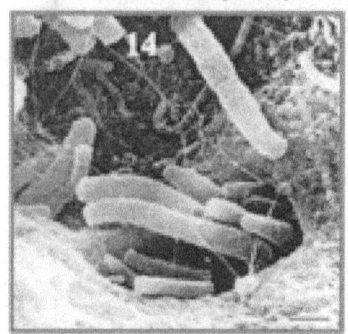 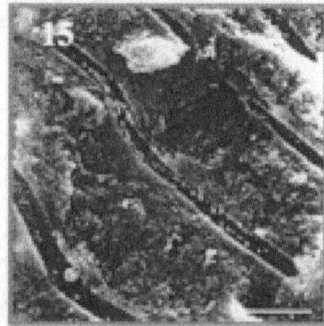

"Figure 14 Filamentous bacteria invading the dentinal tubules at their orifices in the bottom of a resorption lacuna."

"Figure 15 Longitudinally fractured dentinal tubules in the radicular dentin area corresponding to the exposed subgingival root surface. Bacteria are present in the dentinal tubules."

190

Effect of Increasing Volumes of RCT Extract O
[γ^{32}P]2N$_3$ATP Photolabeling of Cdk2, P53 & H-R

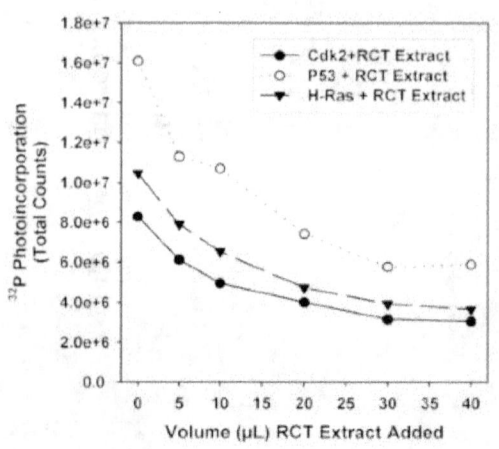

This one produced a pretty flat graph curve with the most inhibition in the first half of the test.

426

CDK2 is noted here with the solid line with black circles at the bottom. CDK2 with root canal extract showed 26% inhibition at 5 ul and 63% inhibition at 40 ul. Thus one root canal shuts down 63% of the immune system. Most of that is focused on the acupuncture meridian attached to that tooth.

Having poisonous mercury coming from your teeth is one problem. Another problem just as severe is having an infected tooth. The teeth that are always infected are root canal teeth, but any cavity or infection under a crown releases the same toxins.

The following interview is from Dr. Joseph Mercola: www.mercola.com

Effective Non-Drug Non-Surgical Solutions for Chronic Illnesses
Dr. Joseph Mercola
1443 W. Schaumburg Rd.
Schaumburg, IL 60194-4065
'phone 847-985-1777
ROOT CANALS POSE HEALTH THREAT - AN INTERVIEW WITH GEORGE MEINIG, D.D.S.

Dr. Meinig brings a most curious perspective to an expose of latent dangers of root canal therapy - fifty years ago he was one of the founders of the American Association of Endodontists (root canal specialists)! So he's filled his share of root canals. And when he wasn't filling canals himself, he was teaching the technique to dentists across the country at weekend seminars and clinics. About two years ago, having recently retired, he decided to read all 1174 pages of the detailed research of Dr. Weston Price, (D.D.S). Dr. Meinig was startled and shocked. Here was valid documentation of systemic illnesses resulting from latent infections lingering in filled roots. He has since written a book, "Root Canal Cover-Up EXPOSED - Many Illnesses Result", and is devoting himself to radio, TV, and personal appearances before groups in an attempt to blow the whistle and alert the public.

MJ Please explain what the problem is with root canal therapy.

GM First, let me note that my book is based on Dr. Weston Price's twenty-five years of careful, impeccable research. He led a 60-man team of researchers whose findings - suppressed until now rank right up there with the greatest medical discoveries of all time. This is not the usual medical story of a prolonged search for the difficult-to-find causative agent of some devastating disease. Rather, it's the story of how a "cast of millions" (of bacteria) become entrenched inside the structure of teeth and end up causing the largest number of diseases ever traced to a single source.

MJ What diseases? Can you give us some examples?

GM Yes, a high percentage of chronic degenerative diseases can originate from root filled teeth. The most frequent were heart and circulatory diseases and he found 16 different causative agents for these. The next most common diseases were those of the joints, arthritis and rheumatism. In third place - but almost tied for second - were diseases of the brain and nervous system. After that, any disease you can name might (and in some cases has) come from root filled teeth.
Let me tell you about the research itself. Dr. Price undertook his investigations in 1900. He continued until 1925, and published his work in two volumes in 1923. In

1915 the National Dental Association (which changed its name a few years later to The American Dental Association) was so impressed with his work that they appointed Dr. Price their first Research Director. His Advisory Board read like a Who's Who in medicine and dentistry for that era. They represented the fields of bacteriology, pathology, rheumatology, surgery, chemistry, and cardiology.

At one point in his writings Dr. Price made this observation: "Dr. Frank Billings (M.D.), probably more than any other American internist, is due credit for the early recognition of the importance of streptococcal focal infections in systemic involvements."

What's really unfortunate here is that very valuable information was covered up and totally buried some 70 years ago by a minority group of autocratic doctors who just didn't believe or couldn't grasp - the focal infection theory.

MJ What is the "focal infection" theory?

GM This states that germs from a central focal infection - such as teeth, teeth roots, inflamed gum tissues, or maybe tonsils - metastasize to hearts, eyes, lungs, kidneys, or other organs, glands and tissues, establishing new areas of the same infection. Hardly theory any more, this has been proven and demonstrated many times over. It's 100% accepted today. But it was revolutionary thinking during World War I days, and the early 1920's!

Today, both patients and physicians have been "brain washed" to think that infections are less serious because we now have antibiotics. Well, yes and no. In the case of root-filled teeth, the no longer-living tooth lacks a blood supply to its interior. So circulating antibiotics don't faze the bacteria living there because they can't get at them.

MJ You're assuming that ALL root-filled teeth harbor bacteria and/or other infective agents?

GM Yes. No matter what material or technique is used - and this is just as true today - the root filling shrinks minutely, perhaps microscopically. Further and this is key - the bulk of solid appearing teeth, called the dentin, actually consists of miles of tiny tubules. Microscopic organisms lurking in the maze of tubules simply migrate into the interior of the tooth and set up housekeeping. A filled root seems to be a favorite spot to start a new colony.

One of the things that makes this difficult to understand is that large, relatively harmless bacteria common to the mouth, change and adapt to new conditions. They shrink in size to fit the cramped quarters and even learn how to exist (and thrive!) on very little food. Those that need oxygen mutate and become able to get along without it. In the process of adaptation these formerly friendly "normal" organisms become pathogenic (capable of producing disease) and more virulent (stronger) and they produce much more potent toxins.

Today's bacteriologists are confirming the discoveries of the Price team of bacteriologists. Both isolated in root canals the same strains of streptococcus, staphylococcus and spirochetes.

MJ Is everyone who has ever had a root canal filled made ill by it?

GM No. We believe now that every root canal filling does leak and bacteria do invade the structure. But the variable factor is the strength of the person's immune system. Some healthy people are able to control the germs that escape from their teeth into other areas of the body. We think this happens because their immune system lymphocytes (white blood cells) and other disease fighters aren't constantly compromised by other ailments. In other words, they are able to prevent those new colonies from taking hold in other tissues throughout the body. But over time, most people with root filled teeth do seem to develop some kinds of systemic symptoms they didn't have before.

MJ It's really difficult to grasp that bacteria are imbedded deep in the structure of seemingly-hard, solid looking teeth.

GM I know. Physicians and dentists have that same problem, too. You really have to visualize the tooth structure - all of those microscopic tubules running through the dentin. In a healthy tooth, those tubules transport a fluid that carries nourishment to the inside. For perspective, if the tubules of a front single-root tooth, were stretched out on the ground they'd stretch for three miles!

A root filled tooth no longer has any fluid circulating through it, but the maze of tubules remains. The anaerobic bacteria that live there seem remarkably safe from antibiotics. The bacteria can migrate out into surrounding tissue where they can "hitch hike" to other locations in the body via the bloodstream. The new location can be any organ or gland or tissue, and the new colony will be the next focus of infection in a body plagued by recurrent or chronic infections.

All of the "building up" done to try to enhance the patient's ability to fight infections - to strengthen their immune system - is only a holding action. Many patients won't be well until the source of infection - the root canal tooth - is removed.

MJ I don't doubt what you're saying, but can you tell us more about how Dr. Price could be sure that arthritis or other systemic conditions and illnesses really originated in the teeth - or in a single tooth?

GM Yes. Many investigations start with the researcher just being curious about something - and then being scientifically careful enough to discover an answer, and then prove it's so, many times over. Dr. Price's first case is very well documented. He removed an infected tooth from a woman who suffered from severe arthritis. As soon as he finished with the patient, he implanted the tooth beneath the skin of a healthy rabbit. Within 48 hours the rabbit was crippled with arthritis!
Further, once the tooth was removed the patient's arthritis improved dramatically. This clearly suggested that the presence of the infected tooth was a causative agent for both that patient's and the rabbit's - arthritis.

[Editor's Note - Here's the story of that first patient from Dr. Meinig's book: "(Dr. Price) had a sense that, even when (root canal therapy) appeared successful, teeth containing root fillings remained infected. That thought kept prying on his mind, haunting him each time a patient consulted him for relief from some severe debilitating disease for which the medical profession could find no answer. Then one day while treating a woman who had been confined to a wheelchair for six years from severe arthritis, he recalled how bacterial cultures were taken from patients who were ill and then inoculated into animals in an effort to reproduce the disease and test the effectiveness of drugs on the disease.

With this thought in mind, although her (root filled) tooth looked fine, he advised this arthritic patient, to have it extracted. He told her he was going to find out what it was about this root filled tooth that was responsible for her suffering. "All dentists know that sometimes arthritis and other illnesses clear up if bad teeth are extracted. However, in this case, all of her teeth appeared in satisfactory condition and the one containing this root canal filling showed no evidence or symptoms of infection. Besides, it looked normal on x-ray pictures.

"Immediately after Dr. Price extracted the tooth he dismissed the patient and embedded her tooth under the skin of a rabbit. In two days the rabbit developed the same kind of crippling arthritis as the patient - and in ten days it died.

"..The patient made a successful recovery after the tooth's removal! She could then walk without a cane and could even do fine needlework again. That success led Dr. Price to advise other patients, afflicted with a wide variety of treatment defying illnesses, to have any root filled teeth out."]

In the years that followed, he repeated this procedure many hundreds of times. He later implanted only a portion of the tooth to see if that produced the same results. It did. He then dried the tooth, ground it into powder and injected a tiny bit into several rabbits. Same results, this time producing the same symptoms in multiple animals.

Dr. Price eventually grew cultures of the bacteria and injected them into the animals. Then he went a step further. He put the solution containing the bacteria through a filter small enough to catch the bacteria. So when he injected the resulting liquid it was free of any infecting bacteria. Did the test animals develop the illness? Yes. The only explanation was that the liquid had to contain toxins from the bacteria, and the toxins were also capable of causing disease.

433

Dr. Price became curious about which was the more potent infective agent, the bacteria or the toxin. He repeated that last experiment, injecting half the animals with the toxin-containing liquid and half of them with the bacteria from the filter. Both groups became ill, but the group injected with the toxins got sicker and died sooner than the bacteria injected animals.

MJ That's amazing. Did the rabbits always develop the same disease the patient had?

GM Mostly, yes. If the patient had heart disease the rabbit got heart disease. If the patient had kidney disease the rabbit got kidney disease, and so on. Only occasionally did a rabbit develop a different disease - and then the pathology would be quite similar, in a different location.
MJ If extraction proves necessary for anyone reading this, do you want to summarize what's special about the extraction technique?

GM Just pulling the tooth is not enough when removal proves necessary. Dr. Price found bacteria in the tissues and bone just adjacent to the tooth's root. So we now recommend slow-speed drilling with a burr, to remove one millimeter of the entire bony socket. The purpose is to remove the periodontal ligament (which is always infected with toxins produced by streptococcus bacteria living in the dentin tubules) and the first millimeter of bone that lines the socket (which is usually infected).
There's a whole protocol involved, including irrigating with sterile saline to assure removal of the contaminated bone chips, and treating the socket to stimulate and encourage infection-free healing. I describe the procedure in detail, step by step, in my book [pages 185 and 186].
MJ Perhaps we should back up and talk about oral health - to PREVENT needing an extraction. Caries or inflamed

gums seem much more common than root canals. Do they pose any threat?

GM Yes, they absolutely do. But let me point out that we can't talk about oral health apart from total health. The problem is that patients and dentists alike haven't come around to seeing that dental caries reflect systemic - meaning "whole body" - illness. Dentists have learned to restore teeth so expertly that both they and their patients have come to regard tooth decay as a trivial matter. It isn't.

Small cavities too often become big cavities. Big cavities too often lead to further destruction and the eventual need for root canal treatment.
MJ Then talk to us about prevention.

GM The only scientific way to prevent tooth decay is through diet and nutrition. Dr. Ralph Steinman did some outstanding, landmark research at Loma Linda University. He injected a glucose solution into mice - into their bodies, so the glucose didn't even touch their teeth. Then he observed the teeth for any changes. What he found was truly astonishing. The glucose reversed the normal flow of fluid in the dentin tubules, resulting in all of the test animals developing severe tooth decay! Dr. Steinman demonstrated dramatically what I said a minute ago: Dental caries reflect systemic illness.

Let's take a closer look to see how this might happen. Once a tooth gets infected and the cavity gets into the nerve and blood vessels, bacteria find their way into those tiny tubules of the dentin. Then no matter what we do by way of treatment, we're never going to completely eradicate the bacteria hiding in the miles of tubules. In time the bacteria can migrate through lateral canals into the surrounding bony socket that supports the tooth. Now the host not only has a cavity in a tooth, plus an underlying infection of supporting tissue to deal with, but the bacteria also exude potent systemic toxins. These toxins circulate throughout the body triggering activity by the immune system - and probably causing the host to feel less well. This host response can vary from just dragging around and feeling less energetic, to overt illness - of almost any kind. Certainly, such a person will be more vulnerable to whatever "bugs" are going around, because his/her body is already under constant challenge and the immune system continues to be "turned on" by either the infective agent or its toxins - or both.

MJ What a fascinating concept. Can you tell us more about the protective nutrition you mentioned?

GM Yes. Dr. Price traveled all over the world doing his research on primitive peoples who still lived in their native ways. He found fourteen cultural pockets scattered all over the globe where the natives had no access to "civilization" - and ate no refined foods.

Dr. Price studied their diets carefully. He found they varied greatly, but the one thing they had in common was that they ate whole, unrefined foods. With absolutely no access to tooth brushes, floss, fluoridated water or tooth paste, the primitive peoples studied were almost 100% free of tooth decay. Further - and not unrelated - they were also almost 100% free of all the degenerative diseases we suffer - problems with the heart, lungs, kidneys, liver, joints, skin (allergies), and the whole gamut of illnesses that plague Mankind. No one food proved to be magic as a preventive food. I believe we can thrive best by eating a wide variety of whole foods.

MJ Amazing. So by "diet and nutrition" for oral (and total) health you meant eating a pretty basic diet of whole foods?

GM Exactly. And no sugar or white flour. These are (and always have been) the first culprits. Tragically, when the primitives were introduced to sugar and white flour their superior level of health deteriorated rapidly. This has been demonstrated time and again. During the last sixty or more years we have added in increasing amounts, highly refined and fabricated cereals and boxed mixes of all kinds, soft drinks, refined vegetable oils and a whole host of other foodless "foods". It is also during those same years that we as a nation have installed more and more root canal fillings - and degenerative diseases have become rampant. I believe - and Dr. Price certainly proved to my satisfaction - that these simultaneous factors are NOT coincidences.

MJ I certainly understand what you are saying. But I'm still a little shocked to talk with a dentist who doesn't stress oral hygiene.

GM Well, I'm not against oral hygiene. Of course, hygiene practices are preventive, and help minimize the destructive effect of our "civilized", refined diet. But the real issue is still diet. The natives Dr. Price tracked down and studied weren't free of cavities, inflamed gums, and degenerative diseases because they had better tooth brushes!

Root Canals and Infected Bone

It's so easy to lose sight of the significance of what Dr. Price discovered. We tend to sweep it under the rug - we'd actually prefer to hear that if we would just brush better, longer, or more often, we too could be free of dental problems.

Certainly, part of the purpose of my book is to stimulate dental research into finding a way to sterilize dentin tubules. Only then can dentists really learn to save teeth for a lifetime. But the bottom line remains: A primitive diet of whole unrefined foods is the only thing that has been found to actually prevent both tooth decay and degenerative diseases.

One of the problems with root canals is that they often spread their infection into the surrounding bone. This is a huge problem since infections in bone are so hard to cure. They are often called "cavitations". Unfortunately these infections cannot be seen with standard dental x-rays. One can only see them with digital x-rays or 64-slice CAT scans. The hole in the photo is where a root canal has been removed. You can see the blackened infected bone that surrounded the root canal.

Generally one cannot measure the voltage coming from a root canal tooth. However, one can measure the voltage coming from a tooth if it has metal in the form of a filling or crown. Teeth, like the rest of cells, are designed to run at

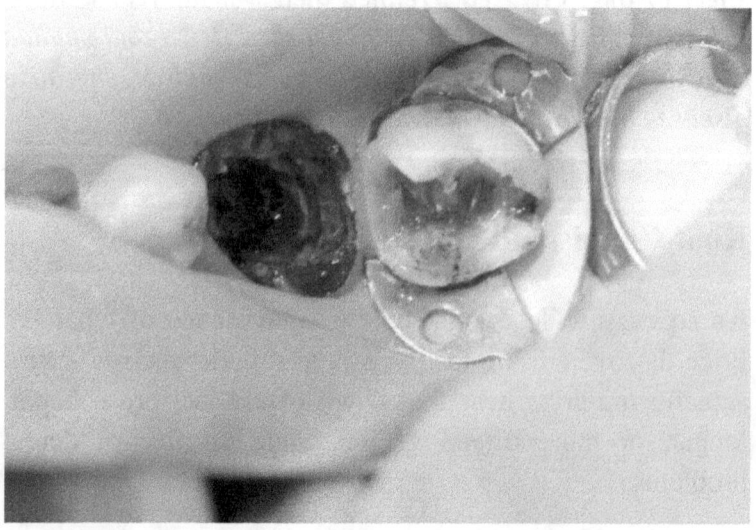

-20 to -25 millivolts. You can take a voltmeter that measures in millivolts. Place one electrode on the cheek and one on the metal of the tooth. If you measure more than 100 millivolts, either that tooth or one of its neighbors is infected.

Measure Voltage From Dental Fillings That Are Metal

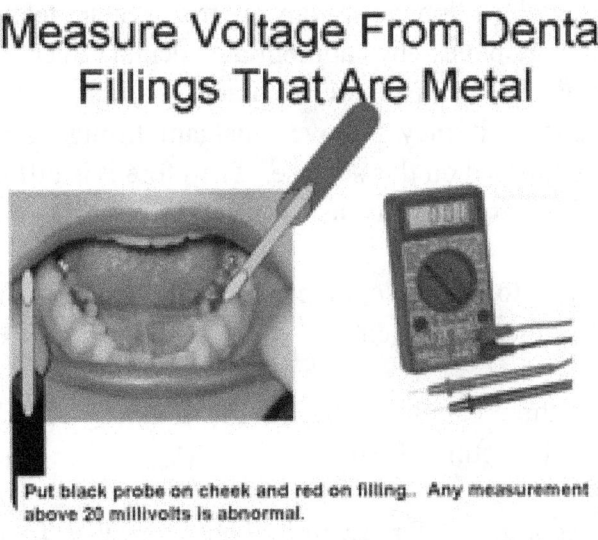

Put black probe on cheek and red on filling. Any measurement above 20 millivolts is abnormal.

219

Tennant

I have a friend that is an oncologist. I looked at 20 of his cancer patients. What I found was that 70% of these patients had a root canal in the same acupuncture meridian as their primary cancer. All but one of the rest had an infected crown in the same meridian as their primary cancer.

In my own practice, I have seen only two patients where I could not find a dental connection to the meridian associated with their cancer. One was a heavy smoker.

These numbers are too small to prove the connection between dental infections and cancer. We can only hope that someone will fund a large study to prove or disprove the connection. In the meantime, it makes sense to remove infections from your teeth and jaws.

We find a similar connection between chronic diseases and dental infections just as Weston Price, DDS described in 1939. The majority of patients I see that have been sick for years have dental infections and most improve dramatically when the infection is removed from their teeth and surrounding bones by appropriate dental intervention. Unfortunately, dentists are routinely harassed by their dental boards if they remove amalgam fillings and root canal teeth based on this science. Therefore it is difficult to find dentists to help you when you are sick from your teeth.

Please go to www.youtube.com and listen to http://www.youtube.com/watch?v=7StVJAkctZU

This is a three part series by Dr. Dawn Ewing called Oral Obstacles to Optimal Health.

I also recommend Dr. Ewing's book Let The Tooth Be Known...Are Your Teeth Making You Sick? It is available from www.senergy.us or 972-580-0545.

10 Allergies

Allergies plague most people at one time or another. For some, it is an annoying runny nose. For others it is the inability to live outside of a special room. For a few, it is sudden death.

What could cause our immune systems to perform in such an abnormal way?

Allergies are the interaction of antibodies and other chemicals made by our immune system. These antibodies believe that the proteins we are eating, breathing, or coming in contact with are dangerous to us and they are trying to destroy them. In the process, they make us sick.

Antibodies (also known as **immunoglobulins**, abbreviated **Ig**) are **gamma globulin proteins** that are found in blood or other bodily fluids of vertebrates, and are used by the immune system to identify and neutralize foreign objects, such as bacteria and viruses. Antibodies are produced by a kind of white blood cell called a **plasma cell**.

In placental mammals there are five antibody isotypes known as IgA, IgD, IgE, IgG and IgM. They are each named with an "Ig" prefix that stands for immunoglobulin, another name for antibody, and differ in their biological properties, functional locations and ability to deal with different antigens.

1. IgA: Found in mucosal areas, such as the gut, respiratory tract and urogenital tract, and prevents colonization by pathogens. Also found in saliva, tears, and breast milk.

441

2. IgD: Functions mainly as an antigen receptor on B cells that have not been exposed to antigens.[11] It has been shown to activate basophils and mast cells to produce antimicrobial factors.

3. **IgE: Binds to allergens and triggers histamine release from mast cells and basophils, and is involved in allergy. Also protects against parasitic worms.**

4. **IgG: In its four forms, provides the majority of antibody-based immunity against invading pathogens. The only antibody capable of crossing the placenta to give passive immunity to fetus**.

5. IgM: Expressed on the surface of B cells and in a secreted form with very high avidity. Eliminates pathogens in the early stages of B cell mediated (humoral) immunity before there is sufficient IgG.

Note that IgG and IgE are prominent in allergy. IgG is involved with food allergies and IgE with inhalation allergy.

Traditional medicine focuses on the information given above and uses a variety of drugs like antihistamines, decongestants, and steroids to mitigate the symptoms of allergies. Sometimes avoidance of the allergen and/or "allergy shots" are used to attempt to desensitize patients.

It is rare to find a traditional physician that recognizes the role of iodine in the prevention and cure of allergies. We discussed the role of iodine in the formation of stomach acid

You cannot be well unless you have adequate stomach acid. The human is designed to never ever absorb proteins!

in the nutrition chapter as it relates to body voltage. Now we will discuss how iodine relates to allergies.

442

The human body is designed so that NO complete protein will be absorbed into the system. The reason is that when the body makes a protein, it knows that it is not an enemy because it made it. However, when a protein that the body did not make is found, it is assumed that it is a foreign invader like a virus, bacteria, fungus, etc. It therefore makes 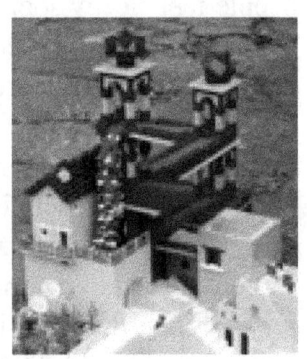 antibodies against that protein and attacks it with the purpose of destroying it.

Proteins are made up of small units called **amino acids.** Think of a Lego as an amino acid. The multiple things you can build from Legos are called proteins.

When you eat a protein, stomach acid must break the proteins down into amino acids. As the digested food reaches the small intestine, the amino acids are absorbed so the body can make and repair proteins.

However, if you don't have enough stomach acid, whole or partially digested proteins reach the small intestine and are absorbed. The body recognizes these as foreign since it didn't make them. **Thus you become allergic to the foods** 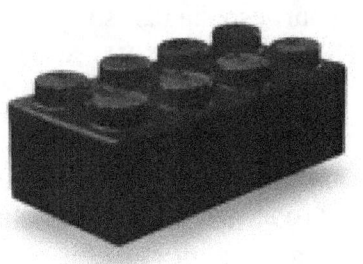 **you normally eat!** Now about 20-40 minutes after each meal, you body thinks it is being attacked by a foreign protein and attacks it. Thus it is like having a mini case of the flu after each meal! This is why so many people feel sleepy soon after they eat. They say, "I ate too much and it made me sleepy!" The reality is that their body is attacking the proteins they just ate.

The reason for this allergy is lack of stomach acid. So why don't you have enough stomach acid? Making stomach acid requires iodine, zinc, vitamin B1, water, salt, and carbon dioxide. Americans that don't eat sea weed regularly are deficient in iodine. The amount of iodine in table salt is about 1/1000 of what you need, there is no iodine in sea salt, and our soils are devoid of iodine. About 80% of the population is deficient in zinc. Thus most people have allergies because they can't make stomach acid!

If one of the undigested proteins is used in the formation of a cell, the immune system will still attack it.

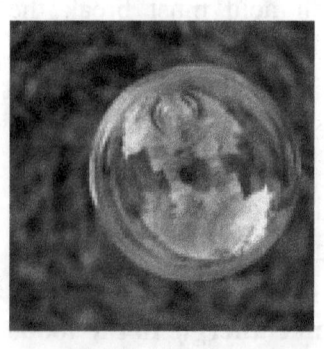

When you don't have enough stomach acid, the digestive process in your stomach creates gas bubbles. These bubbles are coated with stomach acid much like soap coats a bubble. The gas bubble causes you to belch or simply rises up into your esophagus where you taste the acid. It burns your esophagus so you feel discomfort or overt pain. This is called GERD or gastro-esophageal reflux disease.

Since it is assumed you have too much stomach acid (and indeed you do have it in the wrong place---the esophagus) you take antacids or drugs that stop acid production. Your

GERD stops. However, now you are developing allergies since you can't digest your proteins!

Without stomach acid you can't adsorb zinc even is you take it. Thus you will become deficient in zinc when you shut down stomach acid production if you weren't deficient already. There are over 350 biochemical reactions that rely on zinc including the production of neurochemicals. If you take drugs that shut down your stomach acid, you will become depressed because you can't make serotonin. So now you are a depressed person with allergies and chronic fatigue. Now you start antidepressant drugs. These work temporarily but have been shown to increase the amount and frequency of depression when taken long term. They also diminish your sexual performance/desire. Your spouse gets tired of you and your emotional ups and downs, your runny nose, migraine headaches, explosive diarrhea, and lack of sexual interest/performance. You can figure out the rest.

Remember this downward spiral started because of the lack of iodine, zinc, salt and vitamin B1. The drugs don't solve the problem---they cover up the problem and create several more problems.

When your immune system is constantly in attack mode, it uses a lot of voltage and adrenalin. Soon your adrenals wear out. You should assume that if you have allergies, your adrenals are tired and dysfunctional. To feel better, you will be drawn toward CATS = caffeine, alcohol, tobacco, and sugar. They give you temporary relief, but they place additional demands upon your adrenals. You must avoid them.

Other routes of getting whole proteins into the bloodstream are vaccinations (contain viruses but also eggs, monkey brains, proteins from the original source of the viruses like pigs, etc.) products you put on your skin like creams, shampoos, and breathing in contaminated air.

To overcome this process, you can do a blood test to find out what foods you are allergic to. Traditionally it is advised that you avoid those foods for up to six months. I find that, like antibodies from vaccines, antibodies to foods last for years even if you don't eat those foods. They key is to never absorb proteins---only amino acids. That means you must have adequate amounts of stomach acid to break all the proteins you eat into amino acids.

You must take iodine, zinc, and vitamin B1 so that you can start making stomach acid. Also, while you are correcting those deficiencies, you must take betaine with each meal. This pill from the beet plant makes stomach acid so you won't become allergic to the new set of foods while you are becoming able to make your own stomach acid in a normal way.

The following are symptoms of lack of adrenalin. The adrenal glands are actually two glands in one. The outer part of the adrenals (cortex) makes cortisol and aldosterone. Cortisol affects inflammation and blood sugar. The aldosterone affects blood pressure, particularly the upper number (systolic). The inner part of the adrenal glands (medulla) makes adrenalin.

You should be able to quickly recognize yourself in this list if you have the problem. If you have allergies, you almost certainly will see yourself here.

Men and Women
Low Adrenalin
Easily frazzled
Flying off the handle frequently
Startling easily
Low tolerance for loud noises?
Poor resistance to respiratory infections
Asthma
Longer than normal recovery time from routine illness
Difficulty recuperating from unusual stress such as jet lag?
Being bothered by what are really small, insignificant things
Dizziness upon standing up
Low blood pressure or fainting?
Low stamina for stress
Caving in easily
Preferring to avoid any confrontations?
Sweating or wetness of the hands when nervous?
Sense of always being stressed out
Feeling better right away when stress is resolved?

Men and Women
Low Adrenalin
Excessive sensitivity to chemicals
Increased allergies
Low tolerance for alcohol, caffeine, other drugs, or strong odors
Unusual fatigue, especially in the morning with more energy after meals and later as day progresses
Having better energy at night, when others are winding down (night owl)?
Salt cravings (especially liking or needing salty foods)
Lack of thirst
Markedly low blood sugar/hypoglycemia (can't skip a meal, needing snacks just to function, low fasting blood sugar on testing)
"Tired but wired" feeling
Low reserve (little spare oomph to meet a challenge)
Thin and/or dry skin
Brown spots on the face
Intolerance to exercise

Some of the list above is extracted from the book From Feeling Fat, Fuzzy, or Frazzled by Richard and Karilee

Shamas, www.penguin.com and from the writings of John Lee, MD.

Lack of adrenalin eventually leads to you just wanting to sit in the corner and have people leave you the heck alone! You are grouchy and moody.

Remember that a boy has been defined as a noise with dirt on it--ha! Little girls are known to be noisy chatterboxes that cry. If you are adrenalin deficient, you will have a hard time being around children.

Since adrenalin insufficiency means you are annoyed/angry when you have to interact with anyone, you will not be a good spouse, parent, child, friend, coworker or worker because people are always wanting to interact with you.

Lack of adrenalin can easily be documented with the Ragland test. Measure the blood pressure laying down. Measure it again immediately after standing up. The upper number (systolic) should go up at least ten points. If it doesn't, you are deficient in adrenalin.

Measure the blood pressure a few minutes after sitting up. If the lower number (diastolic) is below 80 and you aren't on blood pressure medications, you are deficient in adrenalin. The blood pressure is often unstable if you are deficient in adrenalin, so the measurement you get a few minutes after standing will be different from either of the two previous measurements.

Adrenalin is made from the amino acid tyrosine, vitamin C, and vitamin B6. Remember that the body's source of amino acids is stomach acid breaking proteins into amino acids including the tyrosine needed to make adrenalin. In addition, the human cannot make vitamin C and thus must

449

consume it. There is very little vitamin C in citrus like orange juice, so that is not adequate.

The following are often recommended as a way to support your adrenal function.

1. Tyrosine 500 mg with each meal.
2. Vitamin C 500 mg with each meal.
3. Pyridoxine (Vitamin B6), 100 mg per dayl.
4. Eat frequent small meals.
5. Increase intake of sea salt.
6. Avoid CATS (caffeine, alcohol, tobacco, sugar)--- they make you feel better temporarily but then drop you.
7. Pantothenic acid (Vitamin B5), 250 mg with each meal.
8. SeriPhos (phosphorylated serine) 1,000 mg taken at bedtime.
9. If your diastolic (lower number) blood pressure is below 80, take licorice 450 mg (one capsule) each morning for week one, 900 mg each morning for the second week, 1350 mg each morning for the third week. Keep increasing each week for six weeks. Then stop for two weeks. You may repeat if you felt better while taking it. Take your blood pressure each week the first thing in the morning. If it is over 140 systolic or 90 diastolic, stop the licorice.
10. DHEA 10 mg daily
11. Pregnenolone, 50 mg daily.

Remember that all organs that secrete something needs iodine to do so. That includes adrenals.

I find that the most predictable way to support the adrenals is with adrenal glandulars. These pills are dehydrated adrenals from animals. They are very similar to desiccated thyroid hormone.   I generally have patients take two on arising and 1-2 at lunch time.

The Cellular Sewage System (Lymphatics)

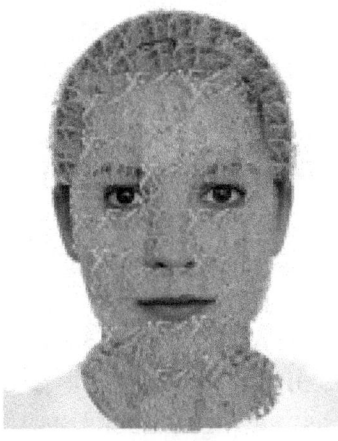

When cells place their garbage at the curb (push it into the extracellular space so it can be removed), most of it is moved into the venous capillaries.   However, proteins are too large to fit there.   Thus we have an entirely separate system to remove waste proteins.

Waste proteins can be considered cellular sewage!

The lymphatic system is dedicated to removing waster proteins.   Thus it is our cells' sewage disposal system. These channels are tubes that connect the extracellular spaces around cells with a large vein that enters the heart just under the clavicles (collar bones).   From here, it goes through the liver, into the bile, into the intestine and is removed from the body with your bowel movement.

What is different about this system is that it has no heart or other pump to move the waste forward.   Instead, the tubes are surrounded by a circular muscle and by stretch receptors.   When the tubes are stretched (such as by walking or moving your arms), they activate the circular muscles. They move the sewage down the tubes much like squeezing a tube of toothpaste.

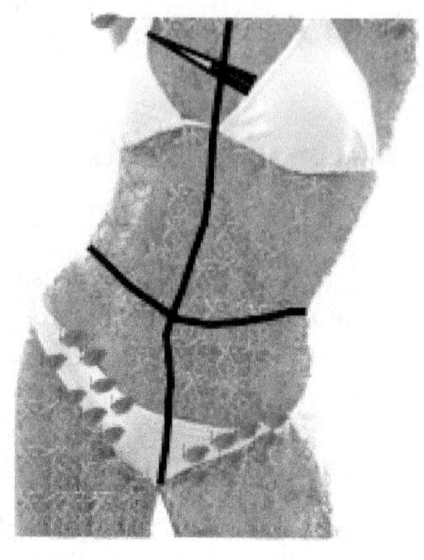

When you are inactive, the sewage isn't moved along the tubes. It can congeal in the tubes. Now your sewage system backs up just the way it can happen when your toilet gets stopped up by something too large to move through the pipes. As the sewage backs up, it floods back into the extracellular spaces just as sewage floods your bathroom floor.

Do you get the image? Your cells are surrounded by sewage. The sewage cannot be eliminated until you unstop the lymphatic tubes just as your toilet won't flush until you move the obstruction on down the pipes.

Sewage is a strong electron stealer. It significantly lowers the voltage in the extracellular space. This is reflected in a consistently low urine pH. That is because urine pH is a reflection of the voltage in your extracellular space. If it is consistently below 6.5, you likely have a stopped up lymphatic system. If someone says, "You are full of s---!" it is likely true.

People often notice that they are gaining weight or can't lose weight. This weight is often sewage instead of fat.

Another way to see if your sewage system is stopped up is to look at the clavicles (collar bones). They should be clearly visible. If you can't see your clavicles, you likely have lymphatic obstruction.

Allergies from Retained Sewage

Imagine what retained sewage does to you immune system. It drives it crazy! All of those damaged proteins are everywhere. It's like you fell into a pit of snakes and are struggling madly to get out. You strike out at anything that moves.

The longer that your lymphatics are obstructed, the more different antibodies you make until you become allergic to almost everything. Now you are called "chemically sensitive".

Surgery and Sewage

From any point on the body, the sewage must pass through a lymph node so that large particles and particularly bacteria can be filtered out before it reaches you blood stream as it flows into the subclavian vein just above your heart. Think of lymph nodes as sponges filled with antiseptics. You could also think of them as sewage treatment plants intended to clean up the sewage water before it comes back to your house.

What happens when a surgeon removes your lymph nodes? They take out some of the lymphatic pipes and their filters. Now how is the sewage supposed to get drained? It can't.

I Need a Plumber!

When you have allergies, you feel tired all the time, you are gaining weight and you can't see your clavicles, you likely need a plumber. Unfortunately, massage therapists can make it worse. Most of them are trained to work 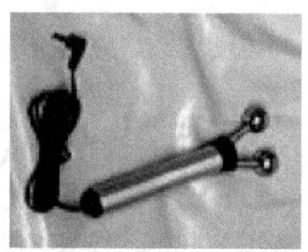 with muscles and not lymphatics. When you do deep massage on tissue filled with sewage, you often rupture the bulging lymphatic channels and the cells that are surrounded by sewage. What you need is a gentle method to contract the circular muscles that surround all lymphatic channels.

The ideal way to accomplish this is electronically. I use the Tennant Biomodulator with an attachment that has two balls on it. By gently following the normal flow of lymphatic sewage with the electrode, the tubes begin to move the sewage along. It is important to be sure the patient is hydrated. One must start where the system flows into the heart just behind the clavicles. Next open the neck channels. Then open the face and head channels. Now start down the body.

As you are opening the channels, it is important to be sure the lymph nodes are able to pass the fluid through them. This can be accomplished by pressing on them like you are pressing the fluid out of a sponge.

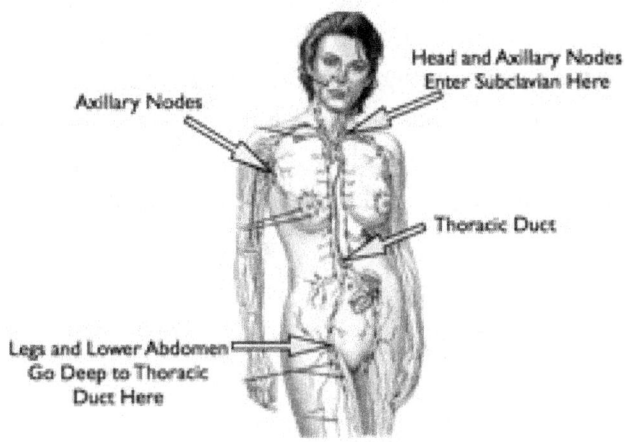

The hardest one to open is the thoracic duct that takes the sewage from the inguinal area to the heart. It runs deep in the body next to the aorta. It requires some training to learn how to do this successfully.

Remember that the channels above the navel run to the nodes in the axilla (armpits) whereas the channels below the navel run to the inguinal region and then deep into the thoracic duct. When the thoracic duct is obstructed, people get fluid retention below the belly button. They think it is strange that they are getting fat just below the belly button and not above it. It's not fat; it's sewage.

The essential oil Bay Laurel is also helpful in getting the lymphatics to drain. So is a mini-tramp.

Asthma

Asthma is often a function of food allergies from lack of stomach acid. It is usually accompanied by adrenal fatigue.

Asthma in children is due to parasites until proven otherwise. Using MMS to kill the parasites, correcting iodine levels, correcting stomach acid and avoiding the foods that the child has become allergic to will commonly eliminate the asthma. Kids with asthma are usually have antibodies to milk, particularly pasteurized milk.

11 Heavy Metal Poisoning

The scientific world has no widely accepted definition for 'heavy metal'. However, it is generally accepted that the term 'heavy' refers to metals with a specific gravity that is at least 5 times the specific gravity of water. The specific gravity of water is 1 at 4°C (39°F). Simply stated, specific gravity is a measure of the density of a given amount of a solid substance when it is compared to an equal amount of water. In general terms, a 'heavy metal' has a specific weight higher that 8 grams per cubic centimeter (g/cm3).

We are particularly interested in the following toxic metallic elements having specific gravities greater than 8 or more times that of water: Cadmium, 8.65; Lead, 11.34; and Mercury, 13.546. Although aluminum is not a heavy metal (specific gravity of 2.55-2.80), it makes up about 8% of the surface of the earth and is the third most abundant element and it is a toxic metal.

http://www.humet.com/acatalog/heavymetals.html

Heavy metals damage mitochondria and therefore destroy cells' ability to function by interfering with voltage. They also inactivate enzymes causing cells to malfunction. The most common metals that cause trouble are mercury, lead, cadmium, and arsenic.

Living organisms require varying amounts of "heavy metals." Iron, cobalt, copper, manganese, molybdenum, and zinc are required by humans. Excessive levels can be damaging to the organism. Other heavy metals such as mercury, plutonium, and lead are toxic metals that have no known vital or beneficial effect on organisms, and their accumulation over time in the bodies of animals can cause serious illness. Certain elements that are normally toxic are, for certain organisms or under certain conditions, beneficial. Examples include vanadium, tungsten, and even cadmium. wikipedia

Lead Poisoning

Lead poisoning may cause
1. Irreversible Neurological Damage
2. Renal Disease
3. Cardiovascular Effects
4. Reproductive Toxicity

The symptoms of acute lead poisoning include:
1. Gastrointestinal problems
2. Constipation,
3. Diarrhea,
4. Vomiting,
5. Poor appetite,
6. Weight loss

The symptoms of chronic lead poisoning include:
1. Neurological problems (reduced cognitive abilities)
2. Nausea
3. Abdominal pain
4. Irritability
5. Insomnia
6. Metal taste in oral cavity
7. Excess lethargy or hyperactivity
8. Headache
9. Seizure
10. Coma
11. Anemia
12. Kidney problems
13. Reproductive problems

In humans, lead toxicity sometimes causes the formation of a bluish line along the gums, which is known as the "Burton's line", although this is very uncommon in young children.

Blood film examination may reveal "basophilic stippling" of red blood cells, as well as the changes normally associated with iron deficiency anemia (m i c r o c y t o s i s   a n d hypochromia).

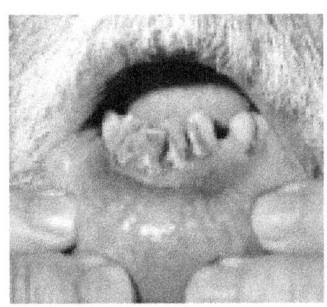

Lead affects the peripheral and central nervous system. The most common sign of peripheral neuropathy due to chronic lead poisoning is painless wrist drop (weakness of the extensor muscles of hand) which usually develops after many weeks of exposure.

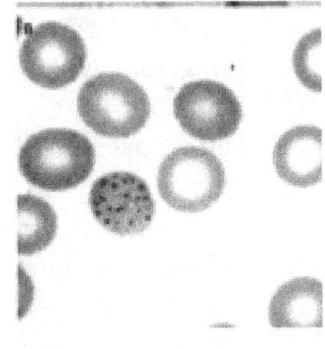

A direct link between early lead exposure and extreme learning disability has been confirmed by multiple researchers and child advocacy groups.
A May 2000 study by economic consultant Rick Nevin theorizes that lead exposure explains 65% to 90% of the variation in violent crime rates in the U.S. and other countries.

Lead has no known biological role in the body. **The toxicity comes from its ability to mimic other biologically important metals, the most notable of which are calcium, iron and zinc. Lead is able to bind to and interact with the same proteins and molecules as these**

metals, but after displacement, those molecules function differently and fail to carry out the same reactions, such as in producing enzymes necessary for certain biological processes.

The majority of lead poisoning occurs in children under age twelve.

The main sources of poisoning:
1. Ingestion of lead contaminated soil.
2. Ingestion of lead dust or chips from deteriorating lead-based paints. Small children also tend to teethe and suck on painted windowsills as they look outside. A piece of lead paint the size of your fingernail will poison you!
3. Drinking water = plumbing and fixtures that are either made of lead or have trace amounts of lead in them.
4. Exposure to metallic lead such as small lead objects, can rarely lead to an increase in blood lead levels if the lead is retained in the gastrointestinal tract or appendix.

Lead can also be found in some imported cosmetics such as **kohl**, from the middle east, India, Pakistan, and some parts of Africa, and Surma from India (kohl is a mixture of soot and other ingredients used predominantly by middle eastern, north African, sub-Saharan African and Asian women, and to a lesser extent men, to darken the eyelids and as mascara for the eyelashes.

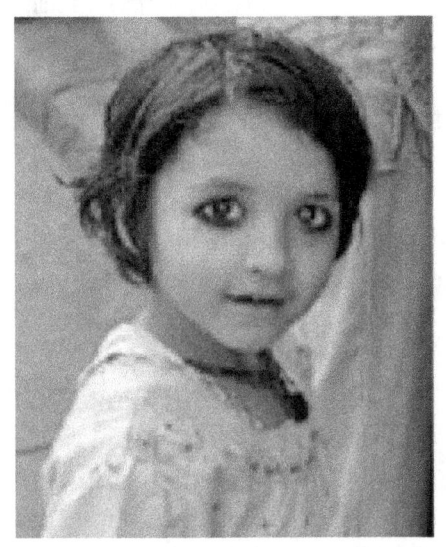

Imported toys, such as many made in China.

There are also risks of elevated blood lead levels caused by folk remedies like azarcon which contains 95 percent lead and is used to "cure" empacho (an impacted stomach)

Lead may be contracted through the mucous membranes through direct contact to mouth, nose, eyes, and breaks in skin.

Most people born before 1950 were exposed to lead in gasoline and paint. It only takes a piece of lead the size of a grain of salt to poison you! Lead was commonly added to gasoline to increase its octane and anti-knock performance. In the U.S. in 1972, the EPA launched an initiative to phase out leaded gasoline. Ethyl Corp's response was to sue the EPA. The EPA won the case, so the TEL phaseout began in 1976 and was completed by 1986. Lead paint was banned in the US in 1977, but many imported toys, jewelry, and other products are still made with lead.
wikipedia

Lead tends to be suppressed in bone by hormones. As your hormone levels decrease, the lead leaches out of bone and often affects the heart in the 40's to 50's = the age of heart attacks!

Mercury Poisoning

Mercury likes fatty tissue like brain, liver, kidneys, and endocrine glands.

According to the World Health Organization, 80% of mercury comes from mercury amalgam fillings in your teeth.

In February 1998, the U.S. Environmental Protection Agency (EPA) issued a report citing mercury emissions from electric utilities as the largest remaining anthropogenic source of mercury released to the air. EPA officials estimated that about 50 tons of elemental mercury are emitted each year from U.S. coal-burning power plants, with lesser amounts coming from oil- and gas-burning units. According to EPA estimates, emissions from coal-fired utilities account for 13 to 26 percent of the total (natural plus anthropogenic) airborne emissions of mercury in the United States.

One-quarter of adults in New York City have elevated levels of mercury in their blood. A study by the city's Department of Health and Mental Hygiene found that mercury was highest in Asians, women, and those with higher incomes.

Heavy metals don't stay in the blood. They quickly move into tissue. If you find heavy metals in a blood test, it means you have a current and ongoing exposure!

The only accurate way to test for heavy metals is with a chelation-urine provocative test. A chelating agent is given IV and then a six hour urine sample is collected and tested for heavy metals. A newer test looks at urine porphyrins. Hair tests are not a reliable way to look for heavy metals.

Materials like zeolite, chlorophyll, cilantro, etc. are not reliable ways to remove metals. They stay in the gut and are not absorbed into the system. Since the metals are deep in your tissue, these agents in your gut cannot access the metals.

One reliable way to remove metals is with chelation. Sweating (infrared saunas), raw garlic, glutathione, etc. are also helpful. It is important to correct levels of glutathione when attempting to remove metals.

In nature, heavy metals are detoxified with fulvic acid. Since you should be taking fulvic to help control your cell membranes and to provide vitamins, minerals, and amino acids, this seems the preferred method.

Environ. Sci. Technol., 2011, 45 (22), pp 9574–9581
DOI: 10.1021/es201323a

It is critical that one look at total body voltage before attempting to remove metals. If your voltages are low, there is a tendency for the metals to be moved from one part of the body to another but not excreted. This often aggravates the situation instead of making it better. Restore the voltage and then correct the heavy metal poisoning.

12 BioModulator

FDA Statement

The Tennant Biomodulator® and certain accessory electrodes are FDA listed by its distributor or manufacturer in these categories:

★ 21 CFR 882.5890 – Neurology transcutaneous electrical nerve stimulator for pain relief

★ 21 CFR 882.5050 – Neurology biofeedback device

Indications for use:

1. Symptomatic relief and management of chronic, intractable pain.
2. Adjunctive treatment in the management of post-traumatic surgical and post-traumatic pain
3. Relaxation training and muscle relaxation

For more information, see www.senergy.us

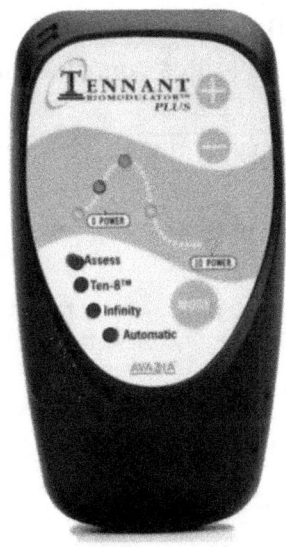

BioModulator®
SlimLine

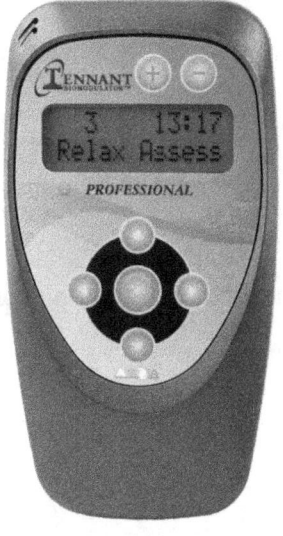

BioModulator®
Pro

Care of the BioModulator:

- Don't turn on if below freezing.
- Clean with alcohol sponge and wipe gently.
- Clean electrode with alcohol sponge between people.
- Do not drop!
- Device can be damaged to the point of non-function if dropped on hard surface.
- Device will be damaged beyond repair if dropped in water or liquids are spilled inside.
- Device uses 2 AA alkaline batteries.
- When ON/OFF switch is in the ON position, device is still powered and battery life is being used.

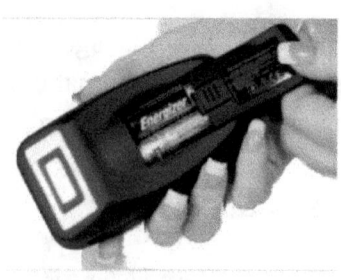

- Initial batteries included with the device have a clear plastic covering. Remove it before placing the batteries in the battery compartment.
- Battery compartment cover slides on/off the device.
- Do NOT force battery cover or push it down. This can cause breakage of cover clips – non-warranty item.

The ON/OFF switch is on the side of the unit.

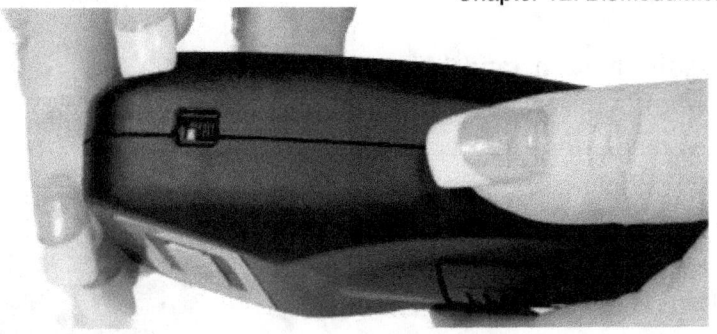

There is an accessory port on the other side of the unit.

The power
is adjusted
with the
plus and minus buttons.

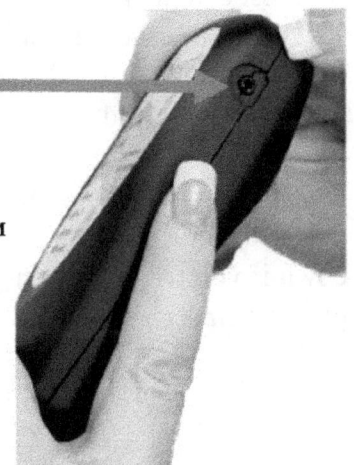

When in Ten-8™ or Infinity™
modes, the LEDs show the
power settings, and are NOT
reflecting the assessed value
as in the Assess or Automatic
mode.

Turn the device on. Press and
hold the (+) button. Watch the LEDs illuminate
progressively up the curve (left to right) as the power level
increases.

467

At the bottom range of each diode, the LED flashes. At the upper end of the range, the LED is solid. As the power increases, the next LED will begin to flash.

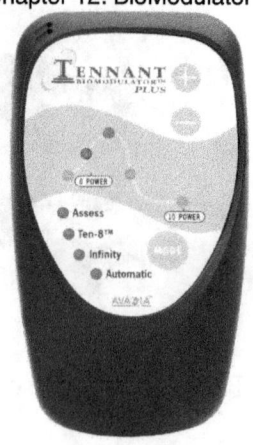

By convention we say that:

● Below-threshold level of energy does not give subjective sensation.
● Threshold level is sensed as slight vibration. This is the most commonly used setting
● Above-threshold level is sensed as comfortable tingling sensation.
● Supra-threshold level is sensed as uncomfortable.

It is better to use too little power than too much. The device operates in volts – cells in millivolts. They will shut down if you use too much power. Let children control the power themselves.

Setting Power
According to Skin Thickness

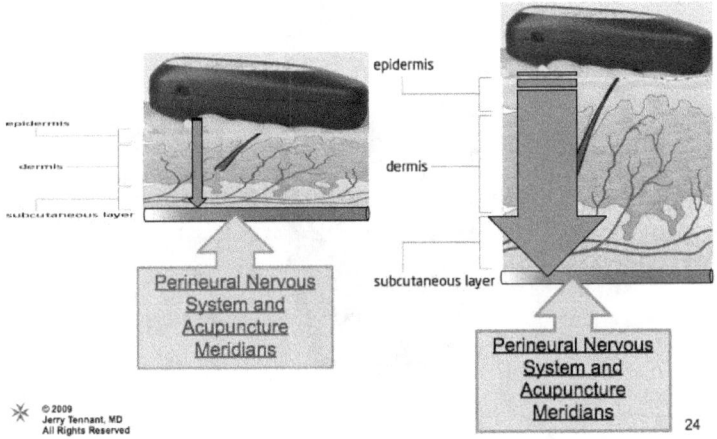

Modes:

● **Assess** – Acts as your "voltmeter" to measure musculoskeletal problems or organ voltage.

● **Ten-8™** – Use for pain and musculoskeletal issues.

● **Infinity™** Use for everything else or alternate with Ten-8™.

● **Automatic (or Automatic Infinity™)** The software measures the voltage and then treats with Infinity for one minute.

Voltage Indications

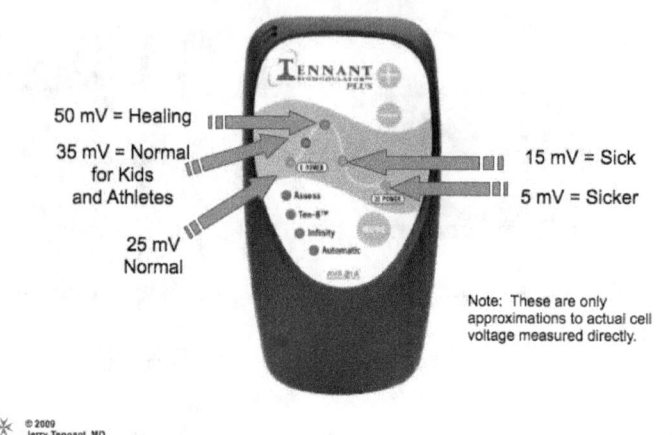

50 mV = Healing

35 mV = Normal for Kids and Athletes

15 mV = Sick

5 mV = Sicker

25 mV Normal

Note: These are only approximations to actual cell voltage measured directly.

33

To use the BioModulator, you must adjust the power for the thickness of skin you wish to measure. Then put it into Assess Mode. Press firmly over the area in question. The lights will tell you the voltage according to the image above. Now measure the BioTerminals described in the chapter of Voltage.

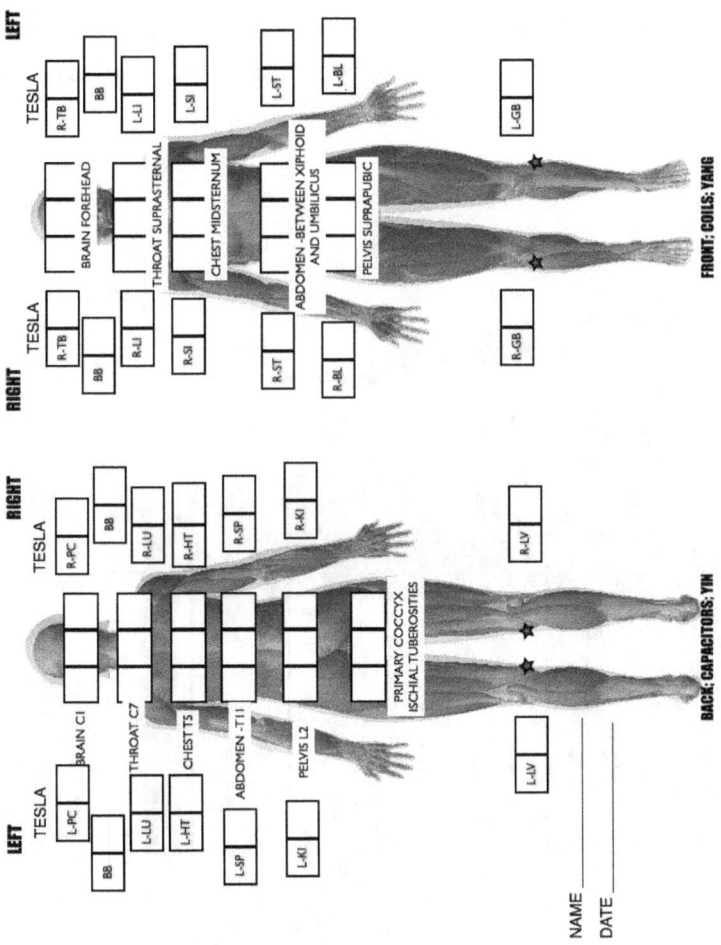

Remember that chronic diseases are characterized by low voltage. Voltages drop before blood tests become abnormal. Blood tests become abnormal before you have symptoms. Wherever you find low voltages, the organs served by those BioTerminals will be struggling now or in the future.

Look at the chart on the next page. It will confirm for you which BioTerminal is associated with various illnesses. It is generally intuitive. For example, eye problems will have low voltage in the skull BioTerminal. Heart problems will have low voltage in the chest BioTerminal. Bladder problems will have low voltage in the Pelvic BioTerminal, etc.

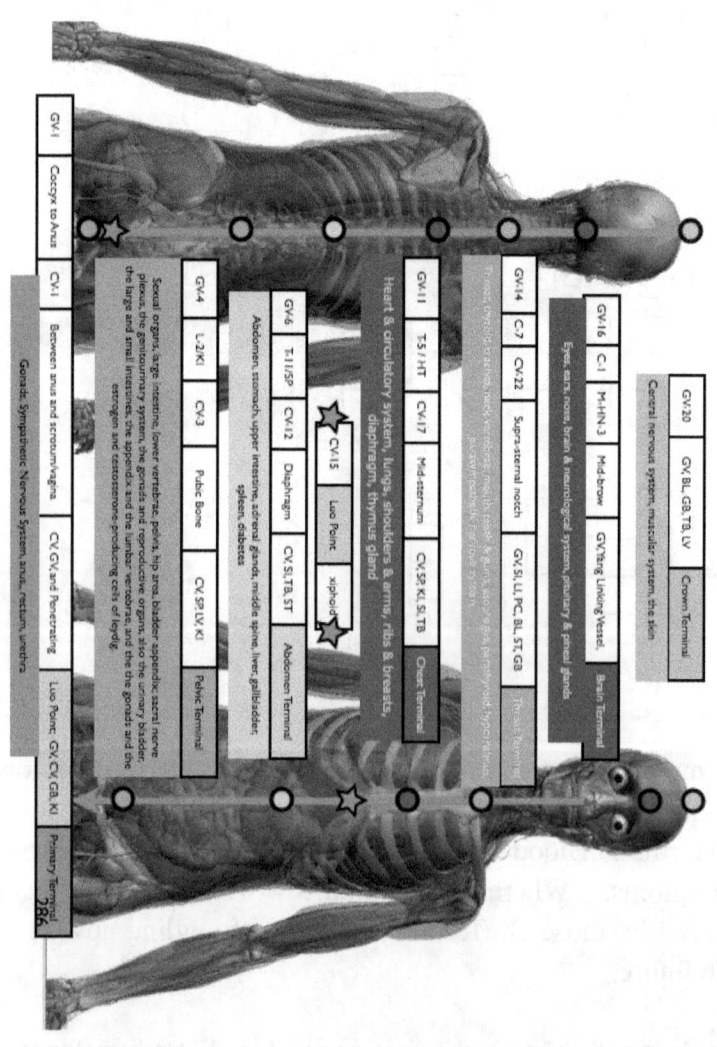

BioTransducer

When we are using the BioModulator on the skin, we are primarily treating by way of the acupuncture meridians or the perineural nervous system. For most things, this works well. However, there is a more efficient way to get electrons into deep or swollen areas. It is with the use of an attachment to the BioModulator called the BioTransducer.

If I put an electrode on each side of my door, electrons will not flow from one to the other because the door is an insulator. If I shine a light on the door, it won't penetrate either. However, if I place a magnet on each side of the door, they will hold onto each other as their magnetic fields interact.

Remember that tissue with low voltage always creates a magnetic field. We call those "stickies" as we move the BioModulator over them.

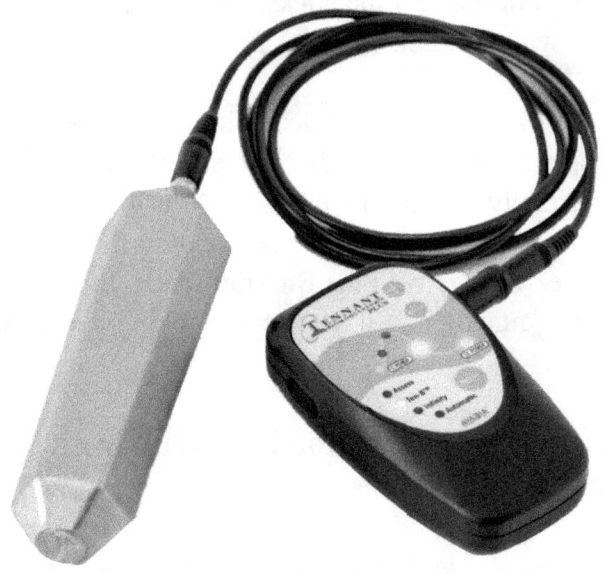

The BioTransducer creates a magnetic field. We modulate the BioModulator frequencies onto the BioTransducer's magnetic field. By doing so, we are able to send the frequencies through solid material like the skull and brain, other bones, and into deep organs like the heart and liver. The BioTransducer thus gives us a more efficient way to get the electrons into deep organs like the brain.

When we move the BioTransducer over an area, when we contact the magnetic field of low voltage, we will feel it stick just the same way we feel a sticky on the skin. When the voltage in the deep organ is corrected, the sticky spot disappears and we know that we have corrected that area.

The trick to learning how to use the BioTransducer is to stop thinking about what you are doing and close out as many external sensory inputs as you can. Dim the lights, turn off the music, stop talking, get relaxed, and just let you hand take the BioTransducer wherever it seems to want to do. Soon you will feel the sticky. With practice, you will soon do it without thinking about it.

It's a little like learning to ride a bicycle. When we first climb on, we are tense and our movements are jerky. We can never really ride until we relax. After we do that, our movements become automatic and we stop thinking about how to ride. So it is with the BioTransducer. You will find the stickies quickly when you stop thinking about where they are.

How is the BioModulator Different from TENS Devices?

Transcutaneous electrical nerve stimulation (acronym TENS) is the use of electric current produced by a device to stimulate the nerves for therapeutic purposes. TENS by definition covers the complete range of transcutaneously applied currents used for nerve excitation although the term is often used with a more restrictive intent, namely to describe the kind of pulses produced by portable stimulators used to treat pain.[1] The unit is usually connected to the skin using two or more electrodes. A typical battery-operated TENS unit is able to modulate pulse width, frequency and intensity. Generally TENS is applied at high frequency (>50 Hz) with an intensity below motor contraction (sensory intensity) or low frequency (<10 Hz) with an intensity that produces motor contraction. [2]

Scientific studies show that high and low frequency TENS produce their effects by activation of opioid receptors in the central nervous system. Specifically, high frequency TENS activates delta-opioid receptors both in the spinal cord and supraspinally (in the medulla) while low frequency TENS activates beta-opioid receptors both in the spinal cord and supraspinally. Further high frequency TENS reduces excitation of central neurons that transmit nociceptive information, reduces release of excitatory neurotransmitters (glutamate) and increases the release of inhibitory neurotransmitters (GABA) in the spinal cord, and activates muscarinic receptors centrally to produce analgesia (in effect, temporarily blocking the pain gate). Low frequency TENS also releases serotonin and activates serotonin receptors in the spinal cord, releases GABA, and activates muscarinic receptors to reduce excitability of nociceptive neurons in the spinal cord. Wikipedia

Micro current is current in millionths of an ampere. An ampere is a measure of the movement of electrons past a point. Microamperage current is the same kind of current your body produces on its own within each cell. This is current in millionths of an amp. It is very small; there is not enough current to stimulate sensory nerves so the current flow cannot be felt. You can tell it is running by watching the conductance meter on the machine. FDA has approved all microcurrent devices for sale in the category of TENS devices. TENS devices are for pain control only and deliver milli-amperage current. ALL TENS devices carry the same warnings precautions and contraindications. Microcurrent devices deliver micro amperage current not milli-amperage current but the warnings for the device are same because all microcurrent devices are approved in the category of TENS devices. http://www.frequencyspecific.com/faq.php

For example, the Tennant BioModulator® is a microcurrent device that has been accepted by the FDA as a Class II TENS device.

Most microcurrent devices use square wave pulses because they have been observed to be more effective clinically.

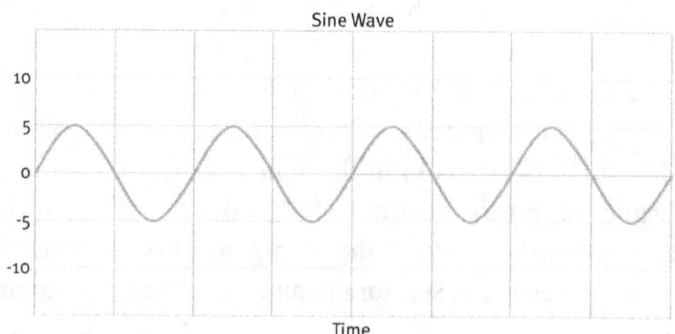

Most TENS devices use sine waves.

Ultra sound creates ultrasonic vibrations and creates heat by vibrating the water molecules in the tissue. It does not provide current nor does it change ATP status. It provides beneficial results by these mechanisms but it is just completely different from microcurrent.

In 1982 Ngok Cheng published, "The Effect of Electric Currents on ATP Generation, Protein Synthesis and Membrane Transport in Rat Skin in Clinical Orthopedics" (volume 171: pages 264-272). This study showed that microcurrent increased ATP production in rat skin by 500%. ATP is the chemical that the body uses for energy. The current also increased amino acid transport into the cell by 70% and waste product removal. The implications for human healing and repair are obvious. ATP production was increased as long as the current was below 500 microamps. When the authors increased the current to 1000 micro amps, or one milliamp, a current range delivered by TENS devices and other types of electrical stimulation therapies, the ATP production was actually reduced.

Pulsed electromagnetic field therapy (PEMFT), also called pulsed magnetic therapy, pulse magnetotherapy, or PEMF, is a reparative technique most commonly used in the field of orthopedics for the treatment of nonunion fractures, failed fusions, congenital pseudarthrosis and depression. In the case of bone healing, PEMF uses electrical energy to direct a series of magnetic pulses through injured tissue whereby each magnetic pulse induces a tiny electrical signal that stimulates cellular repair. Many studies have also demonstrated the effectiveness of PEMF in healing soft-tissue wounds; suppressing inflammatory responses at the cell membrane level to alleviate pain, and increasing range of motion. The value of pulsed electromagnetic field therapy has been shown to cover a wide range of conditions, with well documented trials carried out by hospitals, rheumatologists, physiotherapists and neurologists. There are several electrical stimulation therapy devices, approved by the FDA, that are widely available to patients for use. These devices provide an additive solution that aid in bone growth repair and depression.[3][4]

An LC circuit, also called a resonant circuit or tuned circuit, consists of an inductor, represented by the letter L, and a capacitor, represented by the letter C. When connected, they can act as an electrical resonator, an electrical analogue of a tuning fork, storing electrical energy oscillating at the circuit's resonating frequency. LC circuits are used either for generating signals at a particular frequency, or picking out a signal at a particular frequency from a more complex signal. They are key components in many electronic devices, particularly radio equipment, used in circuits such as oscillators, filters, tuners, and frequency mixers.

Parallel Tuned Circuit (LC Circuit)

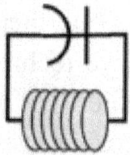

An LC circuit can store electrical energy oscillating at its resonant frequency. A capacitor stores energy in the electrical field between its plates, depending on the voltage across it, and an inductor stores energy in its magnetic field, depending on the current through it.

If a charged capacitor is connected across an inductor, charge will start to flow through the inductor, building up a magnetic field around it, and reducing the voltage on the capacitor. Eventually all the charge on the capacitor will be gone and the voltage across it will reach zero. However, the current will continue, because inductors resist changes in current, and energy to keep it flowing is extracted from the magnetic field, which will begin to decline. The current will begin to charge the capacitor with a voltage of opposite polarity to its original charge. When the magnetic field is completely dissipated the current will stop and the charge will again be stored in the capacitor, with the opposite polarity as before. Then the cycle will begin again, with the current flowing in the opposite direction through the inductor.

The charge flows back and forth between the plates of the capacitor, through the inductor. The energy oscillates back and forth between the capacitor and the inductor until (if not replenished by power from an external circuit) internal resistance makes the oscillations die out. Its action, known mathematically as a harmonic oscillator is similar to a pendulum swinging back and forth, or water sloshing back and forth in a tank. For this reason the circuit is also called a tank circuit. The oscillation frequency is determined by the capacitance and inductance values used. In typical tuned circuits in electronic equipment the oscillations are very fast, thousands to millions of times per second.

1. Robetson et al., Fourth ed.
2. Robinson, Andrew J; Lynn Snyder-Mackler (2007-09-01). Clinical Electrophysiology: Electrotherapy and Electrophysiologic Testing (Third ed.). Lippincott Williams & Wilkins. ISBN 0781744849.
3. Markov, Marko S. "Expanding Use of Pulsed Electromagnetic Field Therapies." Electromagnetic Biology & Medicine 26.3 (2007): 257–274. Academic Search Complete. EBSCO. Web. 10 June 2010.
4. Mooney, V. "A randomized double-blind prospective study of the efficacy of pulsed electromagnetic fields for interbody lumbar

fusions." Spine 15.7 (1990): 708–712. MEDLINE. EBSCO. Web. 10 June 2

The Tennant® BioModulator® has incorporated these principles into a unit capable of interacting with the electronics of human tissue.

The output of the Tennant® BioModulator® is designed to be an LC resonating circuit using microcurrent. When a load (the human body) is placed across the circuit, a unique waveform occurs which then resonates with the body as the

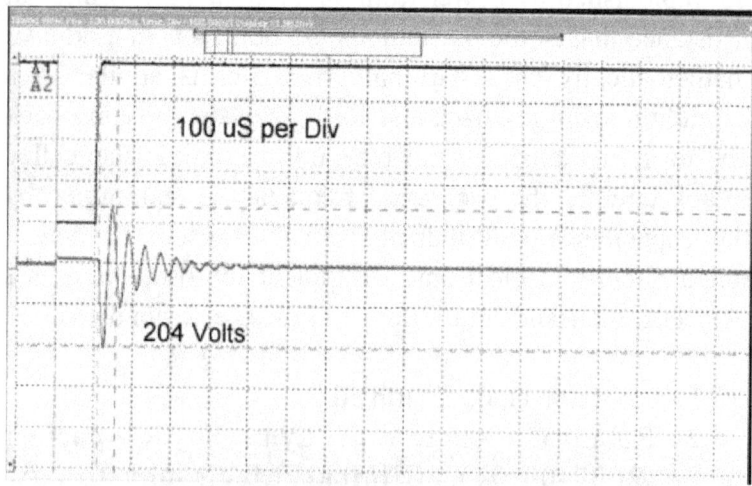

coil and capacitor of the LC circuit oscillate as described above. This creates a biofeedback mechanism that continues until preset proprietary conditions are met. In the process ATP is increased as described above.

The Tennant BioModulator® uses a damped asymmetrical biphasic sinusoidal waveform. This waveform is able to cause transfer of electrons from the device to the cells.

Thus one can see the major differences between the Tennant® BioModulator® (TBM) and a traditional TENS device. The TBM is microamp whereas the TENS is milliamp. The TBM increases ATP whereas the TENS reduces ATP. The TBM has a waveform that changes as the tissue electronics change whereas the TENS waveform is constant, either a sine or square wave. The TBM's design incorporated PEMF whereas the TENS has no such capability. The TBM allows one to measure tissue before and after therapy whereas the TENS units have no such

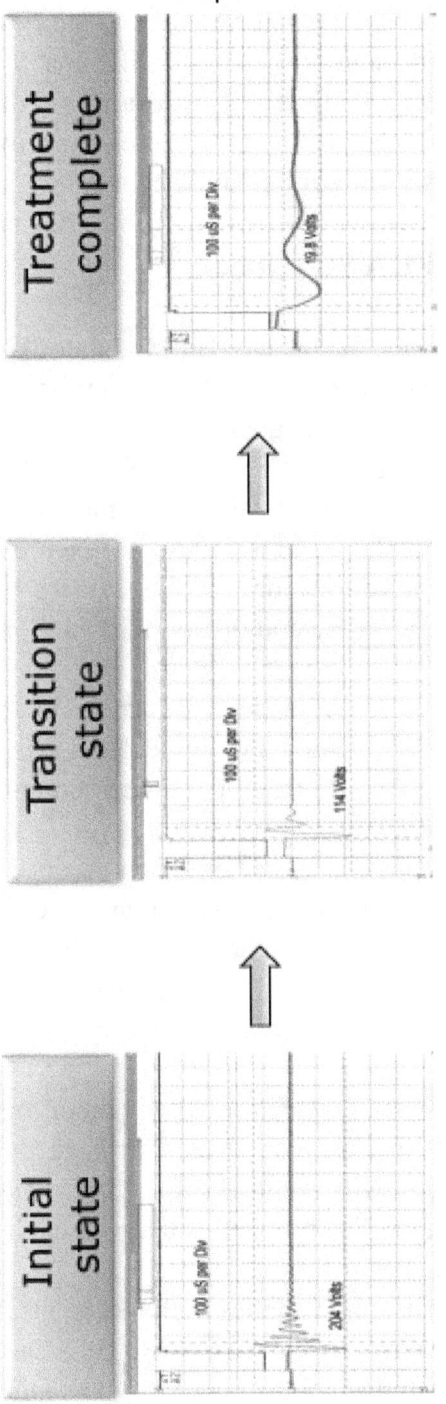

capability. TENS devices are designed to influence nerve transmission using milliamps whereas the TBM using microcurrent (microamps) does not affect nerve transmission but rather improves cellular conditions allowing for natural healing.

FDA Statement

The Tennant® BioModulator® and certain accessory electrodes are FDA listed by its distributor or manufacturer in these categories:

1. 21 CFR 882.5890 – Neurology transcutaneous electrical nerve stimulator for pain relief
2. 21 CFR 882.5050 – Neurology biofeedback device

Indications for use:

1. Symptomatic relief and management of chronic, intractable pain
2. Adjunctive treatment in the management of post-traumatic surgical and post-traumatic pain
3. Relaxation training and muscle relaxation

I have had some criticism because I have not given credit to the Russians, particularly Alexander Karasev and/or Alexander Nadtochi and their colleagues for inventing the basic pattern of the waveform used in the Tennant BioModulator.

When I was in medical school, one of my professors said, "Anytime you think you have developed something new, you will eventually find that some German did it 50 years ago. The problem is that you can't speak or read German."

This logic applies to the Russians that developed the device known as the SCENAR. It is said that Karasev lost some family members to food poisoning in 1973 and that lead him to invent the SCENAR. He then went into business with Alexander Revenko, MD, Alexander Nadtochi, Yuri Gorfinkel, and others. They received a Russian patent for the frequency pattern of the SCENAR in 1989 although the frequency pattern was in use in the US as early as 1845. Several examples of such devices are in a museum in

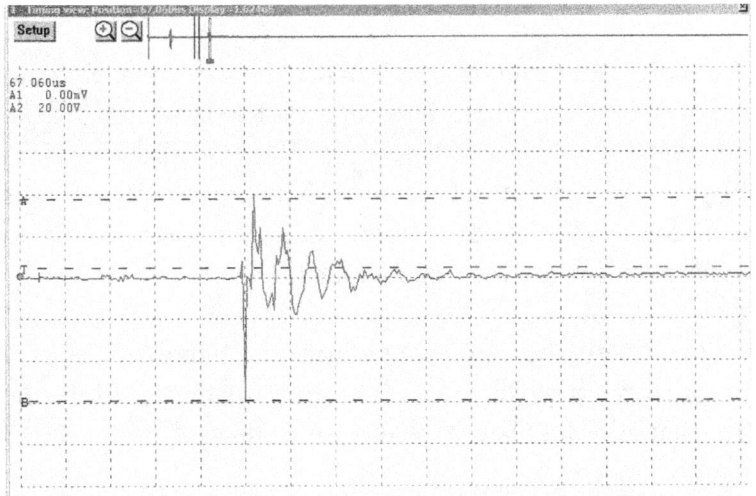

Minneapolis. This graphic shows the waveform in an 1845 device.

I was fortunate enough to personally examine a Rife device originally thought to be manufactured in 1939 in the possession of the Scottish engineer Aubrey Scoon. Some believe it was built in the 1940s by Verne Thompson. It emitted the same basic waveform as the SCENAR and BioModulator.

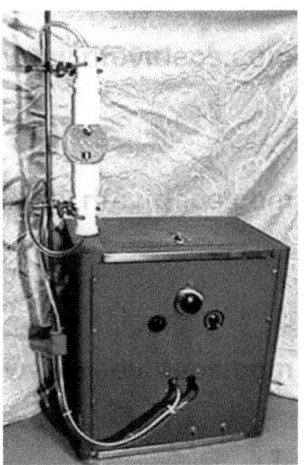

Viktor Schauberger described the basic waveform in the early 1900s and used it (after capture by the Nazis) to make a flying saucer in the 1940s.

Therefore it is my view that Karasev simply rediscovered what other scientists had found before him. I did not steal the waveform from him any more than he stole it from Rife. All of us in science stand on the shoulders of those that came before us.

We did't know exactly how far it is between planets until we sent up the Hubble telescope in 1990. After that an obelisk that is over 3000 years old was discovered in Egypt. On it the exact distances between the planets was recorded. Thus it is with science. We keep having to rediscover things over and over again.

I have taken the basic waveform and modified it in a proprietary way to emit frequency patterns from the Tennant BioModulator® that are not present in any other similar device.

Using the BioModulator

Now let's look at some examples of how one can use the BioModulator to help identify and confirm various illnesses.

A woman had a tooth extracted. The socket became infected and she was placed on antibiotics. Still the area would not heal. She was given different antibiotics, both orally and intravenously. Still the area would not heal. Repeat surgery to remove the infected bone still did not allow the area to heal.

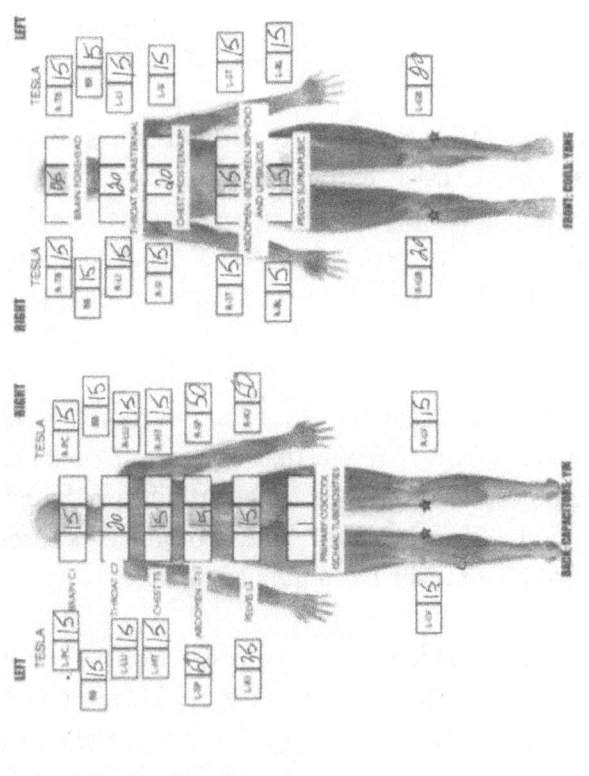

Now let's look at her voltages. What you can see is that most of her voltages are low since they should all be 20 to 25 millivolts. Almost all the voltages to the solid organs are low-voltage. You will recall that the solid organs are attached to the BioTerminals on the back. Also, all but two of the BioTerminals on the front (hollow organs) are low as well.

When the average of these numbers is less than 20, we realized that the patient has low total body voltage. Low total body voltage is hypothyroidism until proven otherwise. Remember that the blood tests are usually misleading.

I looked at her hypothyroidism questionnaire. This questionnaire asks the person to indicate which symptoms of hypothyroidism are present and how severe they are. The maximum score possible is 42. This patient rated 42. In addition, her physical exam was characteristic of hypothyroidism.

Now look at the numbers from the corresponding Tesla circuits. You will see that almost all of these are low. When these are low, you usually find that the adrenals are fatigued. Her adrenal questionnaire scored 48/51, confirming that she has adrenal fatigue.

Now focus on the BioTerminals for the skull. The posterior one is 15 and the anterior one is 5. Thus the voltage to all the organs/structures in the skull is inadequate for healing. Do you remember what voltage it takes to heal? You're right! It's -50 millivolts. Now we know exactly why this person can't heal the infection in her jaw. She simply doesn't have the voltage to do it.

The solution now is easy. Use the BioModulator to insert electrons into the skull BioTerminals. In addition we can use the BioTransducer to use magnetic fields to get the electrons down into the center of the jaw (the acupuncture meridians will take them to the periosteum of the jaw but it will be more difficult for them to get into the center of the infection without the BioTransducer).

While we are actively providing the electrons necessary to heal the jaw, we must also deal with the rest of the body. It will give us the support system necessary to heal. We start correcting the hypothyroidism and the adrenal fatigue with desiccated hormones, iodine, vitamins, minerals, etc., needed to get them functioning as we have discussed in other chapters.

Remember that the immune system needs voltage, iodine, and ozone to kill bugs. We will aggressively start restoring her deficiency of iodine so her "iodine shield" can be restored to prevent new infections.

Remember that sodium chlorite works the same way as the white blood cells kill bugs---oxidation. So we would also use a short burst of sodium chlorite to help kill the infections. She will be full of L-forms because of all the antibiotics she has taken. Remember that sodium chlorite is an electron stealer, so we would not want to use it more than a week or two to attempt to get ahead of the infection. We would use the BioModulator and BioTransducer as much as possible to restore the electrons consumed by the sodium chlorite.

Remember also that low voltage causes low oxygen. We would use hyperbaric oxygen if that were available.

This person perfectly demonstrates what happens when voltage drops. First she became hypothyroid. Fluoride would have had a lot to do with this---also soy consumption and consuming things that act like estrogen. This dropped her voltage so it was hard for her to get her work done. However, her adrenals kept pushing to get her through the day. After a while, they gave up as well.

Low voltage caused by the hypothyroidism allowed the following things to happen:

1. Chronic pain
2. Decreased oxygen
3. Decreased production of ATP
4. Infections including L-forms that never respond to antibiotics

Addition of antibiotics made even more L-forms. They don't respond to anything except changing the voltage of the environment. (Sodium chlorite works by way of voltage change, not biochemically like antibiotics.)

Let's look at another person. This man worked with gasoline and diesel and grease most of his life. He developed cancer of his left kidney. The left kidney was removed but no chemotherapy or radiation was used. Nine years later, he was found to have tumors in his pancreas, left hip, and lungs. He chose not to have chemotherapy or radiation but instead changed his diet and did nutritional things to improve his immune system. He also did a lot of detoxification. Two years later, the lung tumors are gone, the tumor in the left hip is smaller, and the tumor in the pancreas has not changed in size.

Look at his voltages. Most of his body is running at 50 millivolts. His body is actively in a healing mode. Fortunately for him, he is not hypothyroid or hypoadrenal. Otherwise, he could not mount this healing effort.

Note, however, that his voltage is low in the Abdominal BioTerminal. It is 15 both back and front. This of course corresponds with the pancreas. Thus he has not been able to resolve this tumor and is at risk of it growing as long as the voltages are low.

Look at the Pelvic numbers. The voltage is low in the pelvis placing this area at risk. It also explains why he has a tumor in the hip.

This emphasizes the importance of measuring and knowing the voltage numbers. He is feeling great. The only way he knows that he is at significant risk for the tumors growing again is that the voltages are low. Tumors can't grow if the oxygen levels are normal, and oxygen levels are controlled by voltage. He must get the voltages up in the Abdominal and Pelvic BioTerminals. I suggested that he wear the BioModulator 24 hours per day with patches attached to those BioTerminals.

When only one or a few BioTerminals have low voltage, you should suspect a dental infection in the same circuit or in a Tesla that controls that BioTerminal. For example, with low Abdominal BioTerminals, the back Tesla is the

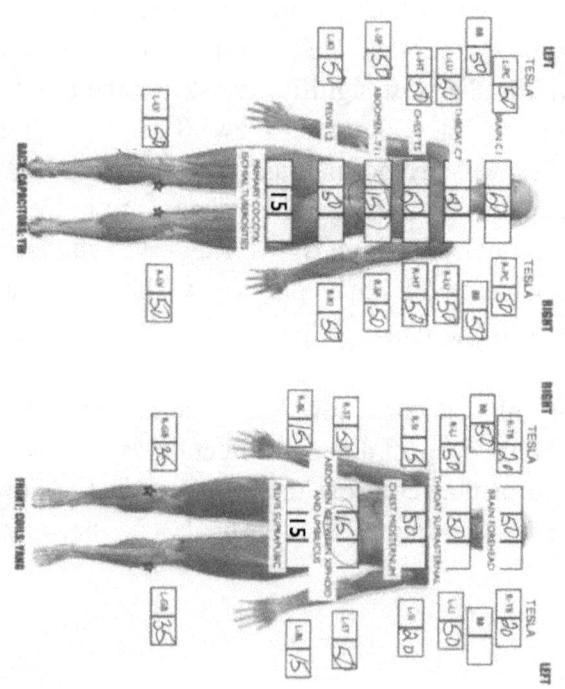

Spleen circuit and the front Tesla is the Stomach. Look for

Loneliness, Acute Grief, Humiliated, Trapped, Inhibited, Greed, Not lovable	Anxiety, Self-Punishment, Broken Power, Hate, Low self-worth, Obsessed	Chronic Grief, Overcritical, Sadness, Controlling, Feeling trapped, Dogmatic, Compulsive, Uptight	Anger, Resentment, Frustration, Blaming, Incapable to take action, Manipulative	Fear, Shame, Guilt, Broken will, Shyness, Helpless, Deep exhaustion	Fear, Shame, Guilt, Broken will, Shyness, Helpless, Deep exhaustion	Anger, Resentment, Frustration, Blaming, Incapable to take action, Manipulative	Chronic Grief, Overcritical, Sadness, Controlling, Dogmatic, Compulsive, Uptight	Anxiety, Self-Punishment, Broken Power, Hate, Low self-worth, Obsessed	Loneliness, Acute Grief, Humiliated, Trapped, Inhibited, Greed, Not lovable
Duodenum Middle Ear, Shoulder Elbow, CNS	Sinus, Maxillary Oropharynx, Larynx	Sinus, Paranasal and Ethmoid, Bronchus, Nose	Sinus, Sphenoid Palatine Tonsil Hip, Eye, Knee	Sinus, Frontal Pharyngeal Tonsil Genito-Urinary System	Sinus, Frontal Pharyngeal Tonsil Genito-Urinary System	Sinus, Sphenoid Palatine Tonsil Hip, Eye, Knee	Sinus, Paranasal and Ethmoid, Bronchus, Nose	Sinus, Maxillary Oropharynx, Larynx	Ileum, Jejunum Middle Ear, Shoulder Elbow, CNS
Heart, Small Int., Circulation/Sex, Endocrine	Pancreas Stomach	Lung Large Intestine	Liver Gallbladder	Kidney Bladder	Kidney Bladder	Liver Gallbladder	Lung Large Intestine	Stomach Spleen	Heart, Small Int., Circulation/Sex, Endocrine

| 1 | 2 | 3 | 4 | 5 | 6 | 7 | 8 | 9 | 10 | 11 | 12 | 13 | 14 | 15 | 16 |
| 32 | 31 | 30 | 29 | 28 | 27 | 26 | 25 | 24 | 23 | 22 | 21 | 20 | 19 | 18 | 17 |

Heart, Small Int., Circulation/Sex, Endocrine	Lung Large Intestine	Pancreas Stomach	Liver Gallbladder	Kidney Bladder	Kidney Bladder	Liver Gallbladder	Spleen Stomach	Lung Large Intestine	Heart, Small Int., Circulation/Sex, Endocrine
Shoulder, Elbow Ileum, Middle Ear Peripheral Nerves	Sinus, Maxillary Ethmoid, Bronchus, Nose	Sinus, Maxillary Larynx, Lymph, Oropharynx Breast Knee	Sinus, Sphenoid Palatine Tonsil Hip, Eye Knee	Sinus, Frontal Ear, Pharyngeal Tonsil Genito-Urinary System	Sinus, Frontal Ear, Pharyngeal Tonsil Genito-Urinary System	Sinus, Sphenoid Palatine Tonsil Hip, Eye Knee	Sinus, Maxillary Larynx, Lymph, Oropharynx Breast	Sinus, Paranasal and Ethmoid, Bronchus, Nose	Shoulder, Elbow Ileum, Jejunum, Middle Ear Peripheral Nerves
Loneliness, Acute Grief, Trapped, Inhibited, Greed, Not lovable	Chronic Grief, Overcritical, Sadness, Controlling, Feeling trapped, Dogmatic, Compulsive, Uptight	Anxiety, Self-Punishment, Broken Power, Hate, Low self-worth, Obsessed	Anger, Resentment, Frustration, Blaming, Incapable to take action, Manipulative	Fear, Shame, Guilt, Broken will, Shyness, Helpless, Deep exhaustion	Fear, Shame, Guilt, Broken will, Shyness, Helpless, Deep exhaustion	Anger, Resentment, Frustration, Blaming, Incapable to take action, Manipulative	Anxiety, Self-Punishment, Broken Power, Hate, Low self-worth, Obsessed	Chronic Grief, Overcritical, Sadness, Controlling, Feeling trapped, Dogmatic, Compulsive, Uptight	Loneliness, Acute Grief, Humiliated, Trapped, Inhibited, Greed, Not lovable

Acumeridian Tooth-Organ Relationships [with Autonomic Neuropeptide Emotion correlations] -- from various sources Dr. Ralph Wilson, N.D.

infected teeth in those circuits using this chart. That would be teeth 2, 3,14,15, 20, 21, 28, or 29. Measure any metal in these teeth with a voltmeter as I described in the dental chapter. If there is a root canal in one of these teeth, you know why the voltage dropped. It must be removed or you will never get the voltages back to normal.

The Pelvic BioTerminal is controlled by the Kidney Tesla on the back and the Bladder Tesla on the front. Look for problems in teeth number 7, 8, 9, 10, 23, 24, 25, or 26 to help explain why this BioTerminal is low. Also remember that if you have a root canal, it will infect the bone and then infect the bone of its next-door neighbors. For example, a root canal in tooth 27 (liver, gall bladder) could take out the kidney, bladder circuit of tooth 26.

This next person is a teenage boy. He developed Crohn's Disease. *Crohn's disease (also known as granulomatous, and colitis) is an inflammatory disease of the intestines that may affect any part of the gastrointestinal tract from mouth to anus, causing a wide variety of symptoms. It primarily*

491

causes abdominal pain, diarrhea (which may be bloody), vomiting, or weight loss, but may also cause complications outside of the gastrointestinal tract such as skin rashes, arthritis, inflammation of the eye, tiredness, and lack of concentration.

Crohn's disease is thought to be an autoimmune disease, in which the body's immune system attacks the gastrointestinal tract, causing inflammation; it is classified as a type of inflammatory bowel disease. Wikipedia

In addition to the Crohn's Disease, this boy has uveitis, an inflammation of the eyes. It is also thought to be an autoimmune disease although uveitis has been thought by many over the years to be associated with infections, particularly fungal infections.

He recently was hospitalized for dehydration from diarrhea. While in the hospital, he contracted Clostridium difficile. We discussed this terrible infection in the chapter on infections.

He has been given large doses of antibiotics. He has developed an anal fistula.

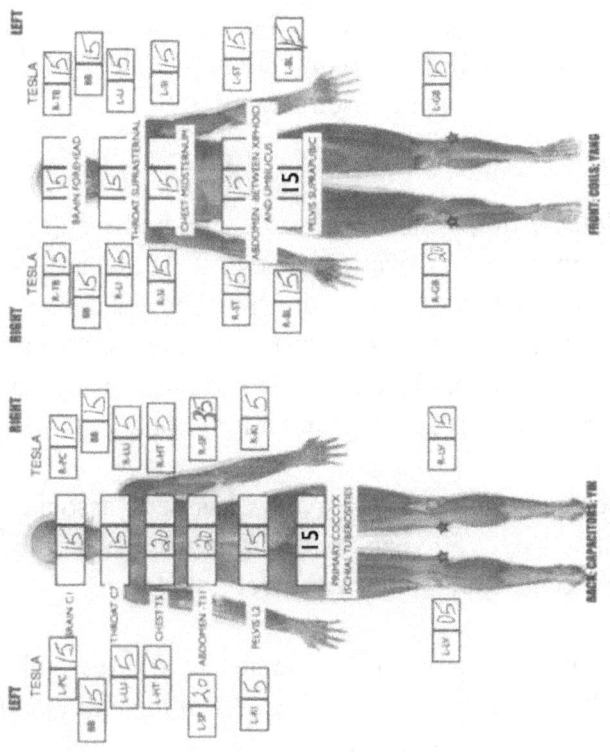

Look at his voltages. Remember that for children or athletes, normal voltage is minus 30-35 millivolts. His readings average 14.6 millivolts. Thus his total body voltage is half what it should be! Now you understand why he isn't getting well.

The primary things that lower total body voltage are hypothyroidism, narcotic drug use, epilepsy drugs, and losing sleep when you have little reserve.

493

This boy's hypothyroidism questionnaire is 17/42. This makes hypothyroidism most likely. The low numbers in his Tesla circuits support his adrenals being worn out as well. With low voltages and low adrenal function, his immune system cannot deal with infections. The heavy use of antibiotics will have created large numbers of L-forms that are resistant to antibiotics.

As voltage drops more and more, the end result is fungal forms that are cell-wall deficient. These are the most pathological forms of infections. They do not respond to antibiotics, cannot be cultured, and are only seen with a phase contrast or darkfield microscope. They can most easily be seen with a Grayfield microscope.

It is of some interest that uveitis has been associated with fungus for over 50 years, but it has always been difficult to prove because the fungus can rarely be cultured!

This boy's diet is primarily canned food. It is full of soy and plastic Trans fats. Soy shuts down the entire endocrine system. Soybeans are high in phytic acid, present in the bran or hulls of all seeds. It's a substance that can block the uptake of essential minerals (calcium, magnesium, copper, iron and especially zinc) in the intestinal tract.

Zinc is called the intelligence mineral because it is needed for optimal development and functioning of the brain and nervous system. It plays a role in protein synthesis and collagen formation; it is involved in the blood-sugar control mechanism and thus protects against diabetes; it is needed for a healthy reproductive system.

Zinc is a key component in numerous vital enzymes and plays a role in the immune system.

Phytates found in soy products interfere with zinc absorption more completely than with other minerals.

Zinc deficiency can cause a "spacey" feeling that some vegetarians may mistake for the "high" of spiritual enlightenment.

One of the problems with canned food is the presence of Trans fats and Canola oil. Canola oil stunts the growth of infants. It is not suitable for human consumption. However, the discussion of Canola is beyond the scope of this book. Trans fats will not make good cell membranes. Cells made with Trans fats cannot hold a charge and cause the voltage to be low. You see that regularly in brain-injured people. The brain replaces itself in 8 months. About six months after a brain injured person is put on canned food containing high amounts of Trans fats, the nervous system stops getting better. A brain made of plastic just doesn't work!

The same is true when other people are put on canned food as their primary diet. Look at this boy's voltage. Part of the low voltage is due to cell membranes made from plastic Trans fats.

Fats of any kind (except coconut oil) cannot be absorbed without bile, so one needs to pay attention to whether the liver is capable of making bile. A liver running on half-normal voltage will not be able to do so. Thus one must supplement bile and digestive enzymes until the voltage normalizes.

I would recommend that this boy wear the BioModulator 24 hours a day while we are changing his diet, and correcting his thyroid function and adrenals, stomach acid, etc.

Crohn's Disease and ulcerative colitis are now believed to be caused by a cousin to the tuberculosis bacteria. It is often quickly resolved with gallium.

Macular Degeneration

Macular degeneration is becoming an increasing problem as people age. Ophthalmologists believe they have two options to treat it. If bleeding isn't present, it's treated with vitamins. If bleeding is present, the eye is injected with drugs intended to shut down blood vessels. Neither work very well. The reason is, of course, that it's all about the voltage in the eye.

What BioTerminal would provide the voltage to the eye? The skull or head BioTerminal of course. It will always be

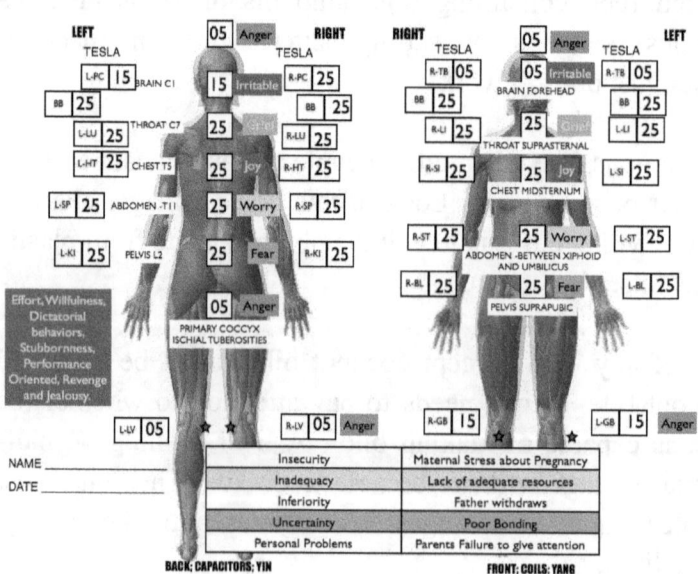

low in people with macular degeneration.

Note in the person above with macular degeneration that the posterior Head BioTerminal has 15 millivolts and the anterior reads 05 millivolts. The Tesla circuits that monitor the Head BioTerminals are the Triple Burner and the Pericardium. Note that the Triple Burner Teslas are reading 05.

The Head gets voltage delivered from the Primary Cable. The Primary Cable is controlled by the Liver and Gall Bladder Teslas. Thus they also affect the structures of the head including the eye. Note that the Liver Teslas are at 05 at the coccyx and at the top of the head (GV-20). Now we know why the person has macular degeneration. The voltage supply is diminished.

Acumeridian Tooth-Organ Relationships [with Autonomic Neuropeptide Emotion correlations] — from various sources Dr. Ralph Wilson, N.D.

Look at the dental chart. This person has a root canal in tooth #6. He has a crown on tooth #22 that measures 180 millivolts with a voltmeter (means there is infection under the crown). This person has low voltage in the eyes because of infection in the teeth that are on the same circuits.

The person was sent to the dentist to pull the root canal tooth including removing any infection in the associated bone. The crown on #22 must be removed and the decay

498

and any mercury under it must be removed and the crown replaced.

The BioModulator is used to restore voltage to the Head BioTerminals. In addition, the BioTransducer is used to place voltage directly on the retina.

Our study of dry macular degeneration showed that if the vision is better than 20/70, we got them all back to 20/20 or 20/25. If there was enough scarring that the vision was worse than 20/70, we did not get back to the vision necessary to read easily (20/50) but the vision did not get worse over the next two years.

Summary

I have attempted to give only a few examples of the usefulness of the BioModulator and a voltmeter in determining the underlying cause of illness = low voltage. You can expand the examples to almost any illness. The location of the illness usually tells you the BioTerminal that will have low voltage. You will quickly learn which Tesla circuits monitors each BioTerminal.

There are a couple of non-intuitive connections for the BioTerminal and Tesla circuits. The large intestine is served partly by the Neck BioTerminal because of the way it is formed embryonically. Other parts are served by the Abdomen and the Pelvic BioTerminals. In addition, the breast is served by the Abdomen BioTerminal and the Stomach Tesla.

There are a few special considerations that are beyond the scope of this handbook. However, the purpose of this handbook is to give one the basic concepts. Training is available for those wishing to learn the nuances.

13 Essential Oils

The universe is all about energy. No matter whether you call the energy chi, prana, electrons, or some other name, the universe is about the interactions of energy.

Voltage is the stored potential to do work. Amperage is the movement of electrons doing work. When electrons move from one place to another, we call that current. Whenever electrons create a current, there is always a magnetic field 90 degrees from the direction of the current.

Electrons forming a current always move in a vortex---not in the flat sine wave like you see in the diagram below. The frequency of a current is the distance between each revolution of the vortex of energy. Frequency is measured in Hertz. One Hertz is one revolution per second. One hundred Hertz is 100 revolutions per second, etc.

People often get confused about the difference between voltage and frequency. One can think of voltage as the power or amplitude of the vortex of energy while frequency is how many revolutions or oscillations the energy makes per second. As you will see, both are important in understanding how cells work.

A key to understanding Energetic Medicine is to understand that each cell is designed to run at a specific voltage and a specific frequency. Generally speaking, disease is caused

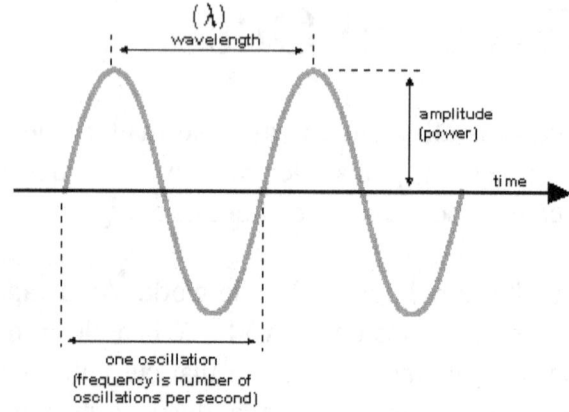

one oscillation
(frequency is number of
oscillations per second)

when cells have toolittle voltage and are running at too low
a frequency.

Oil	MHz	Harmonics	Organ	MHz
Rose	320	160, 80	Thyroid	62-68
Helichrysum	181	91	Lungs	58-65
Ravensara	134	67	Liver	55-60
Lavender	118	59	Thymus	65-68
Wild Tansy	105	53	Heart	67-70
Myrrh	105	53	Stomach	58-65
Melissa	102	51	Spleen	60-80
Sandalwood	96	48	Colon	58-63
Peppermint	78	39	Brain	70-78
Human	62-68			
Galbanum	56	28	Headache	67-88
Basil	52	26	Flu	58
Cancer	<42		Viral Infections	55-60

Oil	MHz	Harmonics	Organ	MHz
Quartz	3.58 MHz, 10 MHz, 14.318 MHz, 20 MHz, 33.33 MHz, and 40 MHz		Cancer	<42

The numbers in this chart are approximate and averages since each oil and each organ operate with hundreds of frequencies that average out to the numbers below.

Note: You will find different frequencies listed for various organs. It depends upon whether the person measuring them found the primary frequency or a harmonic. It is not always easy to tell if you are measuring the primary frequency or a harmonic of that frequency. Also, it depends upon how the frequency was measured. To measure accurately, one must have a room or chamber that is shielded. Otherwise, outside frequencies will contaminate what you are trying to measure. In addition, the equipment that has the sensitivity to measure these frequencies that are operating at around -20 millivolts is expensive and usually only found in laboratories. Some have determined these frequencies using muscle testing called kinesiology. See the following chart. Note that these frequencies are the harmonics listed in hertz and the corresponding sound (note), whereas the frequencies listed above are in megahertz.

ORGAN	FREQUENCY/NOTE
BLOOD	321.9 (E)
ADRENALS	492.8 (B)
KIDNEY	319.88 (Eb)
LIVER	317.83 (Eb)
ORGAN	FREQUENCY/NOTE
BLADDER	352 (F)
INTESTINES	281. (C#)

LUNGS	220 (A)
COLON	176 (F)
GALL BLADDER	164.3 (E)
PANCREAS	117.3 (C#)
STOMACH	110 (A)
BRAIN	315.8 (Eb)
FAT CELLS	295.8 (C#)
MUSCLES	324 (E)
BONE	418,3 (Ab)

http://www.greatdreams.com/hertz.htm

How Do I Measure Cell Voltage and Cell Frequency?

The body has two wiring systems that carry voltage to each organ. Both are made of fibrous tissue since fibrous tissue has the least resistance to the movement of electrons in the body. By having two circuits, if one fails, there is the opportunity for the other to keep the organ working somewhat. One wiring system is called the Perineural Nervous System and is actually a sheath around each nerve. The other is the acupuncture system and is actually the fascial planes of the body.

One can tap into either wiring system to measure the voltage in the organs. It is difficult to use a voltmeter to measure the organ voltage because voltage surges about every six seconds. Thus we commonly use an ohmmeter to measure and then convert that to voltage. There are several devices designed to accurately and reproducibly measure organ voltage like the Nakatani (MEAD) system, the Voll systems, and the Tennant BioModulator. By placing one of these devices onto a wire known to go to each organ, one can know the voltage in that organ.

Cells in the adult human are designed to run at -20 to -25 millivolts and to heal at -50 millivolts. The minus sign means that the voltage is an electron donor. If the voltage drops to the point the solution is an electron stealer, we put a plus sign in front of the voltage. Cancer occurs at +30 millivolts.

Measuring cell frequency is not easy. Although it can be done with sophisticated and expensive laboratory equipment, there are no affordable and reliable instruments to do it in the clinical setting. Hydrogen emits over 100 different frequencies. Oxygen emits over 400 different frequencies. Thus water emits over 500 frequencies. (These frequencies are listed in the Handbook of Chemistry and Physics.) Now imagine the number of frequencies in a complex molecule like serotonin or in an organ like the liver! Each will emit thousands of different frequencies.

There is no frequency generator that can generate so many frequencies at the same time. Thus the idea that a computer chip can drive a frequency generator to emit the "digital signal" of biologically active molecules is simply fanciful.

In 1978, Dr. Helmut Schimmel originated the Vegetative Reflex Test (V.R.T.) or VEGATEST- Method. The system is based on measuring against special test ampoules filled with biologically active substances rather than organ-linked acupuncture points themselves. With each skin measurement point, the response of the person to the test ampoules results in a "yes or no" reading. By using substances in vials, it is an attempt to overcome the limitation of a computer not being able to create these frequencies. Other similar devices like the MORA, Bicom, Dermatron, etc., attempt to follow this method.

Some people attempt to estimate cell frequency using Applied Kinesiology (testing to see if muscles are weak or strong and using the change from one to the other to tell them the answer they seek). Studies have shown this not to be reliable in some cases.

Others say they have devices that measure the frequency by sending "digital signatures of biologically active substances" to the body to see if the body reacts to it. They are not really doing so because there are no devices that can send such signals. Any biologically active substance contains hundreds or thousands of frequencies of variable voltage. We do not have any frequency generators that can reproduce that type of signal. Those that say they are sending such signals are just using a software program that is a random number generator. It randomly assigns numbers to each organ or substance. Such devices never give reproducible results because they aren't really measuring anything. Thus you are told that they are using Quantum physics to hide the fact that they aren't really measuring anything.

Remember that there are no clinical (only laboratory) devices that can accurately and reproducibly measure frequency in the body. Some scientists are working on developing such devices, but to the best of my knowledge, no such device is currently available for purchase to use outside a research center equipped with a Faraday cage to screen out the noise (frequencies that surround us all the time and confuse measurements).

One can see that pain is present or something isn't functioning by what the patient says/feels and/or how much mobility they have in their movements of arms and neck. Each different oil contains hundreds of frequencies. If you apply the frequencies of any given organ, that organ will function better and you see the result or the patient feels the result. In this system, we do not know a specific frequency that we can write down, but we know that that oil or blend of oils contain the frequencies that correspond to a certain organ.

Birch Oil -targets bones
Helichrysum Oil - targets nervous system
Marjoram Oil - targets smooth muscles
Birch Oil -targets skeletal muscles
Lemongrass Oil - targets tendons and cartilage
Cypress Oil - targets the circulatory system
Geranium Oil - targets the emotional system

Treatment of Low Voltage and Low Frequency

Once one determines that the voltage of an organ is low, you will want to correct it. One does that by inserting electrons into one of the wires that carries voltage to that organ, by drinking water that contains electrons (alkaline water), by eating foods that contain electrons (unprocessed foods), by getting into the sun, putting your feet in the dirt, hugging other living things, or by using devices designed to supply electrons like the Tennant BioModulator, low-level lasers, essential oils, homeopathy, exercise, etc.

Correcting frequency is not as commonly understood. For the transfer of electrons to the cell, the electrons must have a frequency (distance between rotations of the vortex of energy) that is the same of the cell. A perfect example of this problem is rose oil. Much is made of the fact that rose oil has the highest frequency of any essential oil. Its frequency is about 320 megahertz. The problem is that no organ in the human is known to operate at 320 megahertz. It can only be effective if a harmonic of 320 megahertz corresponds to the frequency of some organ. Its harmonics include 160 megahertz and 80 megahertz. The human brain operates at 70-78 megahertz. (These numbers are not that precise, so a small variation in numbers is okay.) Thus rose oil can transfer its energy to the brain since 80 megahertz is very close to the 78 megahertz that the brain will accept. So rose oil is effective in helping brains work better not because it has the highest frequency of any oil but because one of its harmonics will transfer energy to the cells of the brain. Peppermint running at 78 megahertz will have a similar effect on the brain as rose oil whose harmonic is 80 megahertz, and peppermint is much more affordable than rose!

Another problem is that, although we might say that peppermint emits a frequency of 78 megahertz, that is the average frequency it emits. Peppermint will actually be emitting hundreds of frequencies that average out to 78 megahertz. The brain will also be running at hundreds of different frequencies that average out to 78 megahertz. Thus a synthetic oil made to smell like peppermint will be emitting one frequency that may or may not be close to 78 megahertz, but it will certainly not be emitting the same hundreds of frequencies that real peppermint oil will emit. Thus it won't work the same.

Look at the table above. Note that the harmonic of lavender is 59 MHz. This is very close to the resonate frequency of many of the organs. Thus we understand why lavender is considered the "universal essential oil", i.e., it is useful for many different things because it resonates with many different organs, particularly lungs, liver, stomach, spleen and colon!

We have the same problem with frequency generators and lasers. Frequency machines like most Rife machines will be emitting a single frequency. Low-level lasers will also be emitting one frequency. Lasers come in specific frequencies. They are usually 380 nanometers, 410 nM, 640 nM, 780 nM, etc. The actual frequency any laser puts out can vary by 20% from the frequency on the label. Again, these are single frequency devices and whether or not that frequency will transfer its energy to the cell is determined by whether it resonates with the cell.

Now you can understand why I created the Infinity Frequency Set in the Tennant BioModulator. It emits a wide range of frequencies and each frequency series it emits is different from the previous ones. Thus it is an effort to duplicate what is found in nature---a wide range of frequencies that will be able to transfer energy to the cells by having the frequencies that will resonate with the various types of cells in the body. Thus it is an effort to have the same effect as applying numerous different essential oils and not having to figure out which oils are needed.

When I began to use essential oils, I found it difficult to memorize the hundreds of oils that are available and figure out which to use for any individual patient. I started out by going through an encyclopedia of essential oils. Under each oil, it would describe the uses for each oil. I put all of these into a database. It took months for me to complete this task. However, then I could sort the database for any illness and find the oils recommended for it. This was only a partial help because now it might list 15 oils for a given illness. Which one should I use?

I then read in David Stewart's book <u>Chemistry Of Essential Oils Made Simple</u> that the terpenes contained in each oil tended to have different effects. The effects described were fairly nonspecific and I wondered how they came to those conclusions. However, I decided to add the chemistry to my database. After completing that, I could now sort my database by the chemical constituents. When I did so, I found that one of the terpenes gave effects that were primarily killing infections and detoxification! Now I had something I could use. I found that another of the terpene family was primarily anti-inflammatory and another was primarily for metabolic problems and brain function. This made a lot more sense than what was in the chemistry book!

In another book, I read that certain terpenes increased the voltage (pH) in cells! Wow! Now I had another way besides the BioModulator to help restore voltage to the cells. Then in another book, I found exactly what I noticed when I sorted my database. A different type of terpenes reduced inflammation.

I knew that to get the energy to transfer to the cells, I needed the correct frequencies for each type of cell. Since there is no clinical way to measure this, it occurred to me that the more of each type of terpene there was in an oil, the more likely it was to have additional frequencies present in that oil. I sorted by database and found the combinations of oils that had the highest percentages of each type of terpenes. I made blends based on this content rather than the usual method of making blends based on octaves or some other method. As far as I know, this approach of blending based on quantity of specific terpenes has never been done before. This is how I arrived at what I called the EER system or the Be Healthy System of oils.

Now the question was, "Would it work?" I would then check the pain/feeling of the patient and the mobility of the patient. I would also look at the blood in my phase contrast microscope before and after. I would also repeat the voltage measurements with my BioModulator device

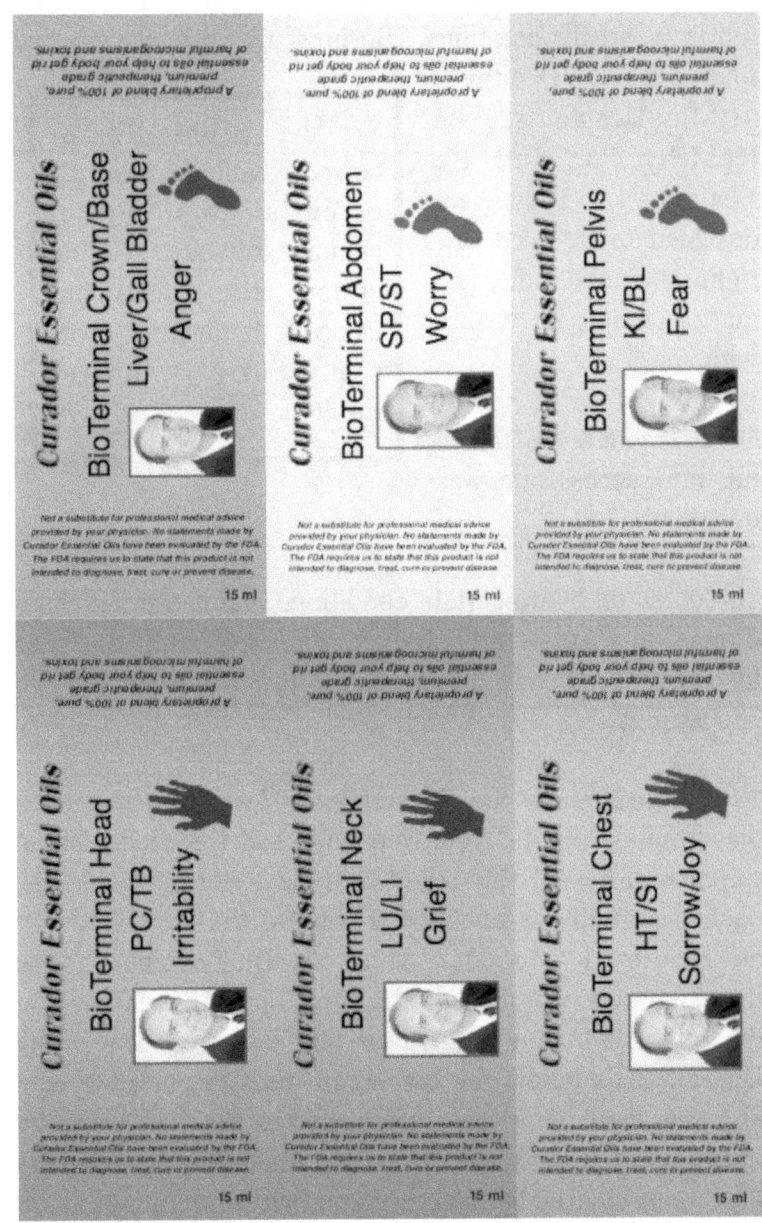

before and after. What I found was that about 70 to 80 percent of the time, the results were remarkable. The rest of the time, it didn't work.

I noticed that in the people where it didn't work, there seemed to be significant emotional overlays. I created a fourth blend for emotions. So now my system contained four blends, Be Healthy #1, Be Healthy #2, Be Healthy #3, and Be Healthy #4. They were designed to be used one right after the other no matter what is wrong with you.

So the BioModulator corrects voltage and the essential oils correct cellular software. Using either gets results but using both together gives exponentially better results.

Once I added the fourth oil, my success rate was over 90%.

Of course there are certain conditions that cause me to go directly to a single oil. If there is a skin problem, I use lavender. For headaches or brain fog, I will go directly to peppermint.

After I understood the BioTerminals, I realized that each was running at a different frequency and I needed a blend for each of them. That resulted in the series of six blends, each designed for each BioTerminal that replaced my Be Healthy 1-4 blends. Since the BioTerminals above the diaphragm pass through the arms, I put a hand image on the oils that you apply to the hands. Since the BioTerminals below the diaphragm pass through the legs and thus their oils should be applied to the feet, I put the image of a foot on those oils. I also included the emotions that are influenced by the corresponding BioTerminal.

When I started using essential oils and got results, I assumed that I was correcting voltage. However, I soon found that the oils did not change the voltage. Further study revealed that the oils were changing the signals coming from the DNA to the proteins in the cells. Thus they were correcting "cellular software". In a computer, a series of zeroes and ones are sent out to tell the hardware what to do. However, the information can become corrupted so that when you press an "A" on the keyboard, a "W" appears on the screen instead. The same thing can happen with cells. In a computer, you correct this problem with software like Norton or McAfee.

Fortunately for us, plants run at the same frequency as human organs. The oils extracted from plants have these frequencies. When you apply essential oils to the human, they act like Norton or McAfee and correct the information being sent from the DNA to the proteins in the cells so that they know what to do.

So the BioModulator corrects voltage and the essential oils correct cellular software. Using either gets results but using both together gives exponentially better results.

Energetic Medicine and Nutrition

It is often overlooked that energy does not replace nutrition. I may get a temporary improvement in a patient that is deficient in iodine if I insert the frequency of iodine, but this will be temporary. The patient must consume iodine to be healthy. So it is with all the nutrients. One must consume all the nutrients needed to make a new cell to be healthy. Using the essential oils or the Tennant BioModulator does not give you license to eat processed, contaminated foods. They will not overcome the poisons created by infected teeth. They help restore the voltage and the frequencies of cells to help them start the process of healing, but without proper raw materials (nutrition) to make new cells, this improvement will be temporary.

Summary

To operate correctly, cells must have both the proper voltage and the proper frequency. Chronic illness is usually characterized by low voltage and a decrease in the frequency of the affected organ. Restoration of health must involve correcting both the voltage and the frequency of each cell and providing the nutrition necessary to make good new cells.

Measurement of the voltage of organs is easy and reproducible with devices like the Nakatani (MEAD) systems, Voll Systems and the Tennant BioModulator. However, there is no clinical device (only expensive laboratory devices) that can reproducibly measure the frequency at which an organ is operating. Thus no clinical device can tell us which oils any specific person needs.

Treatment of low voltage can be done with various electron donors. A predictable way to do so is with the Tennant BioModulator. Treatment of low voltage is difficult as one must find a way to insert frequencies into the organs that correspond to the normal frequencies of those cells. These are not single frequencies but hundreds of frequencies. A pure essential oil is ideal in that each contains hundred of frequencies. However, the trick is to figure out which oil has the appropriate frequencies for any given person. I developed a system of oil blends that have a higher number of frequencies in each blend than a single oil and thus can usually find the oil(s) with the correct frequencies quickly.

14 Emotions

The role of emotions in health has been discussed and disputed for years if not centuries. Most feel that having emotions out of control cause systemic illnesses. This has been called the "Mind/Body Connection".

Perhaps the group that focuses on this concept more than most is the so-called "German New Medicine" as described by Ryke Geerd Hamer, M.D. Dr. Hamer's son was killed and shortly after, Dr. Hamer developed cancer. He began to search his records and found that many cancer patients had an emotional event before developing their cancer.

Hamer describes "The Five Biological Laws of the New Medicine" in which he discusses his theories about how organs are involved with shocking events. Those involved with German New Medicine believe that almost all disease is the result of an emotional event.

Long before Dr. Herd's theories, acupuncturists described the influence of certain acupuncture points on emotions:

Acupuncture Point	Emotion
BL42	pent-up anger.
BL47	treats repressed fear
GB20	obsessive thought patterns
GB21	irritation
GV20-GV26-CV6	shock and overwhelming emotions.
HT3	most important point for anxiety.

Acupuncture Point	Emotion
HT7	overexcitement.
KI6	stage fright or fears
LU1	grief
P6	fear
SP4	anger and rage.
ST36	anxiety
TH15	worry

The Tennant BioTerminals are also associated with emotions:

BioTerminal	Emotion
Main Cable	Anger
Head	Irritability
Neck	Grief
Chest	Joy
Abdomen	Worry
Pelvis	Fear

I used to believe that emotions caused organic problems. For example, anger gives you a headache. Grief makes your neck stiff. Worry gives you a stomach ache. Fear gives you diarrhea.

What made me question those assumptions was noticing that correcting the voltage in the BioTerminals often changed people's emotions. For example, we corrected the voltage in the Chest

BioTerminal for a grumpy woman. She called back to the office to thank us and tell us she was laughing. She reported that she didn't remember the last time she had laughed. We didn't do anything focused on her emotions. We just put electrons into the Chest BioTerminal.

Thus I began to look at whether emotions that were inappropriate were simply low voltage in the part of the brain associated with each individual BioTerminal and acupuncture system. It seems to be true.

Perhaps the most powerful system of dealing with emotions is the

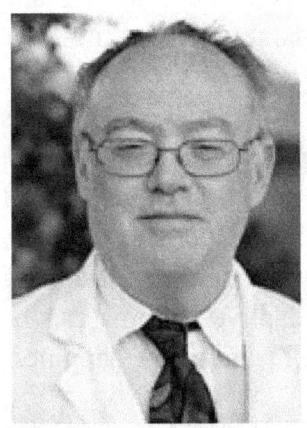

Dr. Joseph A. DiRuzzo

Prenatal Re-Imprinting (PNRI) developed by Dr. Joe DiRuzzo. Most people believe that emotional patterns are learned during the first years of our life and are controlled by our genetics. Psychotherapy is focused on the part of the brain that thinks with the believe that one can change emotions and behavior patterns by understanding them.

We are all aware of the poor outcomes of traditional psychology and psychiatry.

Dr. DiRuzzo began to realize that the basis of emotions are formed in the neural plate. When an egg and a sperm meet, they form two cells, then four, then eight, then 16, then 32. They then form a hollow ball called the **blastula**. The blastula invaginates in one location forming what is called a **gastrula**.

The gastrula with its blastopore soon develops three distinct layers of cells (the germ layers) from which all the bodily organs and tissues then develop:

1. The innermost layer, or **endoderm**, gives rise to the digestive organs, lungs and bladder.
2. The middle layer, or **mesoderm**, gives rise to the muscles, skeleton and blood system.
3. The outer layer of cells, or **ectoderm**, gives rise to the nervous system and skin.

After the gastrula is formed with its three layers, the first structure to form is a thickening of the ectoderm into what is called the **neural plate**. This neural plate will eventually become the brain.

As soon as the neural plate forms, it begins to have Pavlovian responses to its environment. This is where the emotions and personalities form that will guide us throughout our entire life.

The critical contribution of Dr. DiRuzzo is that our personalities are formed during our embryonic/fetal period and they reflect primarily what our mother was experiencing at the time. PNRI asserts that all problems in life are the result of simple maladaptive reflexes (responses) established in utero, under conditions of maternal and/or fetal stress. These maladaptive patterns can be changed by a simple technique, resulting in increased happiness and ease.

With PNRI techniques, one can easily access the areas of the brain where these pre-subconscious memories are stored and constantly playing. With the simple, but elegantly effective techniques, one can often move a person from suicidal depression to happiness in a matter of minutes!

The most frequent cause of depression is the "unwanted baby" syndrome. Often mothers don't want to be pregnant. The

> The critical contribution of Dr. DiRuzzo is that our personalities are formed during our embryonic/fetal period and they reflect primarily what our mother was experiencing at the time.

timing isn't convenient, they don't know if they can afford a baby, the relationship with the father is shaky, they don't want to leave their job, etc. The adrenalin the mother creates from these feelings crosses the placenta and affect the fetus in the same way. Thus the fetus is stressed in the same way the mother is stressed.

With PNRI, one can easily reprogram the recorder that keeps playing over and over in the person's mind that they aren't wanted and that day to day is a constant stress associated with fear.

The most common maladaptive emotions causing suffering are:

Emotion	Mother was Feeling
Feelings of insecurity	Stress about being pregnant
Feelings of inadequacy	Lack of resources for pregnancy
Feelings of uncertainty	Poor parental bonding
Feelings of inferiority	Father withdraws support for pregnancy
Impatience	Bad maternal diet = not enough good nourishment coming to fetus
Various personal problems	Failure of parents to give attention to the unborn child.
1. Relationships	Failure of parents to give attention to the unborn child.
2. Finances	Failure of parents to give attention to the unborn child.
3. Self-esteem	Failure of parents to give attention to the unborn child.

It is difficult to find someone capable of doing Prenatal Re-imprinting. To my knowledge, no one is currently teaching it to medical professionals. In addition, it can be exhausting to the practitioner.

Psych-K

Psych-K is another method I have seen work. It involves the use of muscle testing to identify the primary and other causes of mental fatigue and confusion. It then uses energy to release and retrain memories that are helpful to the health of the person. Certified Psych-K therapists can be found on the internet.

Summary:

We have three components to the human cell:
1. Hardware: this is the cell itself and its mechanical parts. This portion is much like your computer hardware.
2. Electrical system: this gives the cell hardware the power to work. Without a power supply or battery, your computer won't work. Neither will your body.
3. Software: this is the programming that tells the hardware what to do. In your body, it is composed of the subconscious as well as the Information that is received by your cells from your environment or your perception of your environment. This includes your spiritual connections. To some degree, the subconscious is your operating system like Mac OS X or Windows and your perception of your environment is other software like Pages for Mac or Word for Windows.

All of these must be in balance if we are to have health.

Emotions are a constant companion of illness. Most people believe that the emotional makeup of a person cannot be changed.

That simply isn't true.   The following things can dramatically change the happiness and health of people:

1. Change the emotional maladaptations programmed during fetal period with Prenatal Re-Imprinting
2. Correct thyroid levels
3. Correct neurochemicals with phytoplankton
4. Give adrenal support
5. Correct voltages of the BioTerminals

15 Nitric Oxide

One of the things necessary to make cells and keep them working is oxygen. This comes to the cell by way of the hemoglobin in the blood. For the blood to reach the tissue, there must be good circulation. Circulation is accomplished with nitric oxide. Thus have adequate levels of nitric oxide is critical for good health.

Nitrous oxide, commonly known as laughing gas or sweet air, is a chemical compound with the formula N2O. It is used in surgery and dentistry for its anesthetic and analgesic effects. It is known as "laughing gas" due to the euphoric effects of inhaling it.

Nitric Oxide (NO) is a gas that serves as a signaling molecule in every cell in the body.
1. It causes arteries and bronchioles to expand
2. It allows brain cells to communicate with each other
3. It causes immune cells to kill bacteria and cancer cells

Nitric Oxide was discovered in 1772 by a British man named Joseph Priestly, who referred to it as "nitrous air." When he discovered this, it was a colorless and gas and a toxic gas. Nitric Oxide continued to receive the label of being a toxic gas and an air pollutant until over two hundred years later, in 1987, when it was proven to be naturally produced by the body of mammals, including humans. http://itech.dickinson.edu/chemistry/?p=260

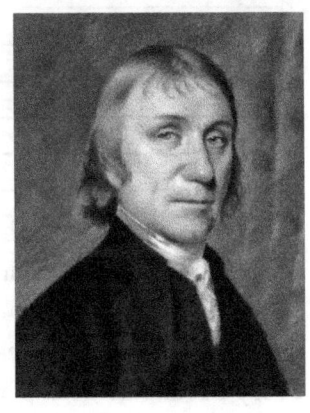

In 1998, the Nobel Prize in Physiology and Medicine was awarded jointly to Robert F. Furchgott, Louis J. Ignarro and Ferid Murad for their discoveries that nitric oxide is a signaling molecule in the cardiovascular system.

In mammals, NO is an important cellular messenger molecule involved in many physiological and pathological processes. Low levels of NO production are important in protecting an organ such as the liver from ischemic damage. However, sustained levels of increased NO production result in direct tissue damage and contribute to the vascular collapse associated with septic shock, whereas chronic expression of NO is associated with various carcinomas and inflammatory conditions including juvenile diabetes, multiple sclerosis, arthritis and ulcerative colitis.

Altitude Sickness	Heart attack
Arteries-flexible	Hypertension
Artery-plaques	Incontinence
Asthma	Insomnia
Bacterial Infections	Kidney Disease
Blood clots	Macular Degeneration
Cancer	Memory Loss
Cholesterol	Obesity
COPD	Osteoarthritis
Depression	Prematures
Diabetes	Sickle cell
Dementia	Stomach Ulcers
Eclampsia	Stress
Erectile Dysfunction	Stroke
Glaucoma	Sun Damage

As you can see in the table, lack of NO (nitric oxide) is a controlling factor in many illnesses that plague us.

On the average, Americans lose 10% of the ability to make NO for every decade of life. This loss of NO plays a significant role in the development of the diseases noted in the table.

NO is biosynthesized from L-arginine, oxygen and NADPH by various nitric oxide synthase (NOS) enzymes. Reduction of inorganic nitrate may also serve to make nitric oxide. There are several things that interfere with this process causing us to lose our ability to make NO.

The process of making NO requires calcium, copper, iron, magnesium, manganese, molybdenum, nickel, selenium, and zinc. It also requires Vitamin B1 (thiamine), Vitamin B2 (riboflavin), Vitamin B3 (niacin or niacinamide), Vitamin B5 (pantothenic acid), Vitamin B6 (pyridoxine), Vitamin B7 (biotin), Vitamin B9 (folic acid), Vitamin B12 (various cobalamins), Vitamin C, Vitamin K1, and Vitamin K2.

Arginine is synthesized from the amino acid citrulline by the sequential action of the cytosolic enzymes argininosuccinate synthetase (ASS) and argininosuccinate lyase (ASL).

Arginine is a conditionally nonessential amino acid, meaning most of the time it can be manufactured by the human body, and does not need to be obtained directly through the diet. The biosynthetic pathway however does not produce sufficient arginine, and some must still be consumed through diet. Individuals who have poor nutrition or certain physical conditions may be advised to increase their intake of foods containing arginine. Arginine is found in a wide variety of foods.   Animal sources: dairy products (e.g. cottage cheese, ricotta, milk, yogurt, whey protein drinks), beef, pork (e.g. bacon, ham), gelatin, poultry (e.g. chicken and turkey light meat), wild game (e.g. pheasant, quail), seafood (e.g. halibut, lobster, salmon, shrimp, snails, tuna).   Plant sources: wheat germ and flour, buckwheat, granola, oatmeal, peanuts, nuts (coconut, pecans, cashews, walnuts, almonds, Brazil nuts, hazelnuts, pine nuts), seeds (pumpkin, sesame, sunflower), chick peas, cooked soybeans, Phalaris canariensis (canary seed or ALPISTE). Wikipedia

A more recent finding is that NO is also made from nitrates and nitrites. Nitrates turn into nitrites in the body which then turn into NO. Don't be confused by the generally held opinion that nitrates and nitrites are poisonous. In the 1950s to the 1970s, there was found an association between nitrates, nitrites and cancer. However, these were Relative Risks as we have discussed in the chapter on medical studies. You will recall that high Relative Risks can really be meaningless and that one should just examine Absolute Risks.

In a summary report, the World Cancer Research Fund and the American Institute for Cancer Research recommended avoiding processed meats based on a meta-analysis showing a link between processed meats and colorectal cancer with a Relative Risk of 21%. In 1994, the National Cancer Institute stated that Relative Risks below 200 percent were not strong enough to make public policy pronouncements about risk factors!

People that eat vegetable diets to lower blood pressure consume nitrates and nitrites five times the amount higher than that proposed by the World Health Organization!. The amount of nitrates and nitrites in your saliva after you eat a spinach salad is much higher than that recommended by the scientific "experts". Does spinach or your saliva cause cancer? Not likely. Moreover, the amount of nitrates and nitrites in breast milk is higher than in any other food or beverage!

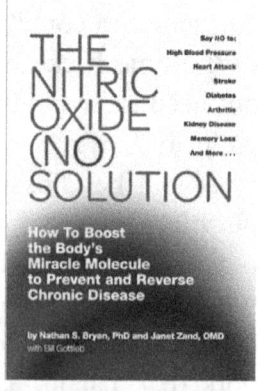

For this reason, a NO Index has been created. It takes into account:
1. The total amount of NO creating nitrate and nitrite in a food

2. The ORAC (oxygen radical absorption capacity) of a food---its amount of antioxidants (electron donors) available to protect the NO

NO Index: This table is from <u>The Nitric Oxide Solution</u> by Nathan S. Bryan, PhD and Janet Zand, OMD. You really must get this book.

One of the things that is new about NO is our ability to easily measure it. Although there are over 1000 medical research studies available about NO, few doctors even think about it because we haven't had a way to measure it. Most doctors therefore have no idea how to correct it.

A test strip is now available that only requires one to spit on the strip.   In one minute, it tells you your levels!   See https://secure.neogenis.com/product-listing.html

There are many supplement companies selling products to increase your NO. However, most of them contain l-arginine. This can be a problem because most people that need to correct their NO levels are over the age of 40, have hypertension, obesity, diabetes, high cholesterol, and/or are smokers. **Such people should not take l-arginine as it can actually increase their risk of a heart attack!**

A study at Johns Hopkins was started giving l-arginine to people that had suffered a heart attack. They found that it didn't improve cardiac ejection fractions or arterial stiffness. However, six people in the l-arginine group died of another heart attack while none died in the placebo group. Therefore the study was stopped and it was recommended that l-arginine NOT be given to anyone that has had a heart attack.

Arginine food sources	Arginine content
Plant products	**(grams /100 gram of food)**
Peanuts, Spanish	3.13
Peanuts	3.09
Almond nuts	2.47
Seeds, sunflower seed kernels, dried	2.40
Walnuts, English	2.28
Hazelnuts	2.21
Lentils, raw	2.17
Brazilnuts	2.15
Cashew nuts	2.12
Pistachio nuts	2.03
Flax seed	1.93
Beans, kidney, all types, mature seeds, raw	1.46
Pecan nuts	1.18
Beans, French, mature seeds, raw	1.17
Soybeans, green, raw	1.04
Tofu, extra firm, prepared with nigari	0.66
Wheat flour, whole-grain	0.64
Garlic, raw	0.63
Muffins, blueberry, toaster-type	0.30
Onion, raw	0.10
Chocolate syrup	0.09
Animal products	
Fish, tuna, light, canned in oil, drained solids	1.74
Chicken, broilers or fryers, giblets, raw	1.19
Salmon, Atlantic, farmed, raw	1.19
Shrimp, mixed species, raw	1.18
Egg, yolk, raw, fresh	1.10
Egg, whole, raw	0.82
Egg, white, raw, fresh	0.65
Pork, fresh, separable fat, raw	0.56
Milk, whole, 3.25% milkfat	0.08

Nitric oxide is synthesized by nitric oxide synthase (NOS). There are three isoforms of the NOS enzyme:

1. Endothelial (eNOS): Signaling molecule--Calcium dependent; produces low levels of gas as a cell signaling molecule

2. Neuronal (nNOS): Signaling molecule--Calcium dependent; produces low levels of gas as a cell signaling molecule

3. Inducible (Immune System) (iNOS)--Calcium Independent; produces large amounts of gas which can be cytotoxic

Nitric oxide secreted as an immune response is secreted as free radicals and is toxic to bacteria; the mechanism for this includes DNA damage. In response, however, many bacterial pathogens have evolved mechanisms for nitric oxide resistance.

If a person doesn't have the cofactors to make NO from l-arginine, it can increase the amount of cytotoxic compounds made by the immune system pathway. This is similar to converting the thyroid hormone T-4 to T-3. If you don't have the vitamins and minerals necessary for the conversion, you make the fake hormone RT3 that keeps your cells from working correctly. If you don't have the cofactors necessary to convert l-arginine, it can be harmful to you! Taking citrulline instead of l-arginine helps solve this.

Another problem is the presence of fluoride. When fluoride is present, it converts NO into the toxic and destructive nitric acid. NO will react with fluorine, chlorine, and bromine to form the XNO species, known as the nitrosyl halides, such as nitrosyl chloride. Nitrosyl iodide can form but is an extremely short-lived species and tends to reform I2.

$$2 NO + Cl2 \rightarrow 2 NOCl.$$

Nitrosyl fluoride reacts with water to form nitrous acid, which then forms nitric acid:

$$NOF + H2O \rightarrow HNO2 + HF$$
$$3 HNO2 \rightarrow HNO3 + 2 NO + H2O$$

Being a powerful oxidizing agent (electron stealer), nitric acid reacts violently with many organic materials and the reactions may be explosive. Wikipedia

An often overlooked fact is that the amino acids in the foods listed are only available if you have stomach acid to convert the proteins that are in the listed foods into amino acids. If you don't have stomach acid, the amino acids are not available and you can't make NO. Remember that to make stomach acid, you need Vitamin B1, iodine, and zinc. Without stomach acid, you can't absorb zinc even if you take it, so you have to take a Betaine tablet with the zinc so it will be absorbed.

So---remember to correct your stomach acid and eat your green vegetables. Correct your vitamin and mineral levels so you can make nitric oxide. It can help prevent glaucoma, macular degeneration, heart attacks, strokes, diabetes, and all the other maladies listed and even improve or restore your sex life!

16 Humic/Fulvic Acid

Fungus and the Planet

Most of us think of fungus as something disgusting in the same category as insects. It's everywhere but you try to avoid it (except for the mushrooms you put on your salad and steak). The reality is

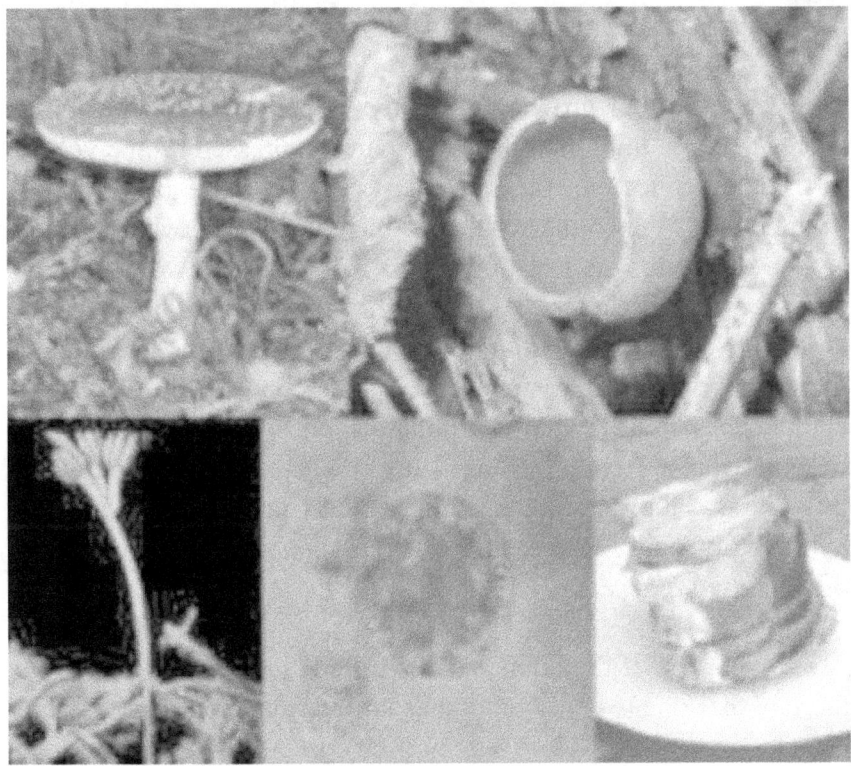

that fungus plays a major role in both health and sickness.

Fungus is the kingdom of organisms that includes yeasts, rusts, molds, and mushrooms. Fungus has characteristics of both plants and animals. They contain cell membranes surrounding a nucleus (like an animal cell) whereas bacteria have no nucleus. They contain no chlorophyll to make energy like plants but they create toxins and enzymes to consume organic material from plants or animals. Fungus reproduces by spores (one-celled reproductive units) that are asexual. Spores cannot be damaged even with extreme heat and can lay dormant for years. They produce energy without the use of oxygen (fermentation) (anaerobic).

The Role of Fungus on the Planet

The reason fungus is present on the earth is to decompose dead organic material. If it were not for fungus, we would all be over our heads in dead leaves and dead animals!

Think about a leaf growing on a tree. It is covered with fungal spores that are doing nothing. They are suppressed by the voltage of the leaf. Since the leaf is living, it contains voltage. If the tree becomes sick, the voltage of the leaf can drop. However, when the season comes for the leaf to drop to the ground, the voltage in the leaf drops significantly. As it does so, this signals the fungus to "wake up" and convert from a spore to its adult form. This fungus does what fungus is designed to do. It converts the leaf to its component parts of vitamins, minerals, and amino acids. These become what we call "dirt" or "soil". The scientific name given this dirt is "humic acid". Humic acid is not a single acid like hydrochloric acid. Rather it is the combination of the components of what used to be a leaf.

A small portion of the humic acid is called "fulvic acid". Fulvic is the key that opens cell membranes so that nutrition can pass into cells.

Now a seed is blown into the dirt. The seed needs nutrients. The fulvic acid in the soil opens the membranes of the seed and allow humic to flow into the seed. If the necessary water is present, it begins to grow. It grows into a plant containing vitamins, minerals, amino acids along with humic and fulvic acid.

The human pulls the plant and eats it. Now the human contains the humic, fulvic, vitamins, minerals, and amino acids needed for cells to work. The fulvic opens the cells of the human so nutrition can flow into the cell. The human is now able to make new cells and grow and repair itself until death finally occurs and the human is returned to dirt the same way the dead leaf was. Fungus renders the human into dirt with its component parts.

The problem of illness starts with pesticides. The pesticides that farmers put on the soil kills the fungus. That means that there is no longer a process to continuously provide soil with humic and fulvic. Eventually the plants won't grow. Then the farmer adds fertilizer so the plants will grow. The fertilizer contains potassium, phosphorous, and nitrogen. These make the plant grow, but they are deficient in vitamins, minerals, amino acids, humic and fulvic. We pull this plant and eat it, but such plants have almost no nutrition. Since these plants don't have humic and fulvic, eventually the human becomes deficient in them as well. Without fulvic, the nutrients taken can't enter the cells and so the cell struggles for nutrition. Disease isn't far behind.

Fungus and Disease

Just as leaves and dead animals are destroyed by fungus as the voltage falls, so the human is filled with fungus. As long as the human's voltage is normal, the fungus is dormant. However, if hypothyroidism, dental infections, lack of stomach acid, and toxins such as fluoride, chlorine, aspartame, Splenda, MSG, antibiotics, and many others that are in our food supply and environment drop our voltage, the fungus wakes up and begins to do what fungus is designed to do. It destroys our cells.

There are about 70,000 species of fungi, 200 of which cause disease in humans. The number of human fungal infections is directly related to the amount of antibiotics (fungal derivatives) consumed by the patient. The more antibiotics consumed means more secondary fungal infections. Antibiotics are consumed as medical therapy and in our food as most meat-producing animals and birds are given antibiotics to increase and speed up their growth.

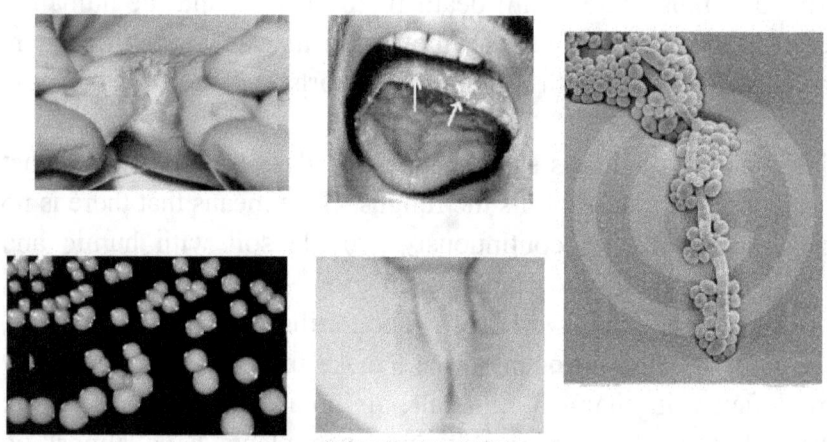

http://www.adhb.govt.nz/newborn/Teaching

The yeast Candida albicans has become the fourth most frequent hospital infection. Eight variations of Candida cause disease in man. Candida usually enter the body by way of the intestine when the guts' good bacteria are killed by antibiotics.

In the 1930s Royal Rife identified material that could be filtered from bacteria through a ceramic filters that only allowed passage of things smaller than 300 microns. He called them "filterable bacteria" because they could cause disease in animals. Particles smaller than 300 microns are now considered to be fungal spores or viruses. Bacteria are around 1000 microns (1,000,000 nanometers) in diameter.

Fungi and bacteria compete with each other for their food supply. Good bacteria in the gut help retard the growth of fungi. Fungi produce "antibiotics" to kill the bacteria. Pharmaceutical companies use fungi to make antibiotics like penicillin.

Examples of Diseases Caused or Aggravated by Fungi

1. Cancer
2. Migraines
3. Crohn's Disease
4. GERD
5. Asthma
6. Chronic Fatigue
7. Leukemia
8. Lymphoma
9. High Cholesterol
10. Hypertension
11. Diabetes
12. Infertility
13. ADHD

Koch's Postulates Remove Fungus from Consideration in Most Infectious Disease

In 1862, Robert Koch, MD, a German doctor discovered the tuberculosis bacteria, Mycobacterium tuberculosis. Notice that its name means "fungal bacteria". Koch developed the standard to determine the cause of infectious diseases. Koch's Postulates say that a microbe must be:

Found in an animal with a disease.

Isolated and grown in culture.

Injected into a healthy animal to produce the disease.

Recovered from the injected animal and found to be the same as the first one.

Fungi are mostly unable to fulfill Koch's Postulates because:

1. They exist in many different forms (spores, mycelia, with and without cells walls, etc.)

2. They are very difficult to culture. They can hide for years as spores until conditions are favorable for them to grow.
3. There are no rapid diagnostic tests to confirm the presence of fungus in the body except live blood analysis with phase contrast or dark field microscopes---not generally used in traditional medicine..
4. Filterable microbes include not only viruses but fungal spores (they may be the same thing)!

Fungus and Cancer

1840s: Louis Pasteur claims each disease is caused by a single external organism.

1840s: Antoine Beauchamp found that microorganisms change from one form to another (pleomorphism).

1840s: Claude Bernard felt that the body's internal environment controlled disease (voltage?).

1872-1968: Gunther Enderlein felt fungi changed from normal to pathogenic inside the body according to the environment.

1899: Dr. Bra (French) announced, "The parasite is fungus-like and is certainly the specific agent of cancer." Nothing more was heard of his announcement.

1925: Dr John Nuzum of Chicago reported consistently culturing organisms that changed shapes from breast cancer.

1925: Dr. Michael Scott of Montana found organism in cancer that changed from stage to stage as coccus, rod, and "spore sac".

1931: Otto Warburg receives Nobel Prize for showing that cancer cells get energy by fermentation the same way fungi do.

1947: Virginia Livingston-Wheeler cultures microbes from all cancers studied.

1950: Drs. Livingston-Wheeler, Wuerthele-Caspe, Jackson, and Diller remove microbes from cancer tissue and use them to cause cancer in animals. They then re-cultured the microbes from the tumors of the animals.

1960: Aflatoxin, (naturally occurring mycotoxins that are produced by many species of Aspergillus, a fungus, most notably Aspergillus flavus) , is discovered in England. It caused the death of thousands of turkeys and was found to cause liver cancer in humans.

1976: Kurt Olbrich develops microscope that can see things <100 nm. He can find fungus in the blood of all patients with cancer two years before they can be diagnosed with CAT scans, MRI scans, etc.

1997: Dr. Mark Bielski states lymphocytic leukemia is always associated with Candida albicans.

1999: Meinolf Karthaus cures leukemia with anti-fungal drugs.

2008: Tullio Simoncini cures cancer with sodium bicarbonate (baking soda) if he can bathe the tumor in it.

An understanding of infectious disease began in the mid 1800s with French scientists Louis Pasteur, Antoine Beauchamp, and Claude Bernard.

- ★Pasteur believed that each disease was caused by an externally acquired single infectious organism.
- ★Beauchamp believed that each disease was caused by infectious organisms that are always in our bodies and changing forms from helpful to pathogenic. He was the first to identify small particles that turned into other forms that he called microzymas.
- ★Bernard believed that the body's internal environment dictated whether infectious disease could occur. He drank a pitcher full of plague bacteria before the medical society to prove it would not harm him.

Prostate Specific Antigen (PSA)

Prostate Specific Antigen is NOT prostate specific! PSA (33-kDa serine protease) is elevated in prostate, breast, ovarian, pancreatic, and colon cancer. PSA is produced by Aspergillus flavus, A. fungigatus, A. oryzae, Ophiostoma piceae, Scedosporium apiospermum (all of the Ascomycete group of fungi). **A high PSA is an indicator of fungus in the blood!**

537

Kolattukudy found that PSA is a "significant virulence factor in invasive aspergillosis, which increased metastatic spread and mortality".

Aspergillus molds are the major producers of aflatoxin. Aflatoxins are the most potent liver carcinogens in the world.

Catchfly Plant and Cancer

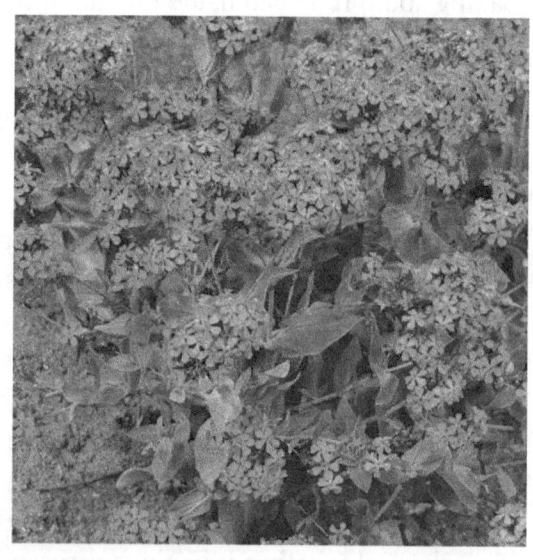

Catchfly plants are any of several plants of the genera Silene and Lychnis, native chiefly to the Northern Hemisphere and having white, pink, red, or purplish flowers and sticky stems and calyxes on which small insects may become stuck. When infected with fungus, the plant's DNA is mixed with fungal DNA so that the fungus takes control of the plant. Instead of producing pollen, the plant begins to produce fungal spores!

The fungus performs a sex-change operation on female catchfly plants, causing them to abort their ovaries and develop stamens -- male sex organs that normally produce pollen. And whatever the gender of its host, U. violacea secretly transforms stamens into spore factories. Dusted with spores instead of pollen, insects lured to the early, long-lasting blossoms unwittingly spread the fungal infection to the next cluster of catchfly they visit.

It apparently has not been studied. However, if this same thing happens in humans, it would explain what is normally called "random mutation" of DNA in cancer patients. Thus as voltage drops, fungus in the human wakes up and infects human cells. It could be that the fungus then takes over the DNA changing the cell into a cancer cell. Making more fungus makes more cancer cells. Since the role of fungus is to decompose dead organic material, it performs this role. However, it is accomplished inside an organism that is still alive until it finally kills the organism.

Fungi in Industry

1. Fungi are used to manufacture:
2. Citric acid (from Aspergillus niger) used in soft drinks
3. Inks
4. Dyeing processes
5. Silvering of mirrors
6. Pharmaceuticals
7. Antibiotics
8. Ephedrine
9. Vitamins
10. Enzymes
11. Alcoholic beverages
12. Bread
13. Cheese

Animal vs. Plant

Animal cells have nuclei and need oxygen for energy production by respiration. Plant cells use carbon dioxide and chlorophyll to make energy and release oxygen. Fungal cells have nuclei but in the yeast form, make energy without oxygen (just like plants) and without chlorophyll (unlike plants) in a process called fermentation.

When you take antibiotics (fungal toxins), they kill bacteria but nothing kills them. The amount of fungal infections in your body is directly related to the amount of antibiotics you have taken.

Candida albicans has become the fourth leading cause of hospital-acquired blood-stream infections. Eight different Candida species infect humans. Probiotics (good bacteria in the gut) compete with fungus for the same food. Probiotics are THE MOST IMPORTANT defense you have against fungal invasion! Fermentation (feeding the fungus) requires sugar and low voltage. **If you crave carbohydrates, you are likely infected with fungus.**

When animals were fed moldy feed, it was noticed that they put on weight faster and in greater amounts! Thus farmers began to give their animals antibiotics (mold products). When you eat farm animals/fish that have been fed fungus, you eat fungus/fungal toxins.

Like other animals, humans put on weight faster when they consume antibiotics either as a prescription medication or in meat from animals that were fed antibiotics.

Patients who are allergic to penicillin have very few antibodies against penicillin in their blood. **People who are allergic to penicillin are filled with fungus/fungal toxins**. A small addition of more fungus (penicillin tablet) causes the body to be overwhelmed with rashes and can lead to death.

Conidia (Spores That Have Lost Cell Membrane and Entered Cells)

1. Conidia (fungal spores without shell) and viruses are very similar:
2. Can only live inside a cell or sac.
3. Trigger disease.
4. Can remain quiescent for years.

5. Can form buds, break off, and infect other cells.

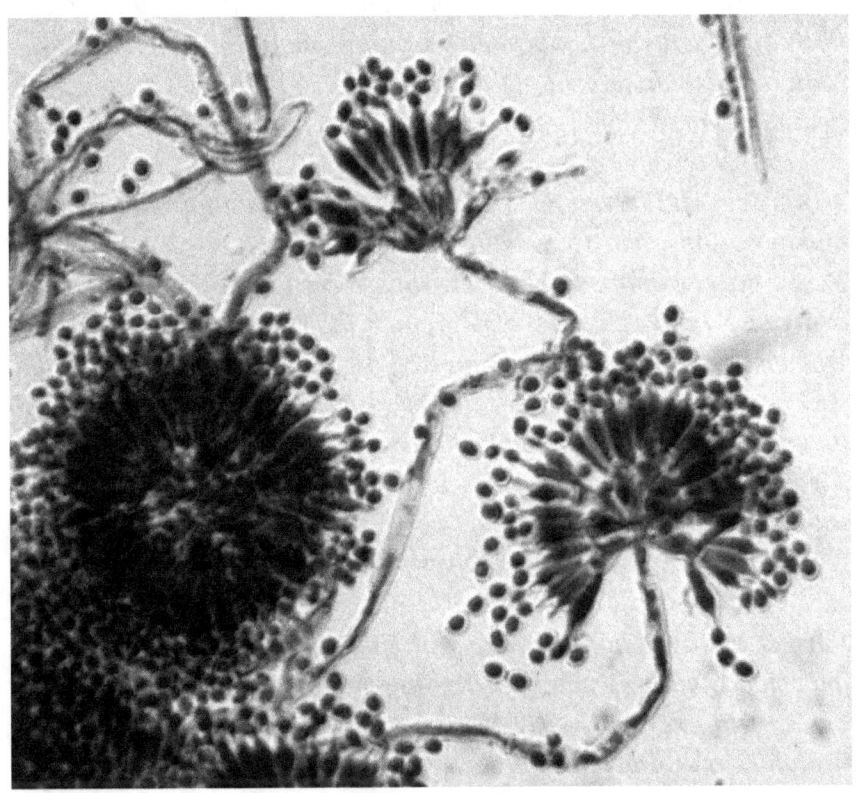

Corn and peanuts are generally infected with fungus and contain the fungal toxin aflatoxin. Penicillin and most antibiotics are fungi that kill or inhibit bacteria. When you take them they kill the bacteria but remain behind in your system.

Taking Antibiotics Increases the Risk of Cancer and Other Diseases

Prior Medication Use And Health History As Risk Factors For Non-Hodgkin's Lymphoma: Preliminary Results From A Case-Control Study In Los Angeles County. Bernstein L, Ross RK; Cancer Res (1992 Oct 1) 52(19 Suppl):5510s-5515s

Abstract: To determine whether non-Hodgkin's lymphoma (NHL) is related to prior medication use or health history, a population-based case-control study was conducted. A total of 619 male and female residents of Los Angeles County who were diagnosed with NHL between January 1, 1979, and June 30, 1982, were compared to individually age-, race-, and sex- matched neighborhood controls with regard to history of use of 49 different medications, 47 chronic and infectious diseases or other conditions, 15 types of immunizations, and 15 specific allergic reactions.

Based on preliminary analyses, long-term regular use of aspirin and other pain relievers and greater than or equal to 2 months Women who had been immunized against polio by injectable vaccine were at significantly lower risk of NHL than women who had not received this immunization.

Among men, cholera immunization and allergy to nuts and berries were significantly protective. Subjects who had received a yellow fever immunization also had lower NHL risk.

Further analyses of these data will attempt to establish the relative importance of these potential risk factors and to determine whether any are markers of early symptoms of NHL. of treatment with penicillin and other antibiotics were associated with significantly increased risk of Non-Hodgkin's Leukemia.

Other drugs associated with greater risk of NHL were use of digitalis and estrogen replacement therapy by women, use of corticosteroids, and greater than or equal to 2 months of use of tranquilizers.

NHL was strongly associated with a prior history of cancer. Cases more frequently reported histories of kidney infections and anemia than did controls; a history of eczema appeared to be protective against NHL.

This study shows the role of pharmaceuticals in lowering voltage, allowing fungus to produce cancer. Once you understand the role of fungus in disease and the role of voltage in controlling fungus, you begin to understand the paradigm that Healing is Voltage.

We see that fungus has the amazing duality of both preventing disease by creating humic and fulvic acid to provide nutrition to the cells of living things and to cause disease when it finds that cells have low voltage. When the voltage is low enough, fungus causes cancer. All of this is controlled by voltage because voltage controls oxygen levels and oxygen levels control fungus.

Farming practices of using pesticides and fertilizers create foods that have little nutrition. In addition, they don't contain adequate amounts of humic and fulvic to keep the human that eats these foods healthy.

Humic and Fulvic Supplements

I have always tried to understand how the universe works. Since cells are simply a fractal (smaller duplicate of a larger whole) of the universe, if I can understand how the universe works, I can understand how to make a cell work correctly.

Fungus plays an important role in the universe. It is responsible for turning dead organic material into dirt. Were it not for fungus, we would all be covered up with dead leaves and dead animals!

Think about a leaf on a tree. Since the leaf is alive, it contains voltage. Since it contains voltage, it also contains oxygen. Remember that the amount of oxygen in water is controlled by the voltage of the water.

Oxygen controls fungus. Thus the fungal spores that are always present on leaves will be suppressed by the oxygen. Also remember that as oxygen disappears, cell-wall-deficient organisms move toward becoming fungal forms. These cell-wall-deficient are part of every living organism. You may want to revisit the chapter on infections and refresh your understand of what are called L-forms.

Now the leaf falls off the tree as winter approaches. As the leaf loses its voltage when separated from the tree, it also loses its oxygen. This loss of oxygen causes cell-wall-deficient organisms to become fungus and the fungal spores on the leaf to "wake up". Then the fungus does what it was designed to do. It begins the process of turning the leaf back into "dirt". This "dirt" contains a mixture of organic acids called "humic acid". A series of complex acids in the humic is called "fulvic acid". It contains all the known vitamins, minerals, and amino acids.

Now a seed blows into the dirt. With the addition of water, the fulvic opens the cell membrane of the seed allowing the humic to enter the seed. With this nutrition and water, the seed grows into a plant containing the humic/fulvic complexes.

When we eat this plant, our bodies get their necessary humic/fulvic so that our cell membranes are controlled and our cells nourished. The fulvic supplies voltage and the humic provides the vitamins, minerals, and amino acids to make new cells. All that is missing is fats.

Unfortunately, farmers use pesticides to kill the fungus. So after a time, the soil becomes depleted of humic/fulvic so the seeds they plant won't grow. Thus they add fertilizers containing nitrogen, phosphorous, and potassium (NPK fertilizers). This will allow the plants to grow, but they lack much of the nutrition needed for healthy cells. Thus our farming practices allow for more produce but it significantly less nutritious than naturally occurring (organic) produce. Add to that the fact that most of our seeds have a pesticide added to their DNA (genetically modified seeds), and we have a food supply that is less than nutritious and filled with pesticides.

Humic and Fulvic have been called Nature's "Miracle Molecules" ---their nutritional contribution to superior health as Nature's Own nutrient activation and delivery system to the cell is just part of their story.---they also perform many other vital biological functions as well.

In Nature, just one of Fulvic and Humic's functions, is to insure Delivery of Nutrients—all 74+ organic ionic minerals, organic vitamins, amino acids and other phytonutrients—to all living things including human beings. In this capacity they are a FULL SPECTRUM MINERAL AND NUTRIENT SUPPLEMENT DELIVERING ALL 74+ Macro, Micro and Trace Minerals, Organic Vitamins, Amino Acids, and Other Nutrients our bodies need, in their organic ionic forms, and in just the right proportions vitamins and minerals need to work synergistically with each other to support our bodies' intricate design.

The following text about humic/fulvic was written by CareyLyn Carter of Mother Earth Labs. She is a well-known humic/fulvic expert with a background in pharmaceutical research and physiology research at Texas A&M. At Mother Earth Labs, she produces one of the few---if not the only---products bottled in an FDA certified facility with guaranteed parts-per-million far above the quantity claimed by other nutrient manufacturers.

Humic is a term that describes a group of complex organic molecules. Fulvic is just one member of this group. The Fulvic molecules are the smallest (lowest molecular weight) of the Humic group and is one of the reasons it is the most biologically active. Fulvic is a Golden Liquid, whereas Humic is almost black in color. Its smaller size allows Fulvic molecules to more easily pass through cell membranes and carry nutrients inside the cell. A single Fulvic molecule can individually carry up to 60 different vital activated minerals nutrients to our cells.

It is inside our cells that most life-giving and sustaining metabolic functions are carried out and it is inside our cells where nutrients are needed as fuel or participants for these metabolic functions to take place. If nutrients don't make it inside our cells metabolic reactions would be impaired. This is why many supplements seem to lack benefit. This is especially true of inorganic supplements which include most mineral supplements. Most over-the-counter mineral supplements are inorganic unless they also contain Fulvic or Humic.

A large portion of these inorganic mineral supplements are just lost through the intestinal tract and rarely make it out of the intestinal tract into the bloodstream. Liquid inorganic mineral supplements are more easily absorbed, but they are typically not in an organic form our bodies easily recognize and can use. This can be a problem because if inorganic mineral supplements can't be converted through a series of steps to their organic, ionic forms, they are removed from our blood and excreted through our urine and lost, or worse, stored in our fat tissue with other waste as mineral metals (heavy metals) that can't be eliminated and can even buildup and become toxic.

Interestingly, another one of Fulvic's other biological functions, is its ability to remove these heavy metal toxins and other toxins stored in our fatty tissues to protect vital organs and safely escort them out of our body. In the presence of Fulvic, nutrients we receive from our diets or from the supplements we take are transformed into their organic, ionic, "cell-ready" form our cells recognize and can use easily and are transported into the cells.

An electric potential is the electric charge gradient of a membrane. Instead of a uniform charge (neutral or zero charge difference) between inside and outside the cell, a healthy membrane is more positively charged on one side and more negatively charged on the other. This has important biological functions such as more efficient passage of nutrients (in) and wastes (out) across the membrane.

A normal electrical potential enables our cells to carry out all life-giving functions and without this electrical potential, cells are not able to properly function and will die.

The value of maintaining the electric potential of our cells can be shown by an experiment that was done by researchers on a giant amoeba, which is a microscopic single cell animal. Under a microscope the electrical potential of the amoeba, which is normally 20 millivolts (the difference in charge between inside and outside the cell), was depressed to zero. The researchers then noticed astonishing changes as the amoeba became dysfunctional, the outer membrane then ruptured in several places, and internal components began to flow into the surrounding fluid. At that point researchers visually concluded that the form and structure of the amoeba had disintegrated and was for all purposes dead.

Upon increasing the electrolytic charge, the form of the amoeba reconstructed and became active and healthy again. This same test was repeated many times with the same results.

This study determined that likely results could be expected by any loss of electrical potential on the cellular level in our own bodies, such as caused by an unbalanced diet, an acidic pH, low cellular oxygenation, loss of sleep, stress, overwhelming emotions, infections, etc., our cells become weakened, cannot function as effectively and can die.

When our cells are not functioning properly and become weakened and even die, we feel this as loss of vitality. We experience fatigue, illnesses, disease and even death. Humic and Fulvic are vitally important electrolytes to establishing and maintaining a healthy cellular membrane potential. When we receive all these nutrients we naturally feel better and more alive. Equally important to humic and fulvic's role in nutrient activation and delivery to the cells for superior health is fulvic's ability to improve waste and toxin removal from cells and tissues by restoring cellular membrane electrical difference between inside and outside of each cell.

When cell membrane electrical charge gradients are working correctly, nutrients more easily enter our cells and waste products from metabolic reactions (highly acidic) or toxins are more easily transported out of our cells and out of our body.

A primary biological role fulvic performs is providing positive and negative charges as needed to establish and maintain optimum membrane potential. Fulvic is like a battery providing The Spark of Life!

In nature, humic and fulvic's role is definitely not limited to their nutritional contributions, such as transforming nutrients into their "cell-ready" active forms that our bodies can use immediately and actually transporting them to cells where they are needed so all the life-giving and sustaining processes that occur in our bodies can take place, they play a host of other vital biological roles as well....humic and fulvic are considered some of the most biologically active substances on earth and the many biologically important functions they perform are well-recognized.

1. Supercharge the body at the cellular level imparting life-sustaining electrical balance and life-giving energy to our cells—all bodily processes are improved and enhanced in their presence, and they help us to achieve and maintain the most optimal health possible.
2. Improves cell membrane potentials so nutrients the cell needs gets in and acidic wastes and toxins the cell doesn't need gets out and cells are healthier. If cells are healthier, we are healthier.
3. Stimulate immune functions and white blood cell production. The organic micro and trace minerals they carry are essential in the production of immune cells.

4. Promotes blood, cell and tissue oxygenation so oxygen is distributed throughout our bodies, metabolic reactions that rely on oxygen occur more effectively and we feel more energized.

5. Help neutralize acidity and restore pH balance which helps maintain or restore good health and prevent disease.

6. Chelate (bind) heavy metals and other toxins and escort them out of the body,

7. Neutralize all classes of free radicals (they are in a class called super-antioxidants because they neutralize more than one class) that cause extensive damage to cells and tissues,

8. Balance endocrine systems and hormone production,

9. Supports cardiovascular function—improved contractility, improved blood pressure control, and oxidative stress reduction which contribute to the prevention of cardiovascular and coronary heart disease.

10. Improves activity of nutrients received from our diets or through supplements that are part of a health maintenance or restorative program,

11. Nutrients, such as carbohydrates and proteins, are also metabolized more completely.

Humic substances are naturally produced in soils by beneficial microbes. This is where they start their journey that will take them throughout the biosphere to support life everywhere they go. In the soil, humic and fulvic's first task is to transform inorganic mineral rocks and mineral metals into their activated, organic, and ionic (water-soluble) "cell-ready" forms...the only mineral form plants can use ...and the only form we can use, too.

Humic and Fulvic Carry these organic minerals out of the soil into the plant and on to the plant cells where they are needed in just about every metabolic "life-giving and sustaining" process. Humic and fulvic are nature's own nutrient activation and delivery system. Humic and fulvic make it possible for plants receive the nutrition, especially minerals, needed to be healthy and thrive. ...and to carry out a host of vital, life-giving functions.

We rely on these microorganisms and the humic and fulvic they produce just as much as plants to be healthy and thrive also. When we consume plants—humic and fulvic naturally carry all 74+ activated organic, ionic "cell-ready" minerals, the vitamins, amino acids and other nutrients to our cells where they are needed to support all of our metabolic "life-giving and sustaining" processes too...

Because fulvic nutrients are in their organic, ionic natural forms, our bodies have no difficulties using them immediately. We need humic and fulvic along with the 74+ organic, ionic minerals, 13 vitamins, 18 amino acids, and other vital nutrients they naturally carry as much as plants to be healthy and thrive!

If we lived a hundred years ago, just by eating a balanced diet we would receive all the fulvic and humic along with all the minerals, vitamins, and other nutrients they naturally carry and stay healthy and strong. Humic and fulvic also play other vital roles in our bodies, just as they do in plants, and have been called "Nature's Miracle Molecules" because like Sunlight, Air and Water...Life just cannot exist without them.

But we don't live 100 years ago...Our US crop plants contain only a fraction...as much as 80% less of the humic substances, especially fulvic, along with the vitamins, minerals, amino acids, phytochemicals, and other nutrients humic and fulvic naturally carry than they did a century ago according to the US Department of Agriculture, (USDA). This is shocking......and this has far-reaching consequences.

Fertilizers and pesticides used in modern agricultural practices destroy or severely stunt the microorganisms in the soil that produce humic and fulvic. Even organic farming methods that protect the microorganisms deplete the humic and fulvic because they are used by plants faster than they can be replaced naturally. Some organic farmers, especially large growers, are now supplementing soils with organic agricultural humic compounds as part of a sustainable agricultural program.

So, despite even the best efforts to eat a balanced diet, our food sources no longer contain the vitamins, fulvic minerals and nutrients our bodies need to stay healthy and strong. Deficiencies in humic and fulvic create a deficiency in organic vitamins and 74+ organic minerals they naturally carry to us in our food sources. Did you know that our bodies rely on humic and fulvic-activated minerals---minerals are alkaline—(and vitamins as cofactors to minerals) to neutralize acids and maintain a healthy pH balance in our cells and tissues? Normal cellular metabolism produce acids as end-products, also our diets can include highly acidic foods, such as carbonated beverages, or emotional and mental states of anxiety, stress, fear, worry are extreme acid producers.

Deficiencies in fulvic and the alkalizing minerals it carries creates an acidic environment inside our cells because fulvic helps to maintain the electrical potential of the cell membrane that promotes the removal of acidic waste products. These deficiencies are taking a serious toll on our health. So does chronic body acidity and inflammation. In a state of chronic acidity and inflammation, we can eventually become prone to disease. When our bodies are acidic (low-voltage), our tissues become inflamed, cells are damaged and even destroyed, and excessive amounts of free-radicals are produced that further harm cells and tissues. Amazingly, there are now 157 degenerative diseases linked to vitamin and mineral deficiencies with chronic body acidity (low voltage) and systemic inflammation.

When we become deficient in the fulvic-activated minerals our bodies can use to neutralize excess acid, our bodies stay in a state of chronic acidity (low-voltage). This chronic acidity promotes an environment that is a breeding ground for viruses, bacteria, and yeast. Fulvic also assists us in eliminating acidic waste and toxins from our bodies and without it they can buildup in our cells and tissues.

Cancer cells are produced routinely in our body, and can typically be handled by our amazing immune systems and cells. But in a state of chronic acidity, cancer cells thrive and our immune systems become weakened. Our immune cells can become stretched to their limit because they must also address other aspects of chronic acidity, so that cancer cells can proliferate.

The incidence of cancer has skyrocketed since the beginning of the 1960s. The national institute of health (NIH) recently reported that cancer is now expected to affect 1 in every 3 females and 1 in every 2 males compared to 1964 statistics of only 1 in 261 people. The increase in incidence of other degenerative diseases is equally sharp and alarming.

It is also a serious mistake to think that taking vitamin and mineral supplements are going to be effective to bridge the gap. Many supplements are not easily absorbed by our bodies and if they are absorbed they can't be used easily by our bodies (this is especially important as we age). Much of what can't be converted into a form our bodies can easily use, is simply excreted by the body and lost. Many supplement manufacturers now understand this and are including fulvic in their formulas---not very much fulvic, but some is better than none at all. If you see anything above 70 minerals advertised on the label, you'll know the product includes humic or fulvic.

Humic and fulvic naturally carry with them in their structures all the vitamins, over 74 organic, ionic minerals along with elements such as phytochemicals, natural sterols, hormones, fatty acids, polyphenols, and ketones, including flavonoids, flavones, flavins, catechins, tannins, quinones, isoflavones, tocopherols, and others. All of these are vital nutrients our bodies need every day...activated into their organic, ionic forms so our cells can recognize and use them immediately...in just the right proportions...and transported into our cells right where we need them to help keep our bodies healthy and strong.

Each cell in our bodies requires a complex interaction of all the vitamins, over 74 minerals, amino acids and other elements and nutrients to function optimally. They all must be present or things don't work as well as they should. In the case of minerals, for every mineral, such as calcium, there are several other minerals that must be present in the proper amount and in turn, those minerals must have other minerals present, or the mineral will not do the job required by the human body. In addition, vitamins are cofactors to minerals-and they need each other to work.

The mineral wheel diagram shows the complex interactions that minerals have with each other. Note all its interactions with just these 23 minerals. It's already hard enough to imagine the complexity if all 74+ minerals our bodies need were included. You can see that some minerals require other minerals to be present to do their job (single arrows on the lines of the mineral wheel, calcium (Ca) and manganese (Mn) for example). Other minerals interfere with another's bioavailability so it can't be used by the body (double, opposing arrows on the lines of the mineral wheel). Calcium (Ca+2) and magnesium (Mg+2) are good examples that must be present in just the right proportions to be effective. If they are not in proportion the opposite of the intended effect occurs.

Example: Many people think they need to supplement just zinc (Zn), but too much zinc affects copper (Cu) metabolism. If down-regulated for a period of time this can cause anemia because of copper's role with iron (Fe) and the production of hemoglobin, among other things. So, how do you really know you need zinc? How much do you need? How much copper? How much iron? How much of all the other minerals that affect or are affected by supplementing just these three?

Also, minerals must be in their organic, ionic, water-soluble forms before our bodies can use them. Most mineral supplements on the market today are not in these forms and can even buildup as "mineral metals" because they can't be easily transformed or eliminated and become toxic. This is especially true of non-fulvic liquid mineral supplements which are more easily absorbed from the intestines into the blood stream. In the presence of fulvic and humic, all nutrients including those supplements are transformed and their benefit is amplified.

It is noteworthy that one of the biological functions of humic and fulvic is to chelate (bind) and transform into a usable form or remove toxic mineral metals from the body.

The goal of mineral supplementation is to insure all 74+ minerals---macro, micro, and trace minerals—are delivered in their organic, ionic forms, concentrated and in just the right proportion nature intended, along with all the vitamins that act as their cofactors.

It probably goes without saying that a superior-quality humic and fulvic product can only be produced from superior-quality raw materials. High-quality raw materials have a high fulvic content and are free from toxins or impurities such as pollution, chemicals, pesticides, or fertilizers. The best sources are from deposits that were originally beds of ancient freshwater lakes (not salt water) during the late cretaceous period that are distant from large population centers where ground waters are still pure. There are only a handful of these left in the world. Humic and fulvic derived from deposits where marine saltwater bodies once existed are not as good because the average molecular weight of the humic/fulvic molecules is higher so not as active and there are more impurities.

Advances in processes based on nanotechnology have enabled us to extract and purify humic and fulvic from deposits of ancient plant material at concentrations that are truly remarkable while maintaining the activity of the fulvic and humic molecules. Deposits contain a massive quantity of plant material that has been compressed over millions of years. It would be impossible to duplicate this quantity using modern plant sources to produce highly concentrated humic and fulvic that achieves real biological activity.

Humic and fulvic in Mother Earth's Labs' humic and fulvic products are derived from the highest quality humic deposits located in the wilderness Fruitland formation located in the Northwest corner of New Mexico in the United States. It is well known to be among the finest freshwater humic deposits in the world because of its very high humic and fulvic content and its purity. The Fruitland Formation is a pristine, remote mountainous wilderness area in northwest New Mexico.

The quality of raw materials, along with manufacturing processes are reviewed to receive USDA Organic Certification – a quality benchmark that all of Mother Earth Labs' humic and fulvic products have.

There are no known negative side effects or toxicity when taken as recommended, even up to 3 ounces 3 times per day as many do who are facing a health. On the contrary, humic and fulvic work to help neutralize and remove toxic elements from the body.

It is important to remember humic and fulvic are completely natural substances and nature's own nutrient activation and delivery system to the cells throughout our biosphere. If our food sources contained the humic and fulvic and all the minerals, vitamins, and other nutrients they naturally carry as they once did a century ago, we wouldn't need to supplement them.

Mother Earth's humic and fulvic products contain highly-concentrated humic and/or fulvic. Since humic and fulvic help to remove toxic substances that have been stored in tissues, people with excessive amounts of toxic build up experience flu like symptoms for a few days while the body is being cleansed of toxins. If this happens, it is suggested you reduce the dose you are taking until you no longer experience these symptoms and work your way back up slowly. Be patient and give your body the time it needs.

It is important to remember that humic and fulvic can amplify the effects of many supplements and may also amplify the effects of prescription medications. Conversely humic and fulvic are also powerful detoxifying agents and may alter the effective dose of prescription medications because many medications are foreign or toxic substances to the body and can be removed by fulvic from the body thereby reducing a medication's effects.

We advise anyone taking prescription medications to check with their health care practitioner how to best integrate supplements to their health restorative and maintenance regimen. We also understand that many practitioners who practice traditional medicine may be unfamiliar with natural healing supplements and modalities including humic and fulvic's natural healing capabilities to help restore and maintain good health holistically rather than symptomatically.

It is important to note that most practitioners who approve supplements their patients wish to take recommend typically allow a minimum of 2 hours in between taking the prescription and the supplement.

Many of the people who learn about the power of humic and fulvic do so when they are facing a health challenge and looking for allies to help them on their path to restore their good health. Humic and fulvic are very potent allies helping restore natural body functions, boost immune response, and enable our body's own amazing ability to heal itself whenever possible by providing the nutrients it needs and energizing the cells to achieve the balance they need to carry out normal functions.

Because there is no danger of toxic buildup many people can take as much as 3 ounces 3 times per day depending on their need. Mother Earth's humic and fulvic products are very concentrated so it is important to start slowly and work up. If you listen to your body, it will tell you and adjust as needed.

Fulvic acid has the following known effects:
1. Increased energy
2. Ferocious antioxidant and free radical scavenger
3. Chelates heavy metals and body toxins, removing them from the system
4. Makes cell membranes more permeable and transports nutrients into the cells
5. Extends the time nutrients remain active – increasing the availability of essential nutrients
6. Increases metabolism of proteins, contributing to DNA and RNA synthesis
7. Powerful natural organic electrolyte
8. Restores electrochemical balance
9. Increases activity of enzyme systems
10. Rebuild and stimulate the immune system
11. Increases bioavailability of nutrients
12. Dissolves and complexes minerals making them bioavailable
13. Prepares nutrients to inter-react with each other
14. Increases absorption of oxygen and decreases acidity
15. Antibiotic properties
16. Treats open wounds, cuts and abrasions
17. Heals burns with minimum pain or scarring
18. Kills pathogens responsible for athletes foot
19. Acts as a wide spectrum anti-microbial and fungicide
20. Treats rashes, skin irritations, insect and spider bites
21. Neutralizes poison ivy and poison oak

CareyLyn Carter

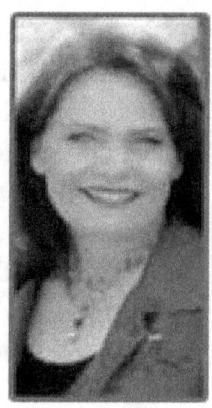

As I mentioned in the beginning of this chapter, the entire universe depends upon humic and fulvic. The sea creatures get it from small plants called marine phytoplankton. We land-based creatures are intended to get it from the plants we eat. However, farming practices have greatly eliminated that source. We have to get it from plankton like the sea creatures or from the deposits mentioned by CareyLyn Carter above.

I have had her create a product with both. I call it Raw Materials since it has most of the nutrients necessary to make new cells. It is deficient in iodine, omega-3 fats, vitamin C, vitamin D3 and vitamin B12/folic so I ask people to take them as well.

Raw Materials is available from my office.

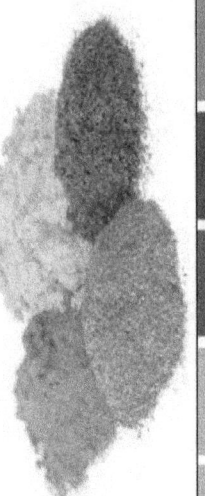
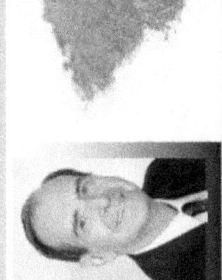

Bile	119, 182, 184, 225, 226, 262-265
Bilirubin	263
Bio-cranial Therapy	7, 8, 12
BioModulator	13, 15, 126, 132, 160, 161, 165, 505, 508, 510-515
BioTerminal	57, 420, 471, 472, 488, 489, 491, 496, 499, 513, 514
BioTerminal System	141
BioTerminals	137, 138, 148, 164, 165, 419, 421, 470, 471, 485, 486, 489, 497, 499, 513, 518
BioTransducer	473, 474, 486, 487, 499
Birch Oil	508
Bladder	119, 136, 144, 145, 153-155, 162, 163, 472, 491, 497
Bladder Tesla	491, 497
Blood	3, 6, 7, 9, 10, 14, 16-18, 20-23, 34, 35, 38-40, 48, 50, 51, 53, 55, 56, 188, 190, 193, 196, 204, 471, 486, 487, 496-210, 215, 219, 221, 223, 228, 231, 238, 243, 244, 256, 259, 260, 263, 265, 267, 273-275, 278, 281, 288, 290, 292, 294-296, 299, 305, 310-313, 317, 318, 321, 322, 459-462, 504, 512, 523, 524, 526
Blood Pressure	190, 204-206, 208-210, 260
Blood Pressure Systolic BP Diastolic BP	206
Bohr, Neils	38-40, 43, 49-51
Bone	4, 6-8, 11, 12, 276, 316, 317

www.ingramcontent.com/pod-product-compliance
Lightning Source LLC
Chambersburg PA
CBHW071352170526
45165CB00001B/8